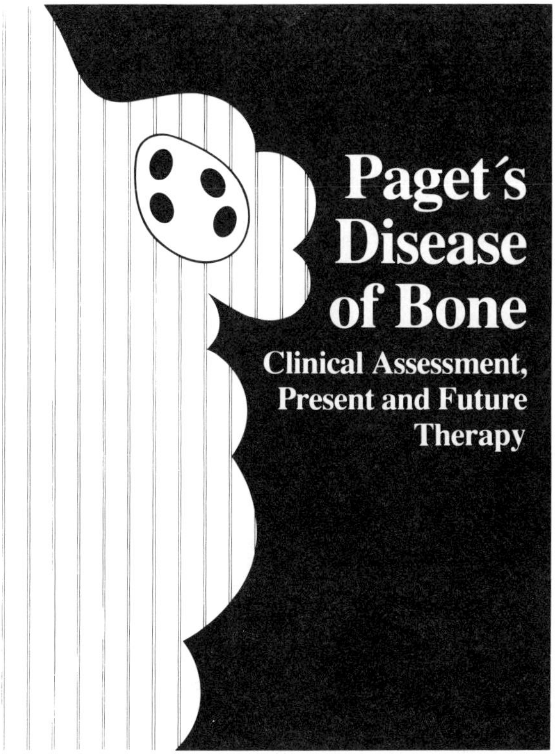
Paget´s
Disease
of Bone
Clinical Assessment,
Present and Future
Therapy

Design on preceding page: In 1877 Sir James Paget published his classic paper "On a form of chronic inflammation of the bones (osteitis deformans)." Microscopic sketches of the bone pathology were prepared by Mr. H.T. Butlin and published in this paper. This design was adapted from Figure 10 drawn by Mr. Butlin. The black represents bone with a scalloped border. The lined adjacent space represents the bone marrow. The multinucleated cell is an osteoclast, which has produced the resorbed surface of the bone. Thus this is a depiction of the earliest event in Paget's disease: increased bone resorption.

Paget's Disease of Bone

Clinical Assessment, Present and Future Therapy

Proceedings of the Symposium on the Treatment of Paget's Disease of Bone, held October 20, 1989 in New York City

Edited by

Frederick R. Singer, MD

Professor of Medicine in Residence
UCLA School of Medicine
University of California at Los Angeles
Director, Bone Center
Cedars-Sinai Medical Center
Los Angeles, California

Stanley Wallach, MD

Professor and Associate Chairman
Department of Internal Medicine
University of South Florida College of Medicine
Tampa, Florida

Elsevier

New York • Amsterdam • London • Tokyo

No responsibility is assumed by the Publisher for any injury and/or damage to persons or property as a matter of products liability, negligence or otherwise, or from any use or operation of any methods, products, instructions, or ideas contained in the material herein. No suggested test or procedure should be carried out unless, in the reader's judgment, its risk is justified. Because of rapid advances in the medical sciences, we recommend that independent verification of diagnoses and drug dosages be made. Discussions, views, and recommendations as to medical procedures, choice of drugs, and drug dosages are the responsibility of the authors.

Elsevier Science Publishing Co., Inc.
655 Avenue of the Americas, New York, NY 10010

Sole distributors outside the United States of America and Canada:

Elsevier Science Publishers B.V.
P.O. Box 211, 1000 AE Amsterdam, The Netherlands

This book is printed on acid-free paper.

Library of Congress Cataloging -in-Publication Data

Symposium on the Treatment of Paget's Disease of Bone (1989 : New York, N.Y.)
Paget's disease of bone : clinical assessment, present and future therapy : proceedings of the Symposium on the Treatment of Paget's Disease of Bone, held October 20, 1989 in New York City / edited by Frederick R. Singer, Stanley Wallach.
p. cm.
Includes bibliographical references and indexes.
Includes index.
ISBN 0-444-01559-0 (alk. paper)
1. Osteitis deformans—congresses. I. Singer, Frederick R., 1939– II. Wallach, Stanley. III. Title.
[DNLM: 1. Osteitis Deformans—diagnostic—congresses. 2. Osteitis Deformans—therapy—congresses. WE 250 1989 S9886p]
RC931.065S96 1989
616.7'12—dc20
DNLM/DLC
for Library of Congress 91-16543
CIP

Current printing (last digit):
10 9 8 7 6 5 4 3 2 1

Manufactured in the United States of America

Contents

Preface

Paget's disease is an old disease historically, but a new disease therapeutically. Human remains unearthed in Lancashire, England, dating from approximately 900 AD, show clear evidence of the affliction. However, it was not until the 1800s that physicians rediscovered the condition, and a little more than 100 years ago that Sir James Paget published a perceptive and accurate description of the disease from the clinical and pathologic points of view. He felt the disease represented an inflammatory condition of the skeleton and hence named it osteitis deformans. The condition again lapsed into anonymity for several decades afterwards, and therapeutic approaches did not evolve until after World War II when several groups, located mainly in the Boston area, began using a variety of agents, including corticosteroids for treatment of this condition. These early attempts at therapy were unsuccessful and the condition remained essentially untreatable until the development of the calcitonins and the bisphosphonates in the 1970s.

In 1978, the Paget's Disease Foundation, a private nonprofit voluntary health agency, was founded to assist individuals afflicted by Paget's disease of bone, to provide education regarding this condition to the medical community, and to encourage research efforts to better understand and treat the condition. An international conference was organized under the aegis of the Paget's Disease Foundation and was held in New York City in October, 1989, ten years after the founding of the Paget's Disease Foundation. The purpose of the conference was to discuss the progress, within the previous ten years, of the clinical assessment of Paget's disease and to place in perspective the status of present therapy and the prospects for future therapy. This book is based on this international conference and details the latest information concerning the diagnosis and treatment of Paget's disease.

Fourteen internationally known authorities on Paget's disease participated in the conference and in the preparation of this unique volume. Dr. Stephen Krane, from Harvard Medical School, reviewed the biology and biochemistry of the condition and the biochemical parameters that can be used to characterize disease activity. Dr. Stephen Teitelbaum of Washington University School of Medicine reviewed the pathologic features of Paget's disease and discussed both the cellular and structural abnormalities characteristic of the disorder. Dr. Ethel Siris of Columbia University College of Physicians and Surgeons discussed the clinical signs and symptoms and indications for treatment, paying special attention to the management of bone pain, intercurrent orthopedic surgery, and complications such as hearing loss, disturbed mineral metabolism, and the deleterious effects of immobilization. Dr. Alex Norman of New York Medical College outlined the radiologic features, the use of radiologic techniques in diagnosis, and the radiologic features of Paget's disease complications, including fractures and secondary tumorogenesis. Dr. Stephen Krane also discussed arthritis management in Paget's disease. Dr. Frederick Kaplan of the University of Pennsylvania School of Medicine discussed the role of orthopedic surgery in the management of patients with complications.

The remainder of the conference was devoted to medical therapies presently available and those projected for future utilization. Dr. Stanley Wallach of the University of South Florida College of Medicine summarized prior experience using porcine calcitonin and the present use of salmon calcitonin. Dr. John Haddad of the University of Pennsylvania School of Medicine provided similar discussion with regard to the use of human calcitonin. Dr. Charles Nagant de Deuxchaisnes of the Catholic University of Louvain, Belgium discussed European experience with new dose forms of calcitonin, especially the nasal spray form that avoids the need for injections. Dr. Frederick Singer of the University of California School of Medicine at Los Angeles discussed the emergence of resistance to calcitonin and the role of antibody formation in the resistant patient.

Several discussants dealt with the use of oral and intravenous bisphosphonates, which are in common use as effective alternatives to calcitonin. Dr. Pierre Meunier of the Faculté Alexis Carrel of the Medical School in Lyon, France discussed his experience with etidronate disodium, the first bisphosphonate to be used as therapy for Paget's disease and the only bisphosphonate available in the United States at present. Dr. Olav Bijvoet of the Medical School at the University of Leiden in The Netherlands discussed his experience using disodium pamidronate, a second generation bisphosphonate. Dr. Peter Burckhardt of Chuv University, Switzerland discussed the use of short-term disodium pamidronate treatment and the results to be expected with this newest way of using the bisphosphonates. Dr. John Kanis of the University of Sheffield, England discussed several third generation bisphosphonates undergoing clinical trials in Europe at present.

Finally, Dr. Will Ryan of Rush Presbyterian St. Lukes Medical School in Chicago discussed the present status of plicamycin treatment, a potent antipagetic agent which can be used when neither the calcitonins nor the bisphosphonates are feasible. He also alluded to the newest agent presently in development, gallium nitrate, which was not formally discussed.

This volume and the conference on which it is based have brought the outstanding progress of the last 20 years in treating Paget's disease into present perspective. It also provided much new material that will assist the reader in understanding and applying present research efforts to future therapies. The joint efforts of basic and clinical investigators, the pharmaceutical industry, governmental and voluntary agencies, and of treating physicians are to be recognized for the successes of the past two decades in addressing this previously untreatable disease.

Frederick R. Singer, MD
Stanley Wallach, MD

Acknowledgments

The editors of this volume wish to extend their sincere thanks to the Paget's Disease Foundation for undertaking the development and management of this fruitful conference, and to the following sponsors for their support of the Symposium: Ciba Geigy Pharmaceuticals, Fujisawa USA-Lyphomed, Merck Sharp and Dohme Research Laboratories, Norwich Eaton Pharmaceuticals, Rhône-Poulenc Rorer, Sandoz Pharmaceuticals, Sanofi Pharmaceuticals, Inc.

The authors are especially indebted to the President of the Board of Directors of the Paget's Disease Foundation, Mr. John B. Johnson, who has been the guiding spirit of the foundation since its inception, and to Mrs. Charlene Waldman, the Executive Director of the Paget's Disease Foundation, who has labored untiringly in the development and management of the conference and has worked yet harder in making this volume a reality.

Special thanks are also due to a number of individuals who were of great importance to the success of the Symposium and this volume. It was the idea of Mr. Walter Oberstebrink, past Chairman of the Paget's Disease Foundation, to sponsor a meeting about the advances in the evaluation and treatment of Paget's disease. Valuable assistance with the preparation of the manuscript was provided by Foundation staff Pamela Champbell and Barbra Schulman and William Dracos, a Duke University student, who served as a summer intern for the Foundation in 1990.

Finally the herculean efforts of my Co-Editor, Dr. Stanley Wallach, in the editing of many of the chapters of this volume, should be publicly recognized.

Frederick R. Singer, MD

Foreword to the Annotated Bibliography

On behalf of the National Arthritis and Musculoskeletal and Skin Diseases Information Clearinghouse (NAMSIC), I am pleased to present a reprint of our publication, *Paget's Disease: An Annotated Bibliography.*

This annotated bibliography contains 190 citations to patient and professional education materials; most have been published since 1984. Its purpose is to provide information sources for physicians, nurses, other health professionals, and patients and their families regarding the diagnosis, treatment, symptoms, and complications of Paget's disease.

I thank the following individuals for their review of this bibliography: Robert Canfield, MD, Columbia University, New York, New York; Stephen Gordon, PhD, National Institute of Arthritis and Musculoskeletal and Skin Diseases, Bethesda, Maryland; Stephen M. Krane, MD, Massachusetts General Hospital, Boston, Massachusetts; Reva C. Lawrence, MPH, National Institutes of Arthritis and Musculoskeletal and Skin Diseases, Bethesda, Maryland; Frederick R. Singer, MD, Cedars–Sinai Medical Center, Los Angeles, California; Ethel S. Siris, MD, Columbia Presbyterian Hospital, New York, New York; Stanley Wallach, MD, University of South Florida College of Medicine, Tampa, Florida; and especially to Ms. Charlene Waldman, Executive Director, Paget's Disease Foundation, Brooklyn, New York.

The bibliography was prepared by Cheryl Harris, NAMSIC staff, and produced for the Institute under contract No. NO1-DK-2290.

The Clearinghouse selects, acquires, and processes documents and other materials in the areas of patient education, public education, professional education, community demonstration programs, and federally funded programs in rheumatic, musculoskeletal, and skin diseases. These materials are available to the public through the Combined Health Information Database (CHID), which can be accessed through the services of a medical librarian or through BRS Information Technology, an online database vendor.

The Clearinghouse also provides a wide range of information dissemination services related to arthritis and musculoskeletal and skin diseases, including responding to public inquiries; publishing a news bulletin, *MEMO*, which is sent to over 9,000 people on the Clearinghouse mailing list; developing bibliographies, fact sheets, and other materials of interest to health professionals and their patients; and distributing professional and patient education materials.

For more information about NAMSIC and our services, please write or call:

National Arthritis and Musculoskeletal and
Skin Diseases Information Clearinghouse
Box AMS
9000 Rockville Pike
Bethesda, Maryland 20892
Telephone: (301) 495-4484

Again, I am honored to be able to contribute to this important text.

Lawrence E. Shulman, MD, PhD
Director, National Institute of Arthritis and Musculoskeletal and Skin Diseases, National Institutes of Health
Bethesda, Maryland

Contributors

Monique Beneton, BSc
Research Assistant, University of Sheffield Medical School, Beech Hill Road, Sheffield, South Yorkshire, S10 2RX England

Derek Bickerstaff, FRCS
University of Sheffield Medical School, Beech Hill Road, Sheffield, South Yorkshire S10 2RX England

Olav L. M. Bijvoet, MD
Professor, University of Leider Medical School, D. Bakkevlaan 61, 2061 EV, Bioemendaal, The Netherlands

Peter Burckhardt, MD
Chief, Department of Internal Medicine, Chuv University Hospital, 1011 Lausanne, Switzerland

Jean-Pierre Dovogelaer, MD
Assistant Professor, Department of Rheumatology, Catholic University of Lovain Medical School; St. Luc University Hospital, Avenue Hippocrate 10, B-1200, Brussels, Belgium

Karla Ginger, BS
Research Assistant, Bone Center, Cedars-Sinai Medical Center, 444 S. San Vicente Boulevard, Los Angeles, California 90048

John G. Haddad, MD

Professor and Chief, Endocrinology Section, Department of Medicine, University of Pennsylvania School of Medicine, 611 Clinical Research Building, 422 Curie Boulevard, Philadelphia, Pennsylvania 19104-6149

Neveen A. T. Hamdy, MD

University of Sheffield Medical School, Beech Hill Road, Sheffield, South Yorkshire, S10 2RX England

John A. Kanis, MD

Reader and Honorary Consultant Physician, Department of Human Metabolism and Clinical Biochemistry, University of Sheffield Medical School, Beech Hill Road, Sheffield, South Yorkshire, S10 2RX England

Frederick S. Kaplan, MD

Associate Professor of Orthopedic Surgery and Chief, Division of Metabolic Bone Diseases, Departments of Orthopedic Surgery and Medicine, 3400 Spruce Street, Philadelphia, Pennsylvania 19130

Stephen M. Krane, MD

Persis, Cyrus, and Marlow B. Harrison Professor of Medicine, Harvard Medical School; Chief, Arthritis Unit, Massachusetts General Hospital, Fruit Street, Boston, Massachusetts 02114

Susan F. Kroop, MD

Instructor, Department of Medicine, Harvard Medical School; New England Deaconess Hospital, 185 Pilgrim Road, Boston, Massachusetts 02215

Eugene V. McCloskey, FRCP

University of Sheffield Medical School, Beech Hill Road, Sheffield, South Yorkshire S10 2RX England

Pierre J. Meunier, MD

Professor of Medicine, Faculte Alexis Carrel, Rue Guillaume Paradin, 690008 Lyon, France; Director, INSERM Research Unit, Department of Rheumatology and Metabolic Bone Diseases, Edouard Herriot Hospital, Lyon, France

Charles Nagant de Deuxchaisnes, MD

Professor, Catholic University of Louvain Medical School; Chief, Department of Rheumatology, St. Luc University Hospital, Avenue Hippocrate 10, B-1200 Brussels, Belgium

Alex Norman, MD
Professor, Department of Radiology, New York Medical College, Elmwood Hall, Valhalla, New York, 10595

Declan O'Doherty, FRCS
University of Sheffield Medical School, Beech Hill Road, Sheffield, South Yorkshire, S10 2RX England

Alain Ravault, MD
Faculte Alexis Carrel, Rue Guillaume Paradin, 690008 Lyon, France

Will G. Ryan, MD
Professor, Department of Medicine, Rush Medical College of Rush University; Director, Osteoporosis Center, Rush Presbyterian–St. Luke's Medical Center, Chicago, Illinois 60612

Frederick R. Singer, MD
Professor of Medicine in Residence, University of California, Los Angeles, UCLA School of Medicine; Director, Bone Center, Cedars-Sinai Medical Center, 444 S. San Vicente Boulevard, Los Angeles, California 90048

Ethel S. Siris, MD
Associate Professor of Clinical Medicine, Department of Medicine, Columbia University College of Physicians and Surgeons, 630 W. 168 Street, New York, New York 10032

Steven L. Teitelbaum, MD
Messing Professor of Pathology, Washington University School of Medicine, St. Louis, Missouri; Pathologist-in-Chief, Jewish Hospital at Washington University Medical Center, 216 S. Kings Highway St. Louis, Missouri 63110

Maniccam Thavarajah, PhD
Research Assistant, University of Sheffield Medical School, Beech Hill Road, Sheffield, South Yorkshire S10 2RX, England

D. Thiébaud, MD
Department of Internal Medicine, Chuv University Hospital, 1011 Lausanne, Switzerland

Stanley Wallach, MD
Professor and Associate Chairman, Department of Internal Medicine, University of South Florida College of Medicine, 12901 North 30th Street, Tampa Florida 33612-4799

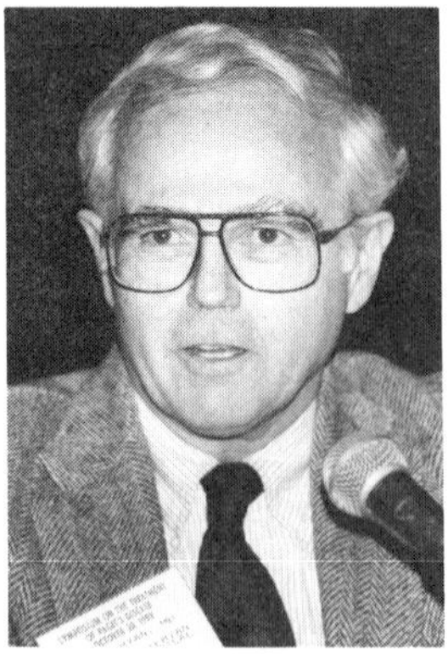

Will G. Ryan

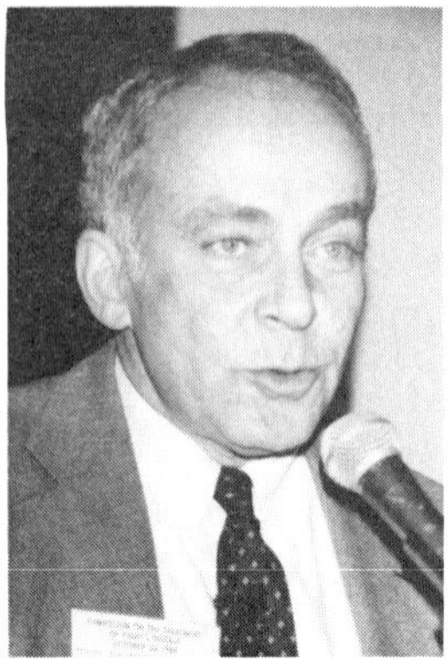

John G. Haddad Jr.

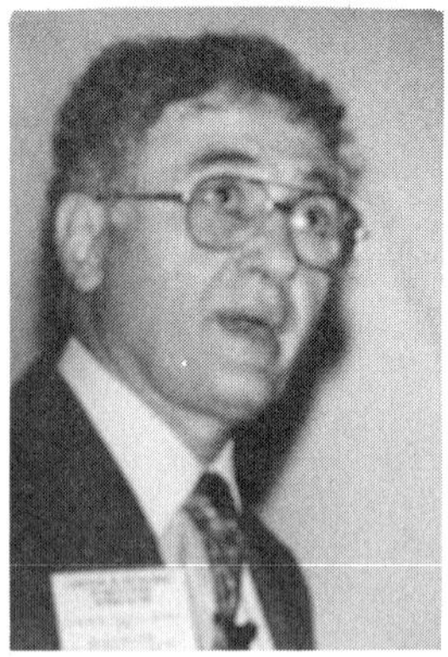

Steven L. Teitelbaum

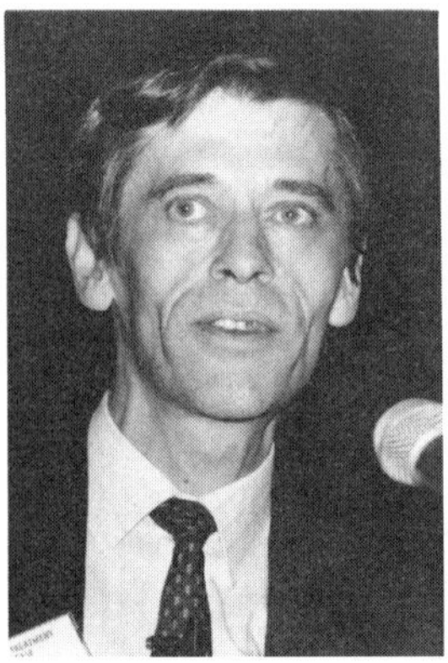

John A. Kanis

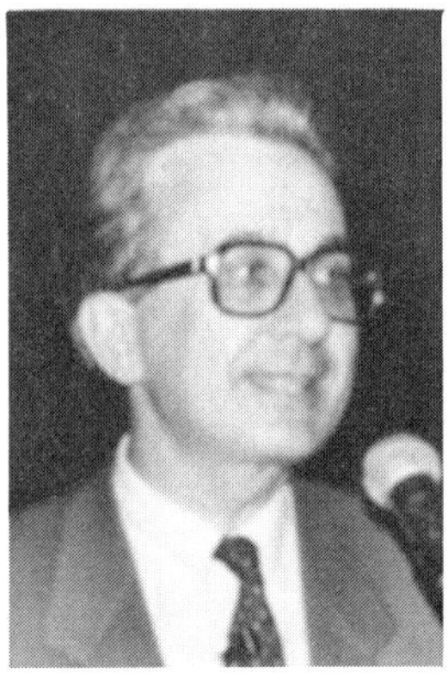

Pierre Meunier

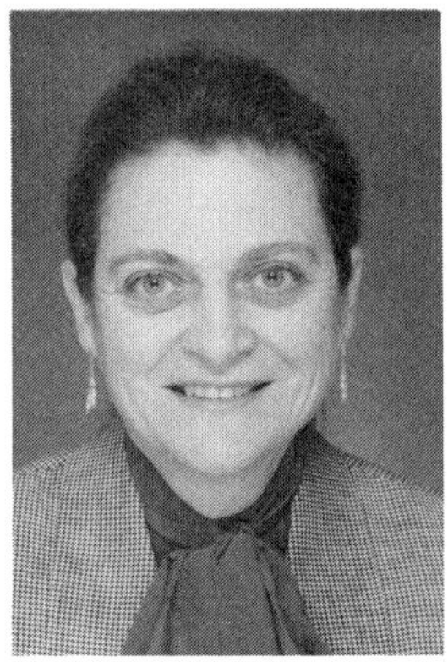

Ethel S. Siris

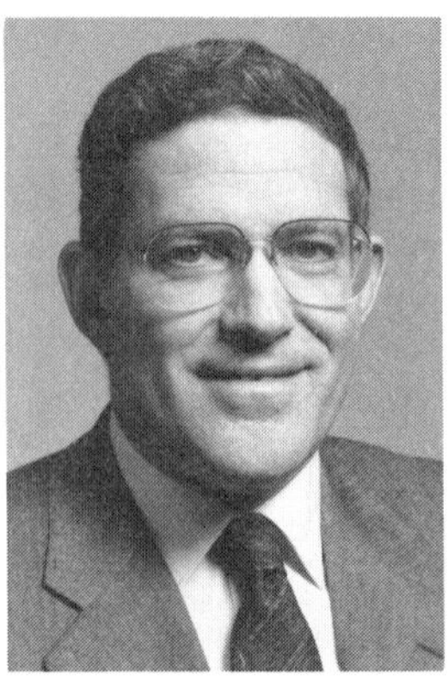

Frederick R. Singer

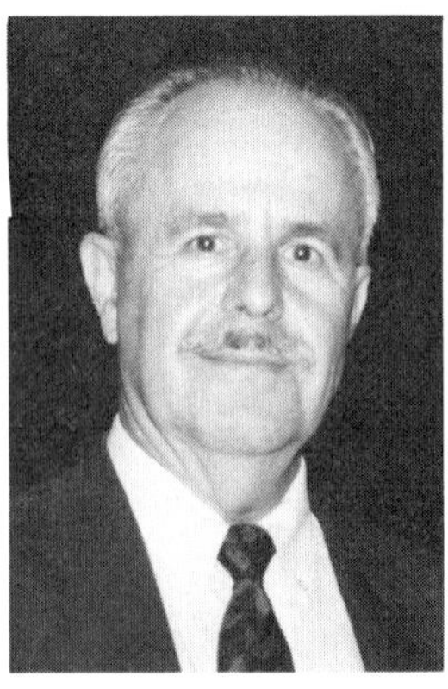

Stanley Wallach

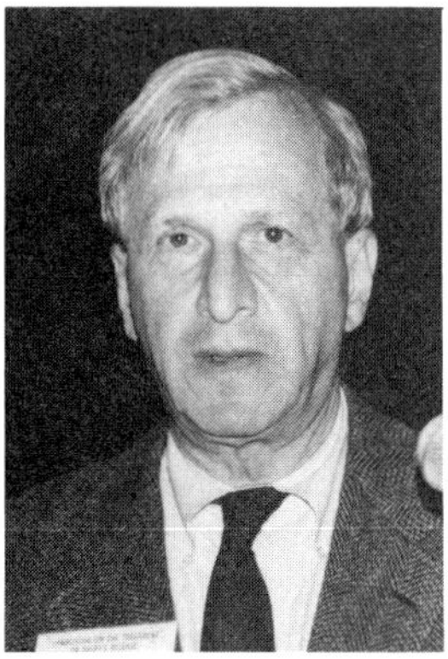

Stephen Krane

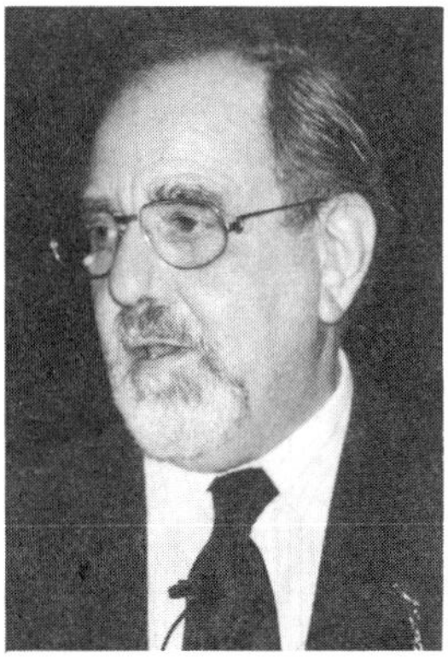

Olav Bijvoet

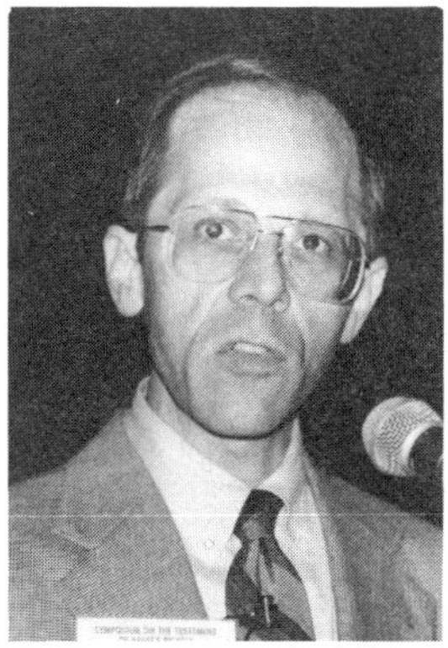

Frederick S. Kaplan

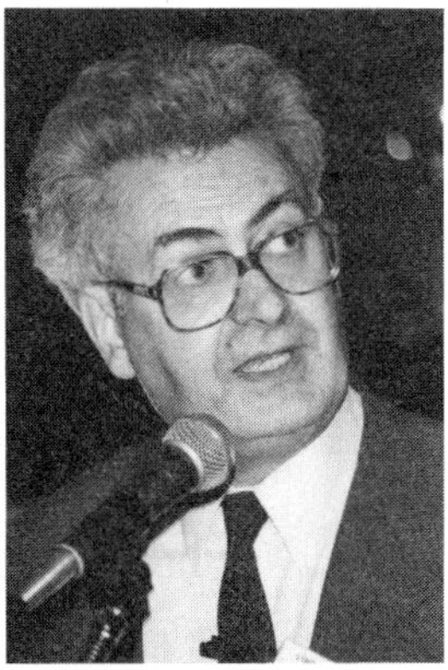

C. Nagant de Deuxchaisnes

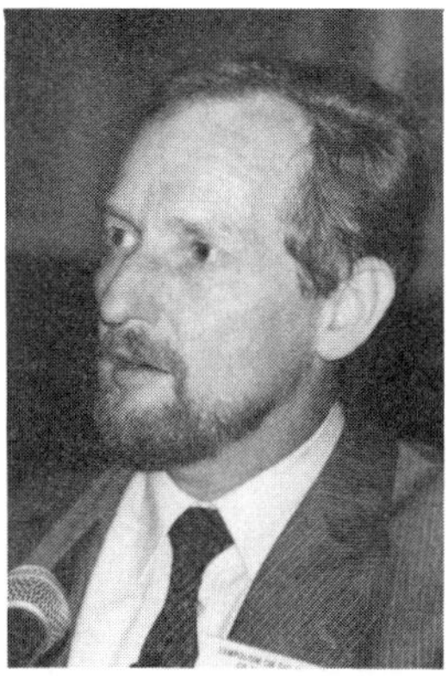

Peter Burckhardt

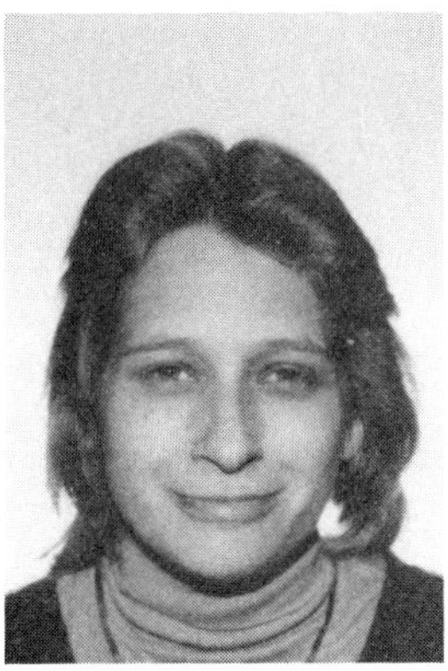

Susan F. Kroop

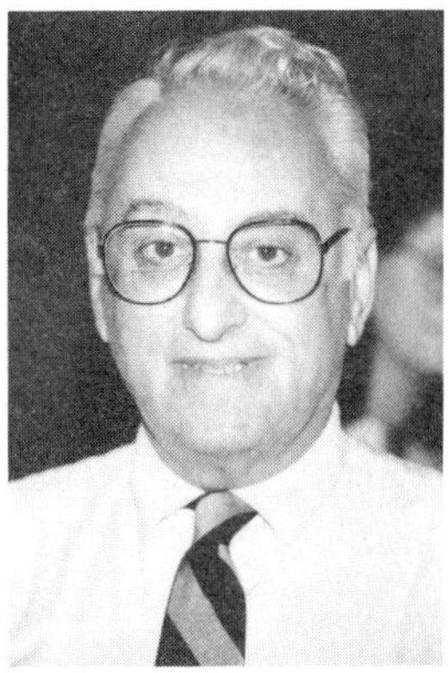

Alex Norman

CHAPTER 1

The Radiology of Paget's Disease

Alex Norman

INTRODUCTION

Paget's disease is characterized by active remodeling of bone; its radiologic characteristics follow the transformation of the gross and microscopic anatomy that occurs in both cortical and cancellous bone. Bone is ultimately remodeled into a coarse trabeculated pattern that when pieced together characterizes the mosaic architecture that distinguishes the condition[1-3] (Figure 1.1). The disease progresses through three distinct phases of remodeling: the early osteolytic or "hot phase," the intermediate or "mixed phase," and ultimately the late sclerotic or "cooled-off phase."

EARLY (OR HOT) PHASE

In the initial stage ("hot phase") of Paget's disease, active osteolytic resorption advances at a rapid pace until much of the original compact cortex is resorbed and replaced by very delicate trabecular structures.[2,3] Only 1% to 2% of patients clinically exhibit a purely lytic stage of involvement,[4] whereas 20% to 30% demonstrate both an osteolytic and an early osteoblastic stage of remodeling.[4-6] The "hot phase" of bone resorption is best illustrated radiographically in long tubular bones and is characterized by an advancing wedge- or flame-shaped segment of bone resorption that progresses from one articular surface and may eventually reach the opposite end of the bone (Figure 1.2). Typically the transition between the

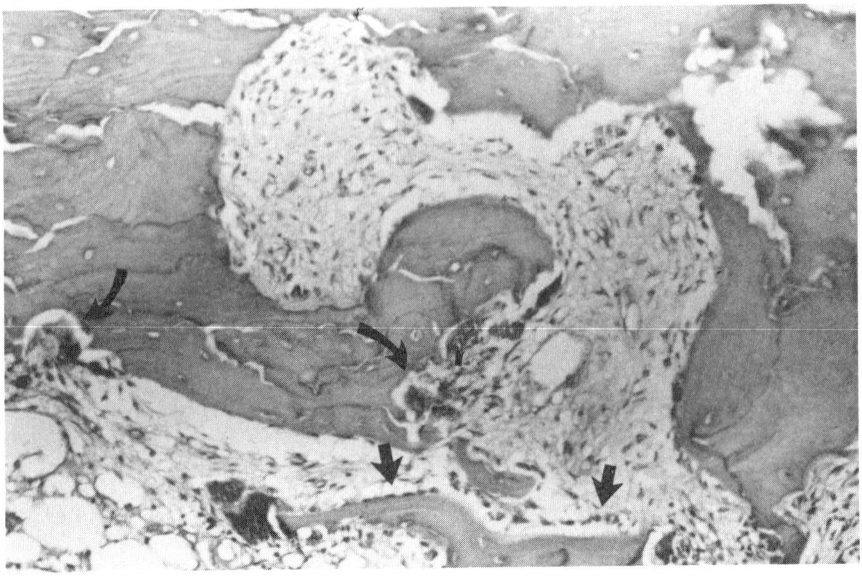

FIGURE 1.1. The histologic features of Paget's disease are illustrated in this photomicrograph. The interplay between osteoclastic resorption (curved arrows) and bone deposition (straight arrows) is demonstrated. The "jigsaw puzzle" of cement lines is the final pattern of pagetic remodeling and the hallmark of the disease.

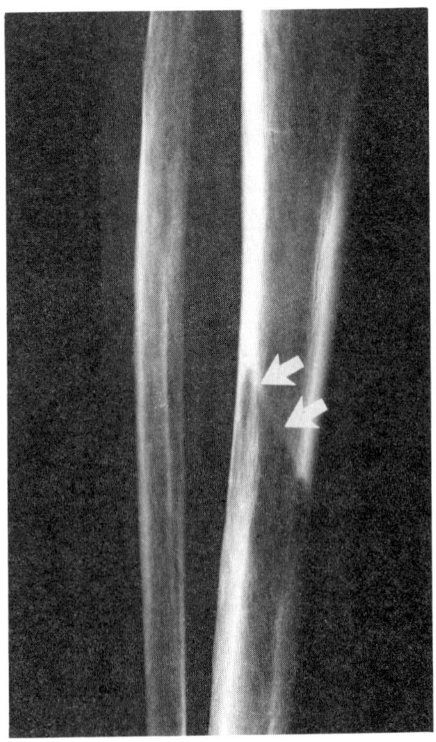

FIGURE 1.2. The initial ("hot") stage of Paget's disease is the "advancing wedge" of resorption that contrasts sharply with the normal bone it is resorbing (see arrows).

normal and lytic bone is sharply defined. The osteolytic stage can sometimes present a problem in diagnosis. Although a bone biopsy can resolve the issue, the procedure should be avoided since it is fraught with the risk of fracture.[5,6]

The transformation between the advancing wedge of pagetic bone and the unaffected cortex is striking. The bone is expanded by periosteal new bone formation on the surface of the cortex. In the extremities the "hot phase" of bone remodeling is relatively short-lived, and in the wake of the osteolytic change comes the coarsely trabeculated new bone response that replaces the old cortex as well as the cancellous bone. The increased density that occurs is impressive and heralds the onset of the intermediate phase of the disease. This process can occur in a single bone or involve multiple sites in the skeleton, such as the pelvis, spine, and sacrum.

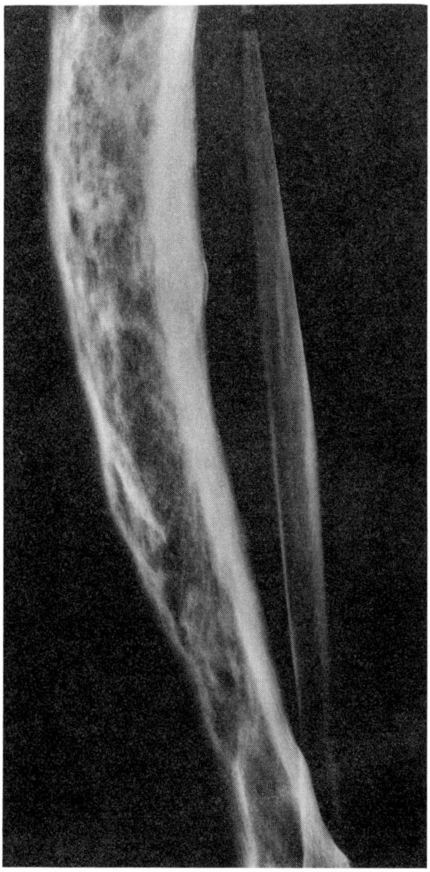

FIGURE 1.3. Classic pattern of Paget's disease in the tibia of a 65-year-old man. The cortices are coarsely trabeculated and thickened, and the bone is broadened and anteriorly bowed. The disease has advanced from the proximal end of the tibia to the opposite end.

INTERMEDIATE (OR MIXED) PHASE

The mixed phase of Paget's disease (osteolytic and osteoblastic) is the stage most frequently seen radiographically. Bone resorption and new bone deposition can be recognized on the radiographs. The cortex is remodeled into a very thick coarsely trabeculated bony structure (Figures 1.3 and 1.4). Widening of the marrow cavity and overall broadening and bowing of the

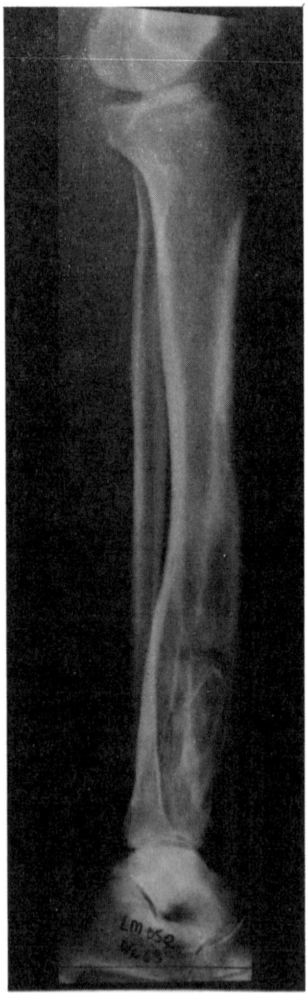

FIGURE 1.4. The tibia of this 54-year-old woman illustrates the intermediate phase of Paget's disease. The lower end of the shaft is coarsely trabeculated, dense, and widened as the disease progresses toward the midshaft.

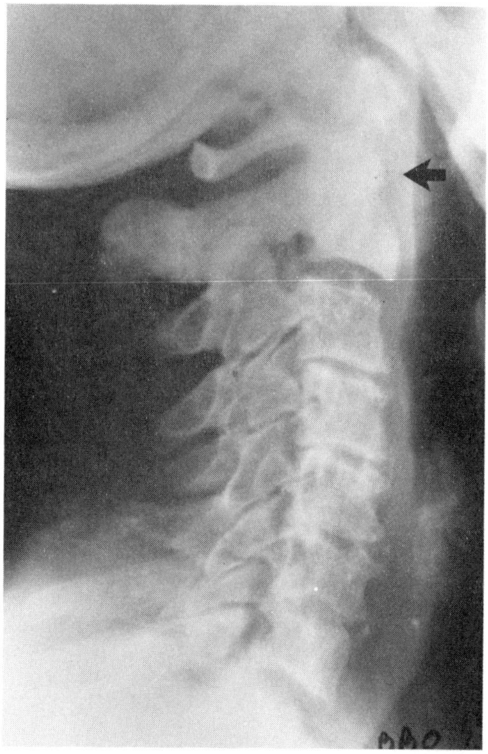

FIGURE 1.5. This "ivory vertebra" was an isolated finding. It was a diagnostic problem and required a biopsy to establish the correct diagnosis of Paget's disease.

bone are common. As Jaffe has mentioned,[2] Paget's disease has a great propensity to undergo reparative change. If this modification progresses, it eventually induces a dense sclerotic change in bone. In the spine this can simulate an "ivory vertebra" (Figure 1.5). The sclerotic changes may be so striking that the question of an osteoblastic metastasis from prostate or breast cancer, Hodgkin's disease, or histiocytic lymphoma must be considered (Figure 1.6).[7,8] In less severe involvement of the spine, infection and discogenic sclerosis may also have to be considered in the differential diagnosis. To see a dense vertebra or other bony area, such as rib or pelvis, as an isolated involvement of bone is rare in Paget's disease, and such cases may require a biopsy to confirm the diagnosis. Fortunately, the pattern of uniform sclerosis of a bone is most often seen with polyostotic involvement of the skeleton and with other lesions' showing a mixed phase, thereby allowing the diagnosis of Paget's disease to be made radiographically.

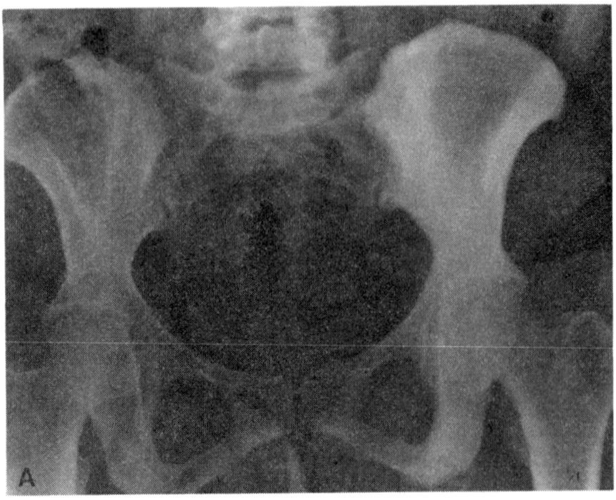

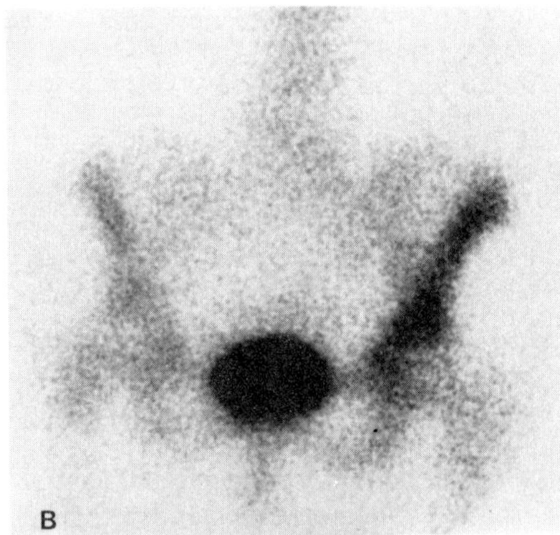

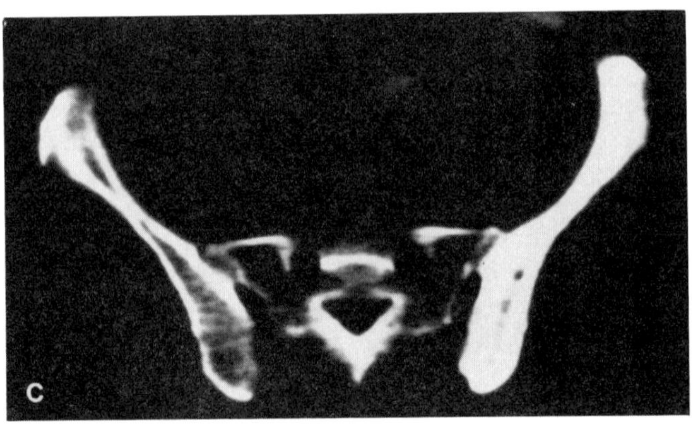

FIGURE 1.6. **(A)** Pelvis of a patient in the reparative stage of the disease with an intense osteoblastic response. **(B)** In the same patient, scintigraphy showed moderate uptake in the left half of the pelvis. **(C)** Computerized axial tomography confirmed the dense sclerotic changes in the left hemipelvis. A biopsy established the diagnosis of Paget's disease.

LATE (OR SCLEROTIC) PHASE

Eventually the process of active bone remodeling slows and the small fragments of the remodeled bone are pieced together by cement lines into a classic mosaic pattern simulating a jigsaw puzzle. Osteoclastic resorption and fibrovascular proliferation in the marrow disappear. What remains is thick, coarsely trabeculated bone with the return of yellow marrow. The cortex is generally enlarged and the medullary cavity is replaced by very coarse, sclerotic trabeculae extending through the bone. This stage is characterized radiographically by changes similar to those of the late intermediate phase.

SKULL

The skull is commonly involved in Paget's disease. The term *osteoporosis circumscripta* was introduced by Schuller,[9] and represents the osteolytic phase discussed earlier in the extremities as expressed in the skull (Figure

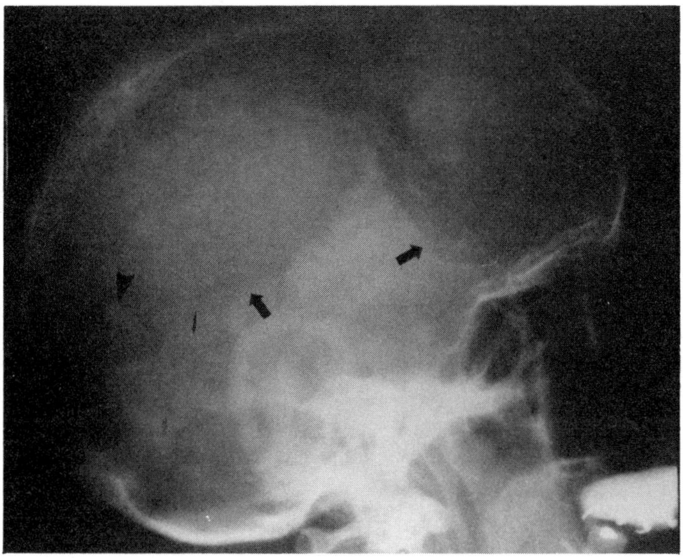

FIGURE 1.7. Osteoporosis circumscripta characterizes the "hot phase" of Paget's disease in the calvaria. Note the collision of two large, circumscribed osteolytic lesions in the calvaria (arrows), which were separate and distinct lesions 7 years before. The cranial sutures did not limit the advancement of the bone resorption. A small focal area of sclerotic bone in the parietal region (arrowhead) heralds the onset of the mixed phase of Paget's disease.

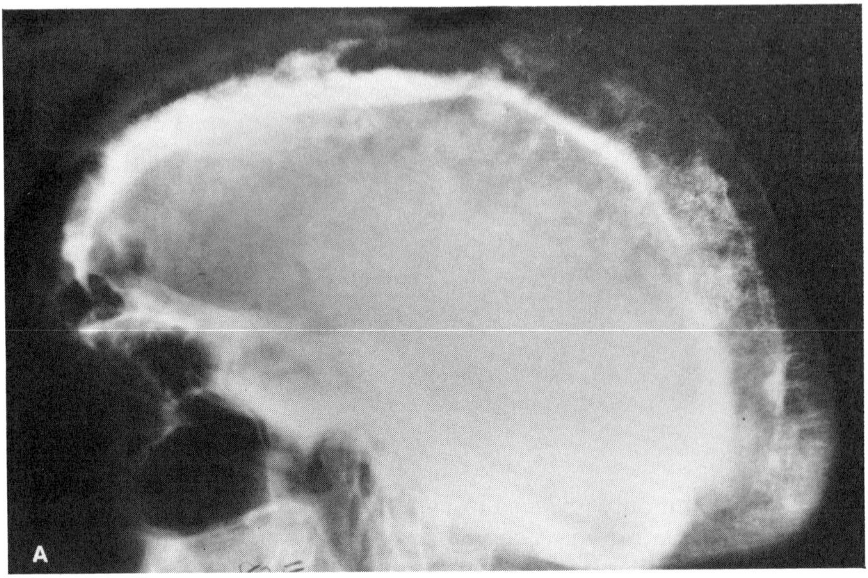

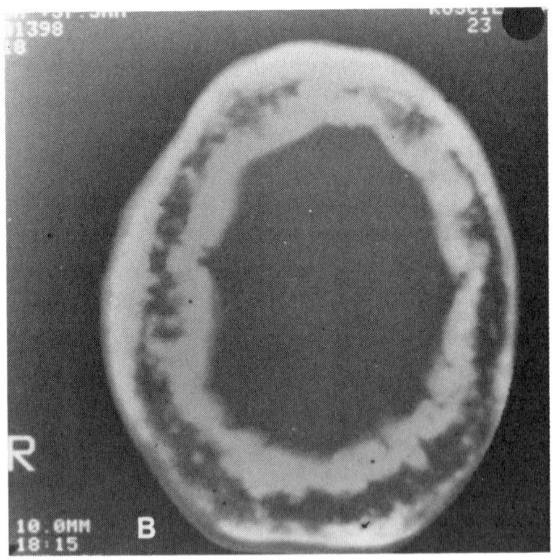

FIGURE 1.8. **(A)** Skull of an 82-year-old woman illustrating striking thickening of the calvarial bone. Invagination of the base of the skull and flattening of the sphenoid-basilar angle are demonstrated. **(B)** The changes in the calvaria are demonstrated on this computerized tomogram. The inner table is thicker and more irregular than the outer. The focal densities of pagetic bone in the diploic spaces are more numerous posteriorly. **(C)** Magnetic resonance (T1 weighted) image of the same patient showing brain compression from the thick inner table (black arrows).

1.7). The circumscribed zone of osteoporosis represents marked resorption of the inner and outer tables of the calvaria. There may be more than one such zone in the skull, but most commonly the frontal bone is affected (osteoporosis circumscripta frontalis).[10] Similar lesions, however, may be seen in the parietal, temporal, and even occipital bones. In time, small

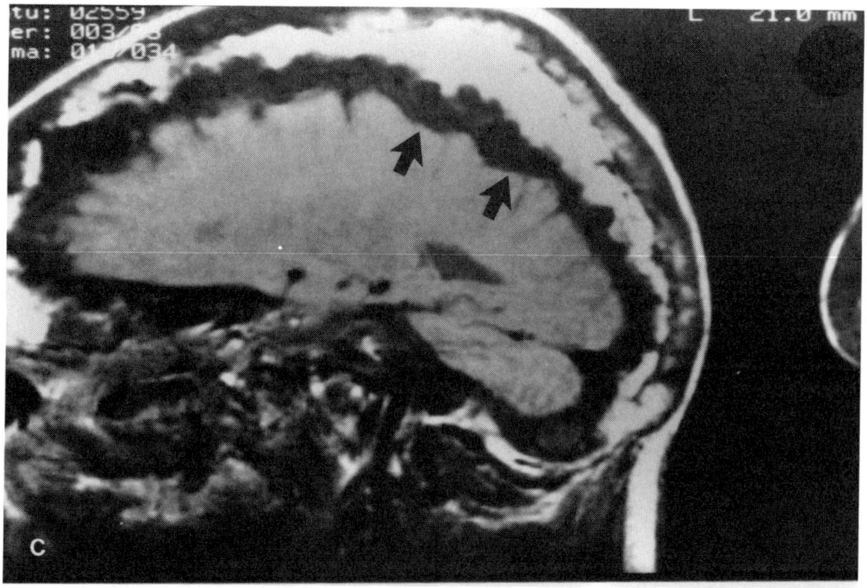

focal radiopacities or islands of newly formed sclerotic pagetic bone (cotton-ball appearance) appear as the disease advances into the phase of osteoblastic remodeling.[1,2] On the other hand, osteoporosis circumscripta can remain unchanged for several years or advance by crossing suture lines to involve the other flat bones of the skull.

When the calvaria is sectioned, it grossly resembles pumice stone.[2] Most of the new bone apposition occurs in the outer table. Less frequently, thick, lumpy bone accretions are seen on the inner table of the skull. Subdural bony masses can encroach on and compress the brain and cause neurologic disturbances (Figure 1.8).

THE VERTEBRAE

Classically, pagetic modification of the vertebral bodies resembles picture framing (Figure 1.9). The vertebrae enlarge and the posterior elements coarsen and encroach on the anteroposterior diameter of the spinal canal. Less often, the vertebra collapses and broadens under the load of weight bearing. Rarely, the bony structure of a vertebral body is totally resorbed and appears as a purely osteolytic lesion with collapse. (Figure 1.10).

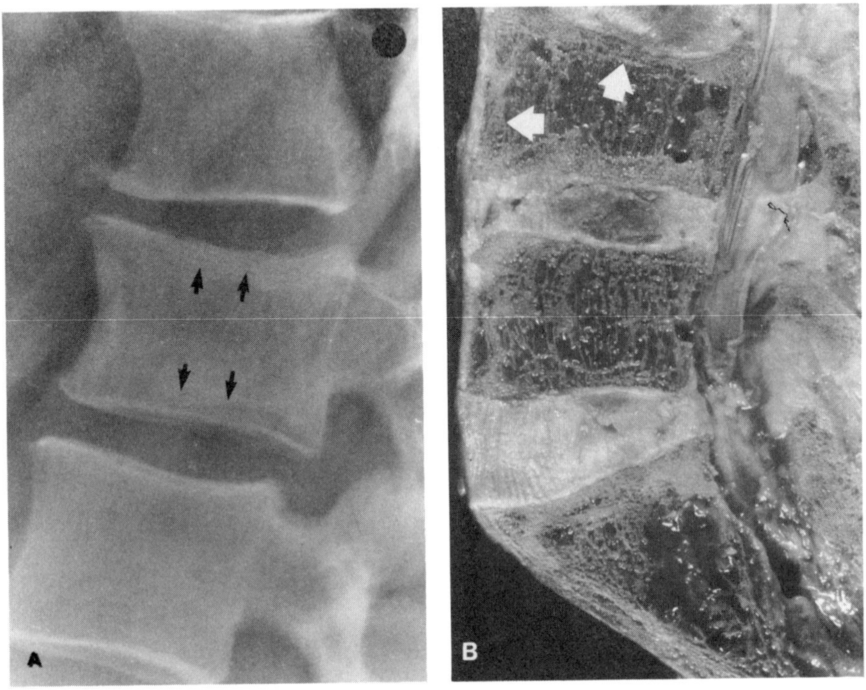

FIGURE 1.9. **(A)** A 72-year-old man was discovered to have monostotic Paget's disease in the second lumbar vertebra in the course of testing. Note the classic appearance of picture framing of the vertebra with coarse trabeculations outlining the vertebral body. The vertebra is slightly larger than the adjacent segments. **(B)** An anatomic specimen illustrating the features that contribute to picture framing of vertebral bodies. Note the coarse trabeculations and sclerosis about the periphery of the lumbar vertebral body (arrows). The thick trabeculae seen in the center of the vertebral body may simulate a hemangioma.

COMPLICATIONS OF PAGET'S DISEASE

Fractures

The most common outcome of the structural weakness of pagetic bone is deformity, usually manifested by convex bowing of long bones, especially of the lower extremities. However, pathologic fracture, either occurring spontaneously or resulting from minor trauma, is also common and may be the first event to draw attention to Paget's disease. Stress or insufficiency fractures (also called fissure fractures) are more frequent than complete transverse fractures and occur as deformities worsen. Fissure fractures can be isolated or multiple, and the number of such fractures in a single bone

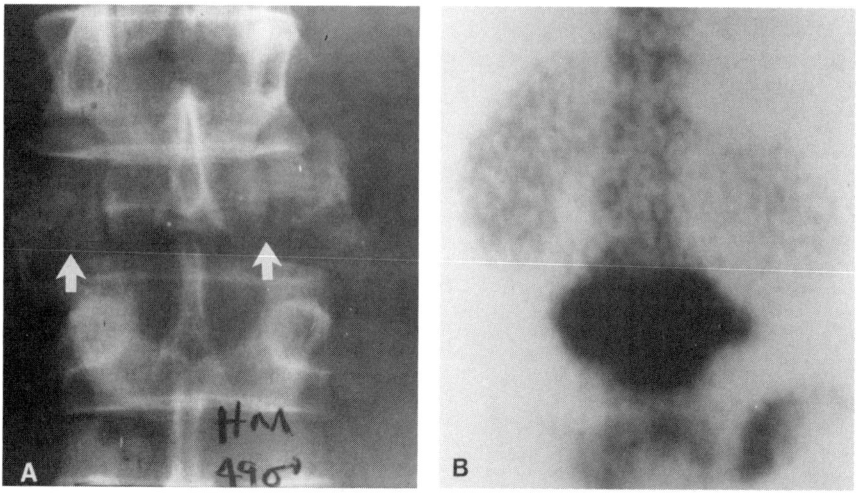

FIGURE 1.10. A 49-year-old man had acute collapse of the third lumbar vertebra, which destroyed the vertebra (arrows). Metastatic bone cancer or multiple myeloma was suspected. A diagnosis of the "hot phase" of Paget's disease was made by bone biopsy. **(B)** A technetium 99 methyldiphosphonate radionuclide bone scan showing intense uptake in the vertebra.

such as the femur can be striking. In one case in our series, a patient had 19 insufficiency fractures on the tension (convex) side of a bowed femur (Figure 1.11).

The incidence of complete fractures has been reported to average more than one per patient.[11] The most frequent sites for pathologic fractures are the femur and tibia. Less commonly, fractures may occur in the spine, humerus, and pelvis. In a personal series of 70 fractures of the femur, Barry[11] reported that 37% of the lesions were in the subtrochanteric region of the femoral shaft, which is the most typical site of injury. The peak age of patients at the time of fracture is the eighth decade and incidence is equal for both sexes.

Fractures occur during all stages of the disease. Those in the femur occur most often during the osteolytic phase. On the other hand, many authors believe that most other fractures occur in the later stages of disease when the bone is more sclerotic (Figure 1.12). The pagetic fracture is classically transverse and has minimal comminution. It resembles the splitting of a banana or the snapping of a carrot.[11] The old adage that fractures heal faster in pagetic bone than in normal bone has not been

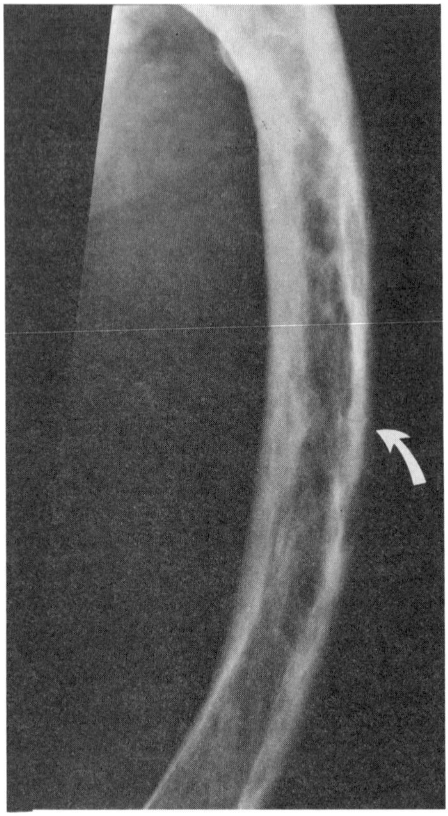

FIGURE 1.11. Femur of a patient with stress (fissure) fractures in the lateral cortex of the midshaft of the femur. The fractures are almost always on the tension (convex) side of the bone.

proved.[12,13] Rather, fractures unite at the same pace as simple traumatic fractures in normal bone.[11,12] There is also no documentation that a pagetic fracture predisposes to the development of a sarcoma. However, an occult sarcoma has been discovered at the sites of pathologic fractures. Hence, a biopsy examination of the site of a fracture is warranted when performing internal fixation.

Tumors

The most serious complication of Paget's disease is sarcomatous degeneration. However, not all tumors are sarcomas. Myeloma, lymphoma, and metastatic bone cancer have been known to coexist with pagetic bone.

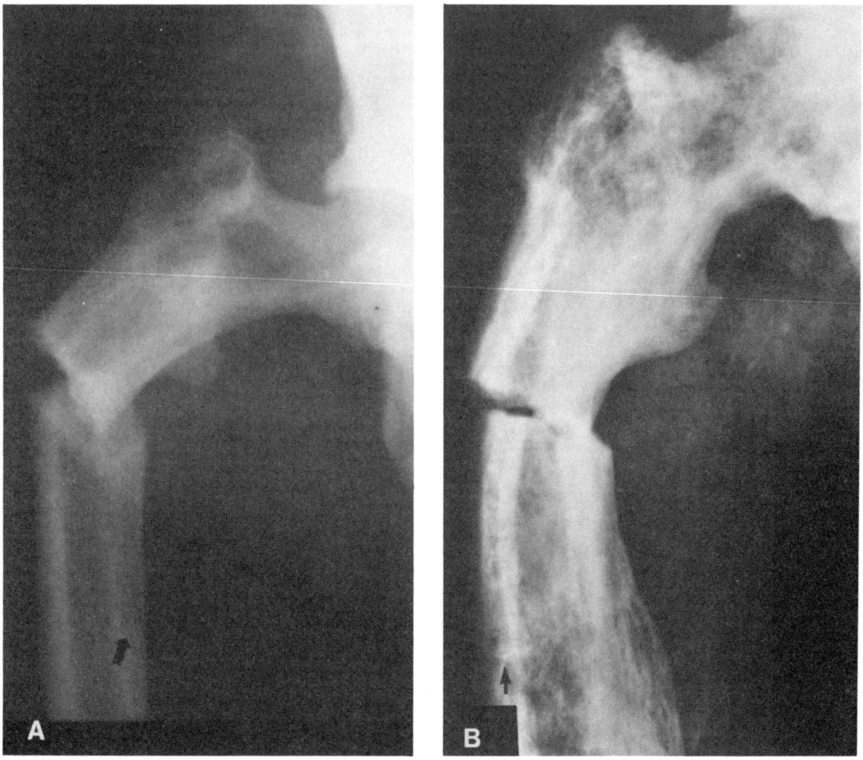

FIGURE 1.12. (**A**) Transverse (banana) fracture in the subtrochanteric region of the femur during the mixed stage of the disease. Note the advancing wedge of resorption along the medial cortex (arrow). (**B**) Another patient suffered the same type of fracture at the same location in the femur. However, the radiologic features are those of late-stage disease. Note the stress fracture along the lateral cortex below the transverse fracture (arrow).

Occasionally Paget's disease can be complicated by a benign tumor, such as a giant cell tumor (Figure 1.13), or an ominous-looking lesion known as a pseudosarcoma of Paget's disease. Also, a large area of bone resorption called a pseudocyst may be mistaken for a malignant lesion (Figure 1.14).

The incidence of Paget's sarcoma is difficult to assess. It has been reported to be as low as 0.15% or as high as 10%.[14] Sarcomas are usually isolated lesions but can be multicentric in origin. The older the patient (60–70 years) and the greater the extent of skeletal involvement, the higher the risk of sarcomatous change. Smith and colleagues[14] at Memorial Hospital reported 85 pagetic sarcomas collected over 55 years (1927–1982). Histologically, the majority of these tumors were osteosarcomas. A small number, however, proved to be chondrosarcomas and fibrosarcomas, and

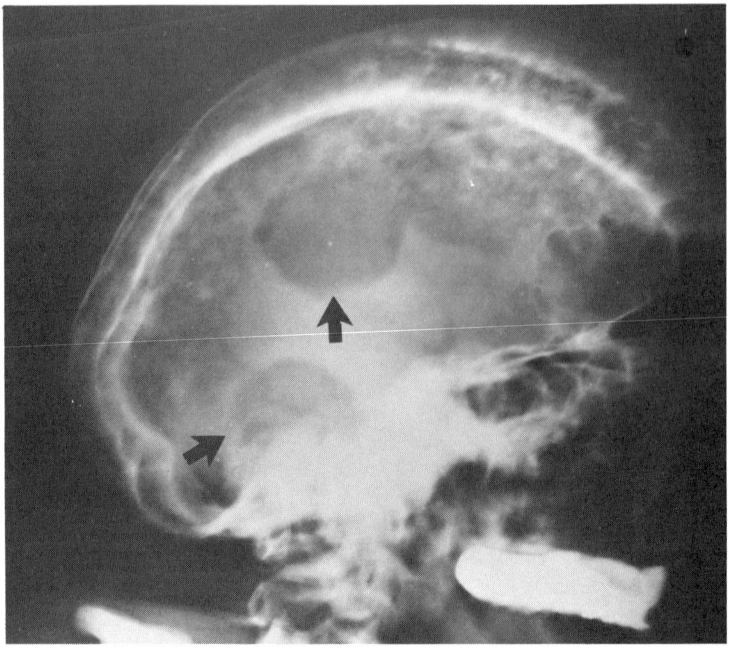

FIGURE 1.13. Skull of a 73-year-old man with extensive skeletal involvement in Paget's disease. Several large destructive lesions in the calvaria proved to be benign giant cell tumors (arrows). He had at least six tumors in the skull that responded to radiation treatment.

one was a malignant fibrous histiocytoma. A few cases were malignant giant cell tumors.

The pelvis and extremities (humerus, femur, and tibia) are the high-risk sites for malignant transformation (Figure 1.15). Although Schmorl's study[15] showed that Paget's disease occurred infrequently in the humerus, the Memorial Hospital study indicated that this bone was at high risk for sarcomatous degeneration (26%); and it was second only to sarcoma of the pelvis (27%).[14,16] Paget's sarcoma of the spine is uncommon. Sarcomatous degeneration can also appear in monostotic Paget's disease. Sarcomatous transformation should be suspected when there is a sudden onset of pain or rapid worsening of previous pain. The presence of a soft tissue mass over the site of spontaneous fracture should create a high index of suspicion of an underlying sarcoma.

Radiologic Features of Paget's Sarcoma

Progressive destruction of pagetic bone is a presumptive finding of a sarcoma. Less frequently, increasing sclerosis or masses of dense amorphous deposits in bone, with or without fracture, also suggest malignant

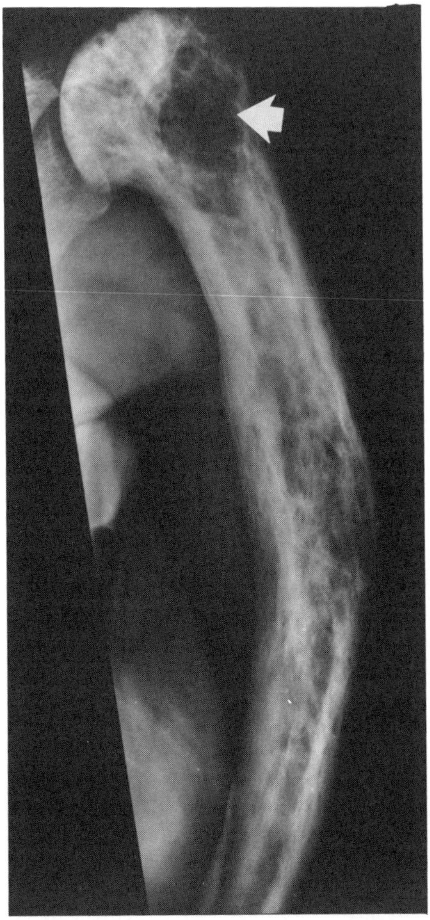

FIGURE 1.14. Mixed stage of Paget's disease in the humerus with typical lateral bowing of the shaft. The osteolytic lesion in the humeral neck is not a malignancy but a "pseudocyst" resulting from active bone resorption.

change. The typical appearance of sarcomatous transformation in Paget's disease is demonstrated by the radiographic occurrence of a large destructive lesion, which extends through the cortex, and the presence of a periosteal reaction or a soft tissue mass. Sarcomas commonly metastasize to the lungs and rarely to other bones. When more than one site of sarcoma is noted, it is more likely that the Paget's sarcoma is multifocal in origin rather than that it has metastasized from another site (Figure 1.16).

Bone scintigraphy in Paget's disease generally shows intense uptake of the injected radionuclide. Although technetium 99 methyldiphosphonate

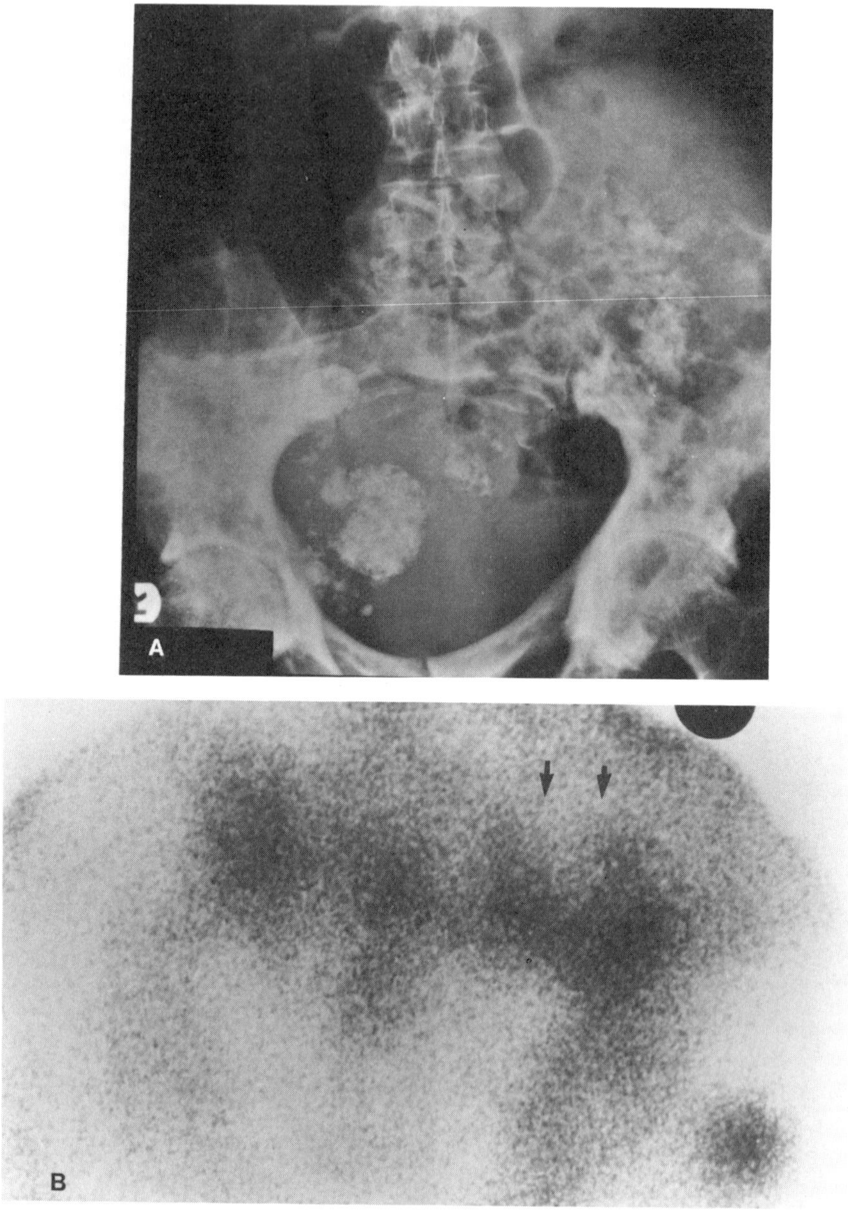

FIGURE 1.15. **(A)** Ilium of a patient with an osteogenic sarcoma; the tumor has destroyed the left iliac crest and extends into the soft tissue **(B)** Technetium 99 methyldiphosphonate bone scintigraphy showing reduced uptake in the tumor (arrows).

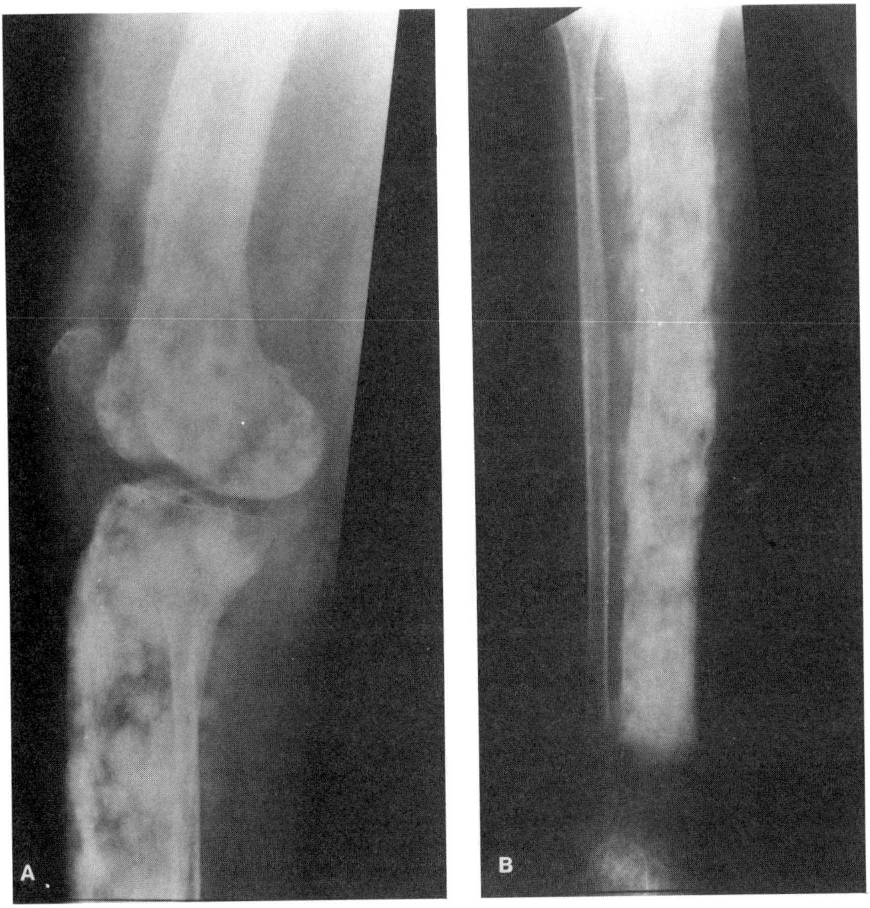

FIGURE 1.16. (A & B) Elderly woman with multicentric osteosarcomatosis in the right femur and tibia. There is extensive sarcomatous bone change extending into the soft tissues of the leg and thigh.

uptake is intense over affected pagetic bone, when a sarcoma occurs reduced activity is often indicated by radionuclide bone scanning. However, if a gallium scan is performed, uptake over the site of a sarcomatous soft tissue mass can be very intense.

Despite the advent of chemotherapy, the 5-year survival rate of patients with Paget's sarcoma is poor. Most patients die within 2 years of the onset of the sarcoma.[3,13,14]

Benign Tumors

Giant cell tumor is a rare complication of Paget's disease. Most giant cell tumors occur in the skull or facial bones (see Figure 1.13), but a few cases have been noted in long tubular bones. When they arise at this site, they usually develop in the shaft rather than at the articular end of the bone, as seen in classic cases of giant cell tumor.[14,16-18] In 1979, Jacobs and colleagues[19] recognized the association of giant cell tumors and Paget's disease and found a familial pattern among Italians whose ancestral roots originated near a small town east of Naples called Avellino. In some cases a multiplicity of giant cell tumors is striking. In one of our cases, a woman of Italian descent had 27 giant cell tumors in the skull.

Another benign lesion that occurs in association with Paget's disease is the "pseudosarcoma" described by Monson and associates.[20,21] Distinguishing the pseudosarcoma from a true malignant transformation can be troublesome radiographically. Pseudosarcomas display a large bony mass and a sizable soft tissue component. Jaffe[2] has suggested that this tumorlike but benign process is the result of an exuberant periosteal reaction. Occasionally a paraspinal pseudotumor of extramedullary hematopoiesis can also be mistaken for sarcomatous degeneration.

REFERENCES

1. Milgram JW: Radiographical and pathological assessment of the activity of Paget's disease of bone. *Clin Orthop* 1977;127:43–54.
2. Jaffe HL: The classic Paget's disease of bone. *Clin Orthop* 1977;127:4–23.
3. Jaffe HL: Paget's disease, in *Metabolic, Degenerative, and Inflammatory Diseases of Bones and Joints.* Philadelphia, Lea & Febiger, 1972, pp 297–308.
4. Eisman JA, Martin J: Osteolytic Paget's disease. *J Bone Joint Surg* 1986;68A:112–117.
5. Seaman WB: The roentgen appearance of early Paget's disease. *Am J Roentgenol* 951;66(4):587–594.
6. Jacobs P: Osteolytic Paget's disease. *Clin Radiol* 1974;25:138–144.
7. Harris DJ, Hons CB, and Fornasier VL: An ivory vertebra. *Clin Orthopaed* 1978; 136:173–175.
8. Jaffe HL: Atypical form of Paget's disease appearing as generalized osteosclerosis. *Arch Pathol* 1933;16:1–26.
9. Schuller A: Ueber circumscripte Osteoporose des Schadele. *Med Klin* 1929;25:631–632.
10. Wilner D, Sherman RS: Roentgen diagnosis of Paget's disease (osteitis deformans). *Med Radiogr Photogr* 1966;42(2):35–78.
11. Barry HC: *Paget's Disease of Bone.* Baltimore, Williams & Wilkins, 1969.
12. Nocholas NA, Killoran P: Fracture of the femur in patients with Paget's disease. *J Bone Joint Surg* 1965;47A(6):450–561.
13. Barry, HC: Fractures of the femur in Paget's disease of bone in Australia. *J Bone Joint Surg* 1967;49A(7):1350–1370.
14. Smith J, Botet JF, Yeh SDH: Bone sarcomas in Paget disease: A study of 85 patients. *Radiology* 1984;152(3):583–589.
15. Schmorl G: Uber Osteitis Deformans Paget. *Virchows Arch Pathol Anat* 1932;283:694–751.
16. Miller C, Rao VM: Sarcomatous degeneration of Paget disease in the Skull. *Skeletal Radiol* 1983;10:102–106.

17. Mirra JM: Pathogenesis of Paget's disease based on viral etiology. *Clin Orthop* 1987; 217:162–170.
18. Schajowicz F, Slullitel I: Giant-cell tumor associated with Paget's disease of bone. *J Bone Joint Surg* 1966;48A(7):1340–1349.
19. Jacobs T, Michelsen J, Polay J, et al: Giant cell tumor in Paget's disease of bone: Familial and geographic cluster. *Cancer* 1979;44:742–747.
20. Monson DK, Finn HA, Dawson PJ, Simon MA: Pseudosarcoma in Paget's disease of bone. *J Bone Joint Surg* 1989;71A(3):453–455.
21. Zadek RE, Milgram JW: Progression of Paget's diseae in the tibia. *J Bone Joint Surg* 1976;58A(6):876–878.

CHAPTER 2

The Biochemistry of Paget's Disease

Stephen M. Krane

The characteristic biological abnormalities of Paget's disease reflect the disordered bone remodeling. It is likely that the initial event in this disease is a focal, intense resorption of existing bone associated with the presence of abnormal large osteoclasts. At the point where the lesions are usually recognized, increased production of woven and lamellar bone is evident, as well as replacement of normal fatty and hematopoietic marrow with a loose fibrous stroma. Coupling of bone formation with bone resorption is evidenced by quantitative histomorphometry and can be confirmed by parallel charges in serum alkaline phosphatase levels and urinary hydroxyproline excretion, as well as by radiocalcium kinetics and measurements of other indexes of matrix protein synthesis and degradation. Although it has been assumed that the formation of pagetic bone is a coupled response to increased resorption, it should be emphasized that all pagetic bone is abnormal. The osteoblastic rate is high, the osteoblastic surface is increased, and the osteoblasts themselves are also probably not normal. The increase in osteoblast function could somehow result from contact of cell membranes of osteoclasts and osteoblasts or stromal cells or through release of some product of osteoclasts. Many of the remodeling events in Paget's disease have been interpreted as consistent with an increased "birth rate" of all of the bone cell populations.[1-6]

Since bone is a two-phase material comprising a calcium/phosphate inorganic mineral phase uniquely organized with respect to its organic matrix, abnormal bone remodeling in Paget's disease would result in changes in the turnover of both phases. Studies of the kinetics of disappearance of tracer doses of radiocalcium indicate that the rates of movement of mineral ions in and out of the skeleton are increased in patients with Paget's disease.[1,5–7] The size of the exchangeable calcium pool and the rate constants of exit from this pool are all increased, and the magnitude of increase is correlated with the extent and activity of the lesions. Although the calculated rates of fluxes of the mineral ions are probably overestimated, the magnitude of turnover calculated from radiocalcium kinetics and independently from matrix resorption are in reasonable agreement.

Although large amounts of mineral ions are removed from the skeleton in extensive Paget's disease, similar amounts would be redeposited without altering plasma calcium or phosphorus concentrations or causing marked changes in urinary excretion of these ions. Indeed calcium balances in pagetic patients are rarely more than 200 mg/d positive or negative despite the occasional enormous turnover. Modulation of bone formation to meet the requirements of bone resorption may therefore represent an important mechanism of calcium homeostasis in Paget's disease.

BONE COLLAGEN

The organic matrix of bone is composed of collagen and noncollagenous proteins.[8] Type I collagen is the most abundant component of the organic matrix of bone and essentially the only collagen type in adult mineralized bone. The manner in which it is deposited is a major determinant of bone structure.

Type I collagen is a heterotrimer containing of two $\alpha 1(I)$ chains and one $\alpha 2(I)$ chain.[9] These chains are synthesized by osteoblasts in bone as precursor procollagen molecules containing both aminoterminal and carboxyterminal globular extensions. Before formation of the collagen fibrils, these extensions are cleaved by specific endopeptidases to yield the helical trimers. There is only one gene encoding each of the chains of type I procollagen. Thus the gene encoding type I procollagen in bone as well as skin (where type I collagen is also abundant) should be the same. So far, there is also no evidence to indicate that the processing of the primary transcript of the type I procollagen genes in skin and bone is different. Therefore, on the basis of primary structure, there are no specific markers that would distinguish skin and bone type I collagen.

Although there are no differences in the primary structure of bone and other type I collagens, the posttranslational modifications of bone collagen are distinct from skin and other soft tissue collagens. The pattern of glycosylation of hydroxylysine residues is clearly different in human skin and bone.[10] The ratio of glucosylgalactosyl hydroxylysine (Hyl[Glc-Gal]) to galactosyl hydroxylysine (Hyl[Gal]) is 0.47 ± 0.01 in normal human bone and 2.06 ± 0.47 in normal human skin, whereas the amount of total glycosylated hydroxylysine is similar in the collagens from these tissues. The pattern of sodium borotritide-reducible cross-links is also characteristic in the collagens from bone compared to those from soft tissues.[11]

Other markers for collagens of skeletal origin are the 3-hydroxypyridinium residues, which are the major cross-links in mature collagens of several skeletal tissues.[11] The major compound, hydroxylysyl pyridinoline (HP), is derived from three residues of hydroxylysine, whereas the less abundant lysyl pyridinoline (LP) is derived from two hydroxylysine residues and one lysine residue.

The most widely used marker for measuring collagen turnover in humans is the excretion of total urinary 4-hydroxyproline.[5,6] Most of the urinary 4-hydroxyproline is present in dipeptides and tripeptides, reflecting the position of this relatively abundant imino acid in the -Y- position of the glycine-X-Y-triplet of the collagen helical sequence. Hydroxylation of prolyl (and lysyl residues in the case of hydroxylysine) takes place on nascent chains, and hydroxyproline and hydroxylysine are not reused for collagen biosynthesis. They are, therefore, potential quantitative markers for measuring collagen breakdown. Unfortunately, the use of hydroxyproline peptides as markers is limited because the small hydroxyproline peptides in the urine represent only a small fraction of the total hydroxyproline released from collagen breakdown. Most of the free hydroxyproline released by cleavage of these peptides is normally oxidized in the liver to form other products.

Although most urinary 4-hydroxyproline is in the form of small dialyzable peptides, the remainder consists of nondialyzable peptides of molecular weight averaging approximately 5,000 daltons.[12,13] These peptides, which were first identified in the urine of patients with Paget's disease, were found to be heterogeneous but with an amino acid composition and other properties of collagen chains in general. At least some of these peptides are rapidly synthesized.

NONCOLLAGENOUS PROTEINS OF BONE

The noncollagenous proteins of bone are a heterogeneous group of molecules.[8] Some are derived from the circulation (for example, albumin and α_2HS-glycoprotein) or from the surface of bone cells and bind to the bone matrix, whereas others are made by bone cells. Alkaline phosphatase, whose activity is elevated in serum of patients with Paget's disease, is a surface component (ectoenzyme) of osteoblasts and is cleaved from the cell surface. Other relatively abundant components are osteocalcin (bone GLA protein or BGP), bone sialoproteins (BSP-I, also known as osteopontin, and BSP-II), osteonectin, and small proteoglycans. Several of these components bind to the mineral phase as well as to the collagen of bone.

Many of these proteins can be measured in serum or plasma by radioimmunoassay and therefore serve as potential markers of bone formation or resorption.[14] A definitive marker of bone formation would be a molecule synthesized exclusively by osteoblasts (normal or abnormal) and not by other mesenchymal cells; blood levels would not be subject to significant modulation by metabolism or urinary excretion. In the case of urinary metabolites, it would be essential that excretion reflect total synthesis. Unfortunately, it is not possible to meet these rigorous criteria with measurements currently available, although there is considerable interest in developing newer technologies. Circulating levels of osteocalcin on the average are increased in patients with Paget's disease.[15,16] Correlations with other indexes of bone turnover (urinary excretion of hydroxyproline or serum alkaline phosphatase) are poor, however, and changes following therapy do not regularly reflect other measurements. It has been proposed recently on the basis of analysis of fragments of osteocalcin in serum and urine, that unique metabolism of osteocalcin in Paget's disease may account for the findings described.[17]

Measurements of levels of other noncollagenous proteins derived from osteoblasts in Paget's disease have not yet proved to be useful. Certainly the value of any measurement of concentrations of a skeletal marker in serum is dependent on the relative rates of multiple processes involved in synthesis; release into circulation; binding to bone mineral, collagen, and/or other matrix components; degradation; and excretion. It is difficult to assign rate constants for most of these processes in humans or even experimental animals without determining metabolic disposition rates. With a molecule such as osteocalcin, which is secreted by osteoblasts but with a portion also deposited in the matrix, the problem is even more complex. No marker would therefore fulfill rigorous criteria to be established as the "gold standard."

COLLAGEN TURNOVER

The intensity and extent of the abnormal bone remodeling in Paget's disease are correlated with increases in bone collagen degradation and synthesis. The increased resorption of pagetic bone collagen is reflected in the elevated rates of urinary excretion of 4-hydroxyproline, hydroxylysine, and hydroxylysine glycosides. The level of excretion of urinary 4-hydroxyproline peptides has generally been found to be proportional to the extent and "activity" of the Paget's disease. Whereas normal adults excrete less than 40 mg/d (300 μmol/d), some individuals with severe Paget's disease may excrete more than 1 g/d (nearly 8 mmol/d).[4–6] This represents only a portion of the total 4-hydroxyproline derived from degradation of bone collagen because of the metabolism of free hydroxyproline. Measurement of hydroxylysine and its glycosides provides a more accurate index of collagen degradation than measurement of hydroxyproline since the former are metabolized to a lesser extent than the 4-hydroxyproline.[18,19] The pattern of their excretion also provides some information as to the source of collagen degradation, in view of their unique proportion in bone collagen compared to other tissue collagens. Thus, the composition or urinary hydroxylysine glycosides in Paget's disease is similar to that of bone collagen. With total hydroxyproline/creatinine ratios greater than 2 μmol/mg (normal < 0.3 μmol/mg), the ratio of urinary Hyl(GlcGal)/Hyl(Gal) was found to be approximately 0.5, similar to that of normal or pagetic bone collagen. When resorption was decreased therapeutically with calcitonin or ethylhydroxybisphosphonate, the ratio of Hyl(GlcGal)/Hyl(Gal) increased, uncovering a source of collagen breakdown other than bone, probably skin or the first component of hemolytic complement, C1q. These results provide further evidence for a primary effect of calcitonin and bisphosphonates in specifically decreasing collagen degradation in bone.

Measurements of nondialyzable urinary hydroxyproline peptides have also provided information about skeletal remodeling in Paget's disease.[12,13] The purification of one of these peptides was reported by Szymanowicz[20] to be of molecular weight less than 1,500 daltons ($>$ca. 15 residues); and it contained one third glycine (Gly) and approximately equal amounts of proline (Pro) and hydroxyproline (Hyp) and could thus be composed of at least five -Gly-Pro-Hyp- triplets. Such a peptide could originate from the minor collagen helix in the aminoterminal propeptide of type I procollagen. In collaboration with Michel van der Rest (unpublished) we used chromatofocusing and high-performance liquid chromatography to purify a similar peptide as well as other collagenlike peptides. We found that some of these other peptides are derived from specific sequences in the helical portion of the $\alpha 1$(I) chains.

Measurements of total nondialyzable hydroxyproline peptides show that their excretion increases relative to the total when bone resorption is acutely decreased with calcitonin.[6] The fact that the total nondialyzable peptides also decrease acutely after calcitonin injection can be interpreted as indicating that there are acute adjustments of bone formation in response to the decreases in bone resorption as additional homeostatic responses in Paget's disease. Chronic therapy with ethylhydroxybisphosphonate, which results in a decrease in urinary hydroxyproline excretion, also results in increases in the ratio of nondialyzable to dialyzable hydroxyproline but a decrease in the total nondialyzable peptides. These results indicate a change in the balance of bone collagen synthesis relative to resorption in favor of increased formation.

The potential value of assays of procollagen peptides as markers for collagen synthesis was first proposed by Sherr and Goldberg[21] and Taubman et al.,[22] who developed antibodies to purified carboxyterminal fragments of type I collagen synthesized by fibroblasts in culture. Because the procollagen peptide extensions of type I collagen are cleaved before fibril formation, measurements of these peptides could be of considerable value were there not extensive deposition in bone matrix or proteolytic cleavage before release into the circulation. The carboxyterminal propeptide of type I procollagen is a heterotrimer of approximately 100 kD, which is stabilized by interchain disulfide bonds. Taubman et al.[23] documented elevated levels of these peptides (which we[24] termed "pColl-I-C") in the serum of patients with Paget's disease compared to normal subjects. The levels of these peptides correlate with the extent and activity of the disease as determined by activity of serum alkaline phosphatase.[22,23] It should be emphasized that the same caveats that apply to osteocalcin apply to the interpretation of changes of procollagen peptides in serum.

The levels of pColl-I-C were decreased when the Paget's disease was treated with dichloromethylene bisphosphonate for 4 to 7 months.[24] The levels of pColl-I-C also decrease within hours of subcutaneous administration of salmon calcitonin. These results suggest that the changes in levels of pColl-I-C following administration of calcitonin or diphosphonates reflect the decrease in bone formation coupled to the decrease in resorption.

Levels of the aminoterminal propeptide of type III procollagen (pColl-III-N) are also elevated in serum from patients with Paget's disease.[24] Although mineralized bone proper exclusively contains type I collagen, type III collagen is found also in bone, predominantly in the blood vessels of the haversian systems and other vascular structures. Type III collagen is also a major component of the loose fibrous stroma that is closely applied to bone spicules in areas of active Paget's disease. The elevated serum levels of peptides derived from type III collagen in Paget's disease probably reflect the synthetic activity of the stromal fibroblasts, which are characteristically abundant in pagetic lesions.

Most of the intramolecular and intermolecular collagen cross-links are derived from the side chains of lysine and hydroxylysine residues that are specifically aligned as a result of the characteristic collagen triple helix and the arrangement of the triple-helical molecules in the fibrils and fibers.[11] In skeletal collagens there are specific 3-hydroxypyridinium cross-links. The predominant hydroxylysyl (HP) pyridinoline is present in several tissues, whereas the minor, lysyl (LP) pyridinoline is present in significant amounts only in bone and dentin. HP and LP are essentially absent from tissues such as skin. Some of these compounds are excreted in human urine.[25] We[26] as well as Robbins and co-workers[27] have measured the levels of the 3-hydroxypyridinium compounds in the urine in Paget's disease and have partially characterized them chemically. These hydroxypyridinium compounds are excreted in the urine in large amounts in Paget's disease, and it is probable, since there is little metabolic degradation, that they will prove to be useful quantitative markers of bone resorption in a variety of conditions.

SUMMARY

1. Biochemical abnormalities in Paget's disease result from the intense remodeling of the skeleton and are reflected in measurements of markers of bone formation and resorption.
2. Assays of available markers of synthesis and degradation of bone matrix are useful in interpretation of pathophysiology and assessment of responses to treatment.
3. Determination of the metabolic disposition of these markers will improve their utility.
4. Studies of Paget's disease of bone have provided and will continue to provide information about physiologic and pathologic bone remodeling of great value to those concerned with metabolic bone disease.

ACKNOWLEDGMENTS

I thank M. Angelo for preparation of the manuscript. Original work reported here was supported by USPHS grants AR-03564 and AR-07258.

REFERENCES

1. Nagant de Deuxchaisnes C, Krane SM: Paget's disease of bone: Clinical and metabolic observations. *Medicine* 1964;43(3)233–266.
2. Paget's disease of bone. Editorial. *Calcif Tissue Int* 1986;38:309–317.
3. Singer FR, Krane SM: Paget's disease of bone, in Avioli LV, Krane SM (eds): *Metabolic*

Bone and Disease and Clinically Related Disorders. Philadelphia, WB Saunders Co, 1990, pp 546–615.

4. Bijovet OLM, Vellenga CJLR, Harinck HIJ: Paget's disease of bones: Assessment, therapy, and secondary prevention, in Kleerekoper M, Krane SM (eds): *Clinical Disorders of Bone and Mineral Metabolism.* New York, Mary Ann Liebert, 1989, pp 525–542.
5. Krane SM: Skeletal metabolism in Paget's disease of bone. *Arthritis Rheum* 1980; 23:1087–1094.
6. Krane SM, Simon LS: Metabolic consequences of bone turnover in Paget's disease of bone. *Clin Orthop* 1987;217:26–36.
7. Krane SM, Brownell GL, Stanbury JB, Corrigan H: The effect of thyroid disease on calcium metabolism in man. *J Clin Invest* 1956;35:874–887.
8. Termine JD: Non-collagen proteins in bone, in Everud D, Harnett S (eds): *Cell and Molecular Biology of Vertebrate Hard Tissues.* Chichester, England, Wiley, 1988, pp 178–202.
9. Ramirez F, De Wet W: Molecular biology of the human fibrillar collagen genes. *Ann NY Acad Sci* 1988;543:109–116.
10. Pinnell SR, Fox R, Krane SM: Human collagens: Differences in glycosylated hydroxylysines in skin and bone. *Biochim Biophys Acta* 1971;229:119–122.
11. Eyre DR: Collagen stability through covalent crosslinking. *Adv Meat Res* 1987;4:69–85.
12. Krane SM, Muñoz AJ, Harris ED Jr: Urinary polypeptides related to collagen synthesis. *J Clin Invest* 1970;49:716–729.
13. Haddad JG, Couranz S, Avioli LV: Nondialyzable urinary hydroxyproline as an index of bone collagen formation. *J Clin Endocrinol Metab* 1970;30:282–287.
14. Epstein S: Serum and urinary markers of bone remodeling: Assessment of bone turnover. *Endocr Rev* 1988;9:437–449.
15. Coulton LA, Preston CJ, Couch M, Kanis JA: An evaluation of serum osteocalcin in Paget's disease of bone and its response to diphosphonate treatment. *Arthritis Rheum* 1988;31:1142–1147.
16. Papapoulos SE, Frolich M, Mudde AH, et al: Serum osteocalcin in Paget's disease of bone: Basal concentrations and response to bisphosphonate treatment. *J Clin Endocrinol Metab* 1987;65:89–94.
17. Taylor AK, Linkhart SG, Mohan S, et al: Presence of a unique fragment of osteocalcin in serum and urine of Paget's disease patients: Possible marker for the disease. *J Bone Mineral Res* 1989;4(suppl 1):S198.
18. Askenasi R, De Backer M, Devos A: The origin of urinary hydroxylysyl glycosides in Paget's disease of bone and in primary hyperparathyroidism. *Calcif Tissue Res* 1976;22:35–40.
19. Krane SM, Kantrowitz FG, Byrne M, et al: Urinary excretion of hydroxylysine and its glycosides as an index of collagen degradation. *J Clin Invest* 1977;59:819–827.
20. Szymanowicz A: Polymorphism of urinary 4-hydroxyproline-containing polypeptides. *J Chromatogr* 1981;225:55–63.
21. Sherr CJ, Goldberg B: Antibodies to a precursor of human collagen. *Science* 1973; 180:1190–1192.
22. Taubman MB, Goldberg B, Sherr CJ: Radioimmunoassay for human procollagen. *Science* 1974;186:1115–1117.
23. Taubman MB, Kammerman S, Goldberg B: Radioimmunoassay of procollagen in serum of patients with Paget's disease of bone. *Proc Soc Exp Biol Med* 1976;152:284–287.
24. Simon LS, Krane SM, Wortman PD, et al: Serum levels of type I and III procollagen fragments in Paget's disease of bone. *J Clin Endocrinol Metab* 1984;58:110–120.
25. Robins SP, Stewart P, Astbury C, Bird HA: Measurement of the cross linking compound,

pryidinoline, in urine as an index of collagen degradation in joint disease. *Ann Rheum Dis* 1986;45:969–973.
26. Eyre D, Ericsson L, Simon L, Krane S: Identification of urinary peptides derived from cross-linking sites in bone collagen in Paget's disease. *J Bone Mineral Res* 1988; 3(suppl):S210.
27. Robins SP, Duncan A, Reid DM, Paterson CR: Urinary hydroxy-pyridinium crosslinks of collagen as markers of resorption in a range of metabolic bone diseases. *J Bone Min Res* 1989;4(suppl 1):S397.

CHAPTER 3

The Pathology of Paget's Disease

Steven L. Teitelbaum

Paget's disease is a common affliction in Western society, being pathologically manifest in approximately 4% of older whites.[1] Although rarely fatal, the disorder may be extremely disabling and painful and lead to marked skeletal distortion.

Although generally viewed as a "metabolic disorder," unlike other such conditions, Paget's disease does not involve the entire skeleton nor does it express itself in a synchronous manner. Rather, the disorder is monostotic or multifocal and asynchronous. Thus, one lesion may represent the end stage of Paget's disease while another may represent the early pathologic event. In light of the multifocal, asynchronous nature of the process, one is unable to generalize about the state of disease in a given individual when viewing a bone biopsy specimen from a particular site. These observations indicate that although the randomly taken ("blind") iliac crest bone biopsy has yielded important cross-sectional (group) information about the natural history[2] and appropriate treatment of Paget's disease,[3] it has little place in the evaluation of a particular patient in whom the diagnosis is established.

NORMAL BONE HISTOLOGY

The pathologic manifestations of Paget's disease involve both the mineral and organic matrices of bone and, as such, reflect the activities of bone cells, namely osteoblasts and osteoclasts. Osteoblasts are the formative cells of the skeleton and, when viewed in nondecalcified microscopic sections, are always found lining a seam of osteoid (that is, bone matrix before its mineralization). The rate of activity of osteoblasts can generally be inferred from their appearance as those that are rapidly synthesizing and mineralizing bone are cuboidal and contain a prominent Golgi apparatus. As the cell becomes less active, it flattens or attenuates, forming a syncytium that separates bone from the general extracellular space and in so doing probably functions to retain more than 99% of the body's calcium in the skeleton.[4,5]

Some of the more useful tools for determining the rate of osteoblastic activity are the tetracyclines.[6] These autofluorescent antibiotics bind to newly deposited bone mineral characteristically located at the interface between osteoid and mineralized bone. Thus, one can identify sites of recent mineralization by administering tetracyclines to patients before bone biopsy and examining the histologic slides by fluorescent microscopy. Most importantly, if one gives two courses of the antibiotic separated by a known period, one can actually quantitate the rate of bone mineralization, which in the steady state parallels formation. This approach has yielded major insights into the rate of skeletal turnover and natural history of Paget's disease.[2]

Osteoclasts are the degradative or resorptive cells of bone and, as we shall see, initiate the pagetic process. They are of hematopoietic origin[7] and are members of the monocyte-macrophage family.[8] Like foreign body giant cells, they are multinucleated and contain an array of lysosomal enzymes.

Osteoclasts are generally found in excavated areas of bone known as resorption bays or Howship's lacunae. They are highly motile and degrade all components of bone[9] by creating at the cell-bone interface a sealed microenvironment that they acidify via a proton transport mechanism identical to that of the renal tubule.[10] Faced with a pH of 4.5 to 5.0, bone mineral is rapidly mobilized and the collagenous component exposed and made available to degradation by an acidic collagenase.[9] Polarization of these proton pumps toward the resorptive microenvironment and their insertion into the plasma membrane are probably responsible for formation of the ruffled border, a pattern of membrane infolding that is the unique resorptive organ of the osteoclast and distinguishes it from other members of the monocyte-macrophage family.[10]

The anatomic consequences of the activities of osteoblasts and osteoclasts should be considered in terms of the four distinct biologic processes of growth, modeling, remodeling, and repair.[11] The first two, growth and modeling, occur only before cessation of epiphyseal (that is, growth plate) closure and respectively represent increasing mass of the skeleton and its sculpting or movement through space. Repair, of course, refers to fracture healing on both gross and microscopic levels and is extant throughout life.

Remodeling, which also continues from birth until death, is the process intimately associated with mineral homeostasis. It, unlike the other three skeletal events, is characterized by an anatomic coupling of the activities of osteoclasts and osteoblasts (Figure 3.1). The process is initiated by the appearance of osteoclasts that resorb a volume of bone, forming a resorption bay. Osteoclasts then leave, and after a period of time osteoblasts that replace all or part of the resorbed bone appear. The site at which tic activity stops and bone replacement begins is marked by a metachromatic line known as the cement line, which ultimately defines the limits of a particular remodeling site. Although there are many thousands of remodeling sites extant in a given individual at a particular time, the process is asynchronous. That is to say, one simultaneously finds sites in the resorptive (osteoclastic), reversal, and formative (osteoblastic) phases of remodeling. In fact, the duration of the formative phase, which in humans approximates 3 months, can be measured by using tetracycline markers.[7]

It is important to realize that remodeling osteoblasts do not necessarily deposit the same amount of bone previously removed by osteoclasts. In

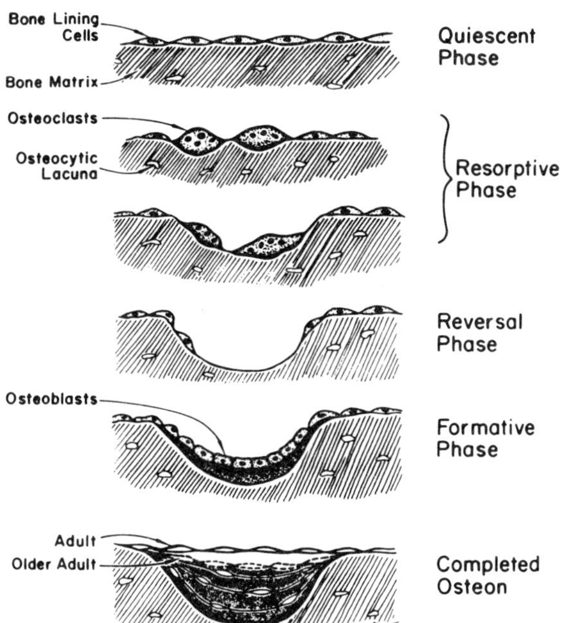

FIGURE 3.1. The sequence of bone remodeling. *Reproduced from Kahn AJ, Fallon MD, Teitelbaum SL: Structure-function relationships in bone: An examination of events at the cellular level, in Peck WA (ed): Bone and Mineral Research Annual II. Amsterdam, Excerpta Medica, 1983, pp 125–174. With permission.*

fact, with age one experiences a net deficit of bone at each completed remodeling site, a phenomenon that is responsible for the ultimate development of osteoporosis.[12] Moreover, the signals initiating bone remodeling and its various phases are unknown but clearly pivotal to understanding the pathogenesis of osteoporosis and, as we shall see, Paget's disease.

PAGET'S DISEASE

Paget's disease is a paradigm of bone remodeling gone awry. Like remodeling, the pagetic process is initiated by the osteoclast, which is clearly abnormal and probably the pathogenetic cell. The osteoclasts of Paget's disease are huge and, when viewed histologically, may be seen to contain hundreds of nuclei (Figure 3.2). (Normal osteoclasts contain approximately five to ten.) Moreover, whereas osteoclasts normally polarize their nuclei toward the antiresorptive side of the cell, they are randomly distributed in pagetic osteoclasts.

The size and appearance of pagetic osteoclasts mirror the speed and avidity with which they resorb bone. They excavate deep Howship's lacunae, and, in fact, their destructive activity may be so great as to lead to development of radiographically apparent, resorptive cavities so large that they may sustain fracture. Thus, the so-called blade of grass lesion represents in actuality the gross expression of the initial phase of Paget's disease, namely resorption.

As the resorptive phase of Paget's disease advances, osteoblasts are progressively recruited into the lesion to begin transition to the formative stage of the disease. Reflecting their enhanced synthetic activity, pagetic osteoblasts are typically large and cuboidal and contain a prominent Golgi apparatus (Figure 3.3). These cells are always found lining osteoid, which is quantitatively increased in Paget's disease. Tetracycline labeling demonstrates that the attendant hyperosteoidosis represents an enhanced rate of bone synthesis and not a mineralization defect (that is, osteomalacia).[1] In fact, the rate of bone synthesis and mineralization may be so great in Paget's disease that tetracycline double labels may encompass as much as one tenth of the total skeleton (Figure 3.4). Given that such a volume generally represents the proportion of bone mineralized during an approximate 2-week period, the rate of synthesis of pagetic bone is generally extremely fast.

Although the pathogenesis of Paget's disease has not been established, the bulk of evidence points to a viral cause. When viewed by electron microscopy (Figure 3.5), pagetic osteoclasts are seen to contain paramyxoviruslike particles.[13] Moreover, these cells express immunoreactive measles

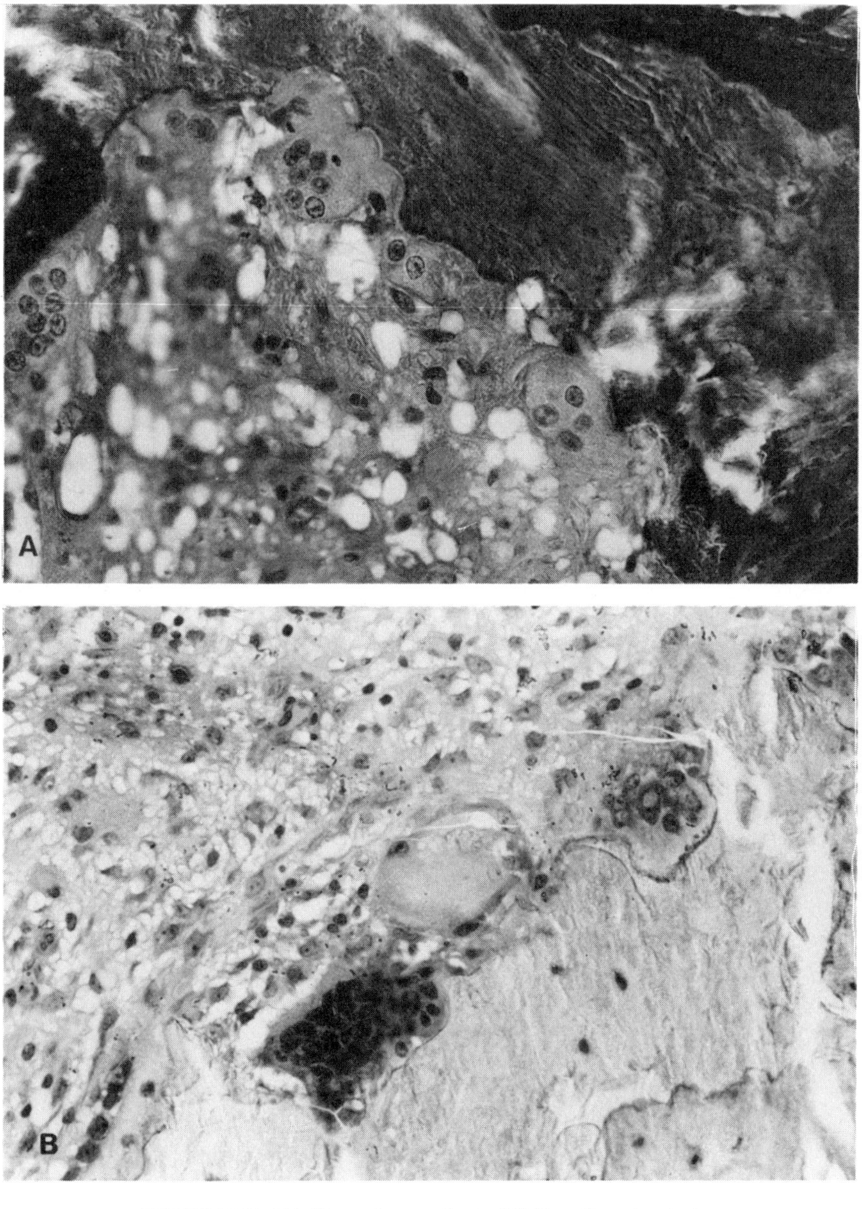

FIGURE 3.2. **(A)** Normal osteoclasts. **(B)** Pagetic osteoclasts.

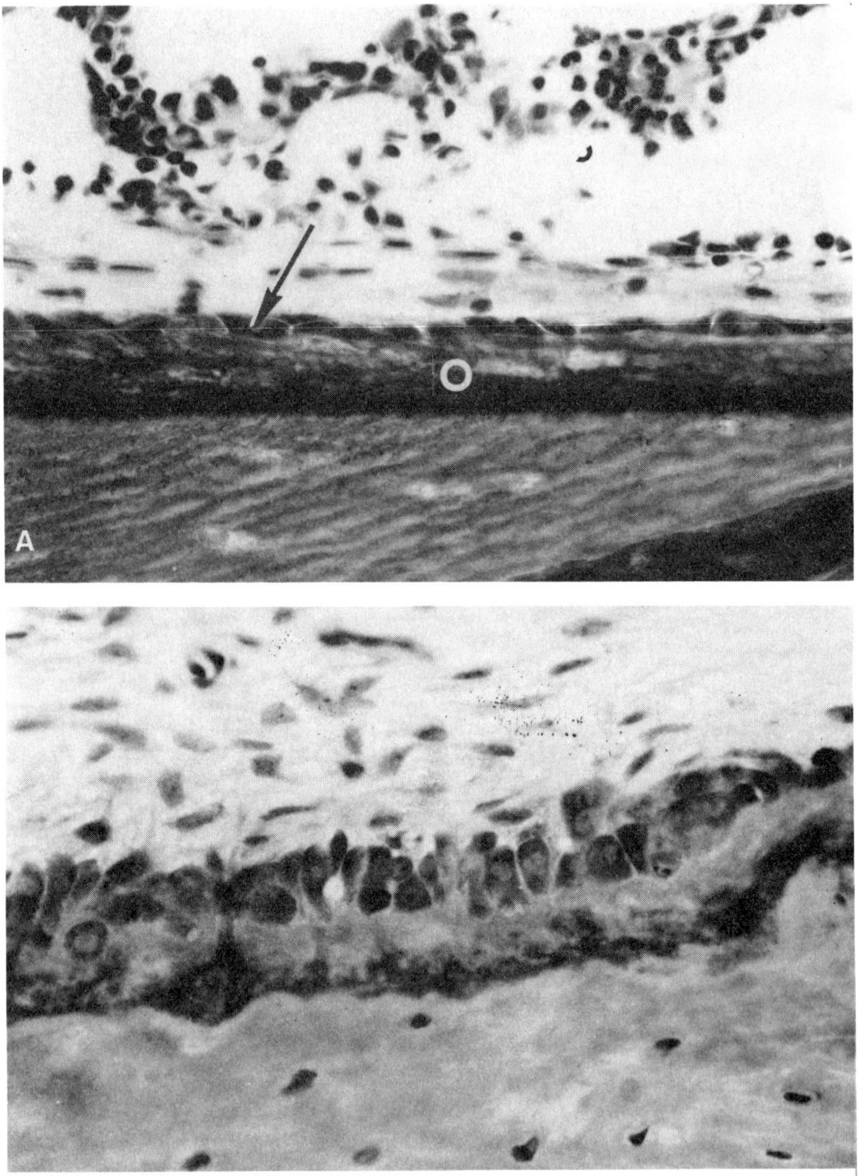

FIGURE 3.3. **(A)** Osteoblasts (arrow) lining an osteoid seam (O) in a normal biopsy specimen and **(B)** osteoblasts lining an osteoid seam in a site of Paget's disease. The perinuclear light area (arrow) is a prominent Golgi apparatus indicative of rapid protein synthesis.

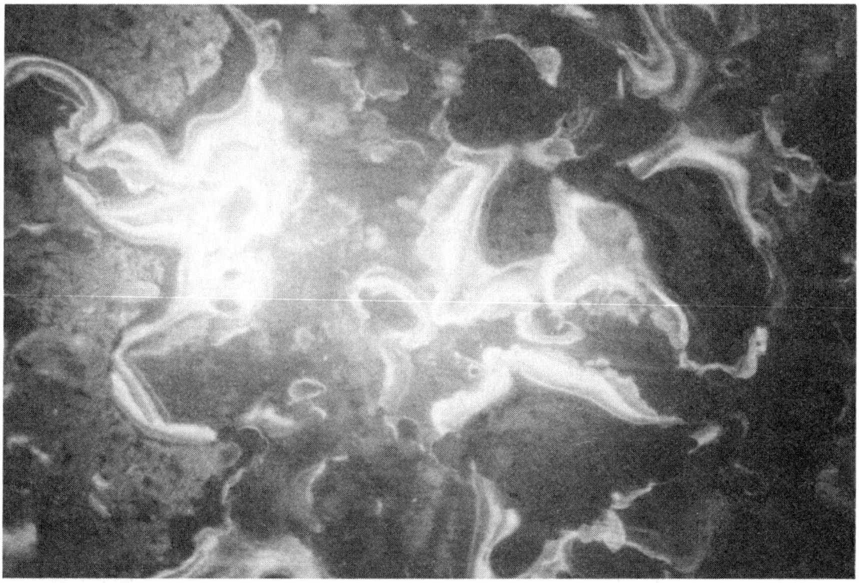

FIGURE 3.4. Extensive tetracycline fluorescence in pagetic bone. The fluorescent bone reflects that it is synthesized and mineralized in the 2 weeks before biopsy.

and respiratory syncytial viral antigens.[14-16] In fact, paramyxoviral infection is typified by formation of syncytial giant cells reminiscent of the bizarre osteoclasts of Paget's disease. Recently, measles virus ribonucleic acid (RNA) has been detected in pagetic bone,[16] and paramyxoviruslike RNA sequences have been isolated from cells cocultured with pagetic bone.[17] It should be pointed out, however, that despite the evidence suggestive of viral origin of Paget's disease, Koch's postulates have not been fulfilled.

OSTEITIS FIBROSA

The compendium of changes attending the transition or mixed resorptive and formative phases of Paget's disease are known as osteitis fibrosa. Although typically associated with hyperparathyroidism, osteitis fibrosa is actually a histologic entity reflecting accelerated remodeling. It occurs not only in Paget's disease but in high-remodeling states such as hyperthyroidism.

Regardless of cause, osteitis fibrosa is characterized by an abundance of osteoclasts, osteoblasts, and osteoid (Figure 3.6), the latter being due to

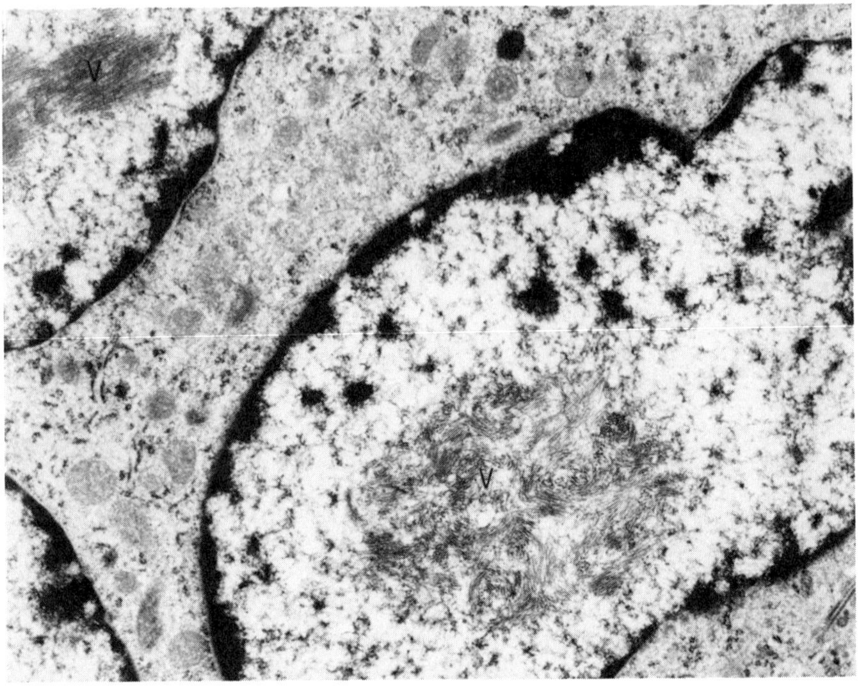

FIGURE 3.5. Viruslike inclusion (V) in nuclei of osteoclasts from patient with Paget's disease. *(Courtesy of Dr. Barbara Mills.)*

accelerated bone matrix synthesis. Remodeling foci are numerous, and most importantly there is peritrabecular marrow fibrosis. The distribution of marrow fibrosis in osteitis fibrosa stands in sharp contrast to that found in idiopathic myelofibrosis in that in the latter, fibrous tissue is randomly distributed throughout the marrow without respect to the bony architecture. The juxtaposition, in osteitis fibrosa, of fibrosis to bone surfaces probably reflects the fact that osteoblasts are derived from fibroblastlike precursors,[18] and their enhanced and rapid recruitment in this condition leads to a large number of such progenitors adjacent to bone.

Thus, Paget's disease in its mixed phase is typically associated with extensive marrow fibrosis that in relatively early stages is peritrabecular in distribution. It should be appreciated, however, that as the lesion progresses, the process may become so extensive as to occupy virtually the entire marrow cavity (Figure 3.7). In this circumstance one encounters a paucity of hematopoietic elements and an abundance of vascular spaces within the marrow.

The rapid phase of pagetic bone formation is also associated with

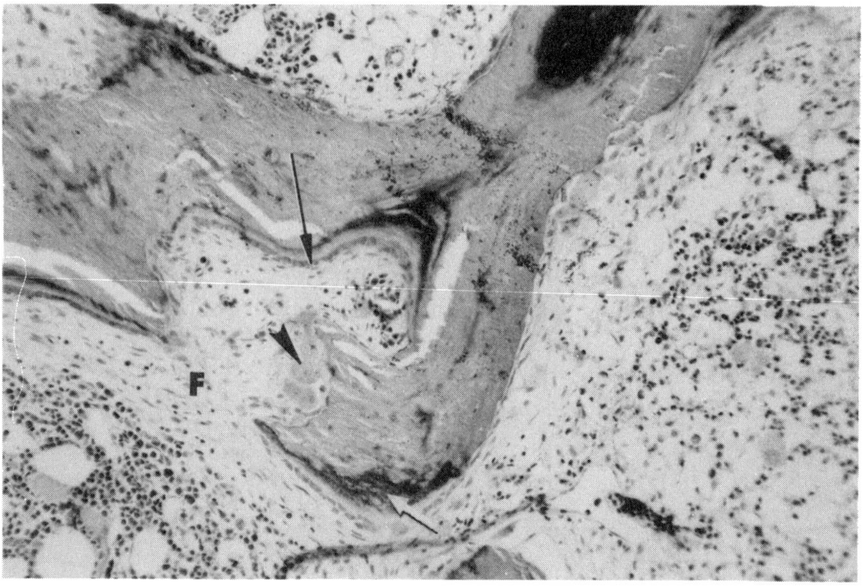

FIGURE 3.6. Osteitis fibrosa. The biopsy specimen was taken from a patient with hyperparathyroidism. Note the abundance of osteoblasts (arrow) and osteoclasts (arrowhead) and the fibrous tissue juxtaposed to the trabecular surface. F, fibrous tissue.

changes in the structure of bone collagen. Normal adult bone is normally in a "lamellar pattern." That is to say, when examined by polarizing or scanning electron microscopy, the bundles are seen to be of uniform size and are arranged in a parallel fashion (Figure 3.8). In states of accelerated formation such as Paget's disease, however, bone collagen is deposited in a "woven" pattern in which both the dimensions and arrangement of the bundles are random and irregular. Thus, polarizing or scanning electron microscopy reveals a haphazard pattern of collagen deposition. Such bone is structurally inferior to its lamellar counterpart and probably contributes to the unusual fractures that often attend Paget's disease.[19]

Thus, remodeling is rapid and irregular in Paget's disease and ultimately leads to severe structural changes. These abnormalities are manifest as marked cortical porosity and, on a microscopic level, increase in the surface/volume ratio of trabeculae. Consequently, the trabeculae are irregular, with most surfaces either covered by osteoid or containing scalloped resorption bays (Figure 3.9), and there is loss of distinction between cortical and cancellous bone.

Reflecting the remodeling cycle, pagetic foci ultimately become devoid of osteoblasts and osteoclasts and "quiescent." This inactive phase of

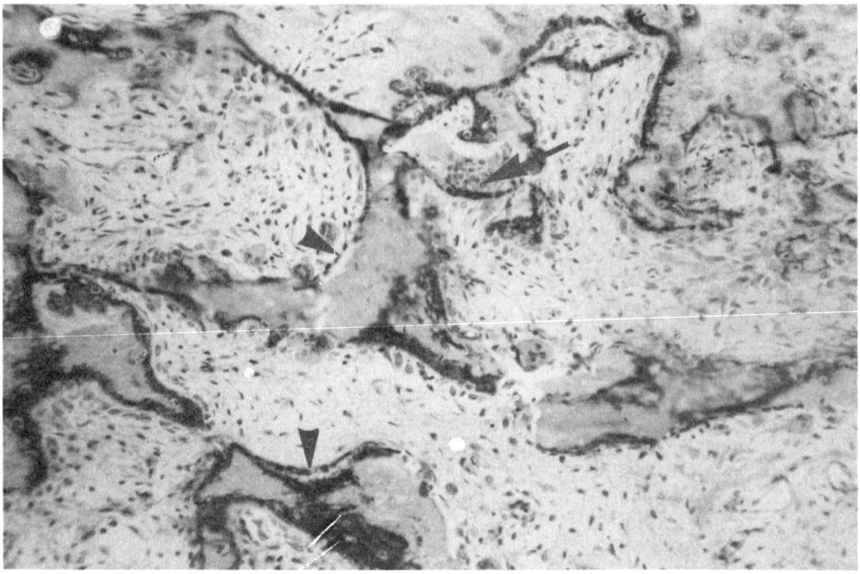

FIGURE 3.7. Mixed phase of Paget's disease in which there is extensive osteitis fibrosa. Note the abundance of osteoblasts (arrowhead) and osteoclasts (arrow). The marrow space is virtually devoid of hematopoietic elements and is replaced by fibrous tissue.

Paget's disease is characterized by an increase in cancellous bone mass due to formation of wide trabeculae. There is also cortical thickening as subperiosteal new bone formation occurs. This combination of events leads to changes in the gross architecture of the bone perhaps most dramatically evident in severe bowing (Figure 3.10).

Mirroring the rapid remodeling that precedes it, the quiescent phase is also characterized by the second unique histologic feature of Paget's disease, its mosaic pattern (Figure 3.11). Reflecting the rapid and disorderly coupling of resorption and formation is an arrangement not unlike a jigsaw puzzle, an abundance of irregular cement lines juxtaposed to each other.

Although Paget's disease may be histologically unique, its appearance may mimic other conditions and its diagnosis can be difficult. For example, any form of osteitis fibrosa may be confused with Paget's disease, and in these circumstances the attendant biochemical changes are particularly helpful. Osteomyelitis, which may be characterized by abundant marrow fibrosis and bone cell proliferation, may also be troublesome, although in this circumstance, the fibrosis tends to be randomly distributed in the marrow and inflammatory cells and necrotic foci are generally present. One must be aware that a mosaic pattern of cement lines may occasionally be associated with osteomyelitis. In difficult diagnoses, recognition of the

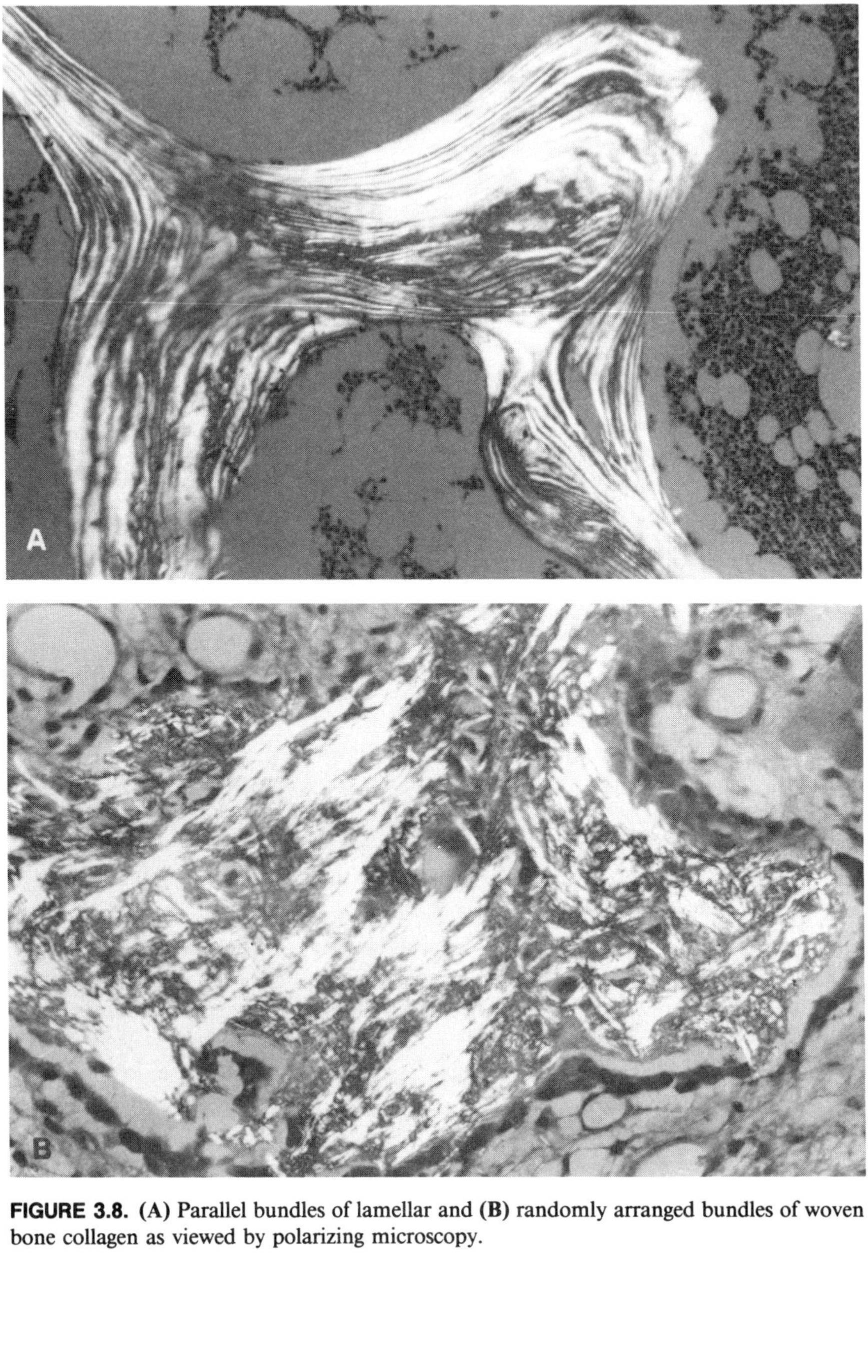

FIGURE 3.8. **(A)** Parallel bundles of lamellar and **(B)** randomly arranged bundles of woven bone collagen as viewed by polarizing microscopy.

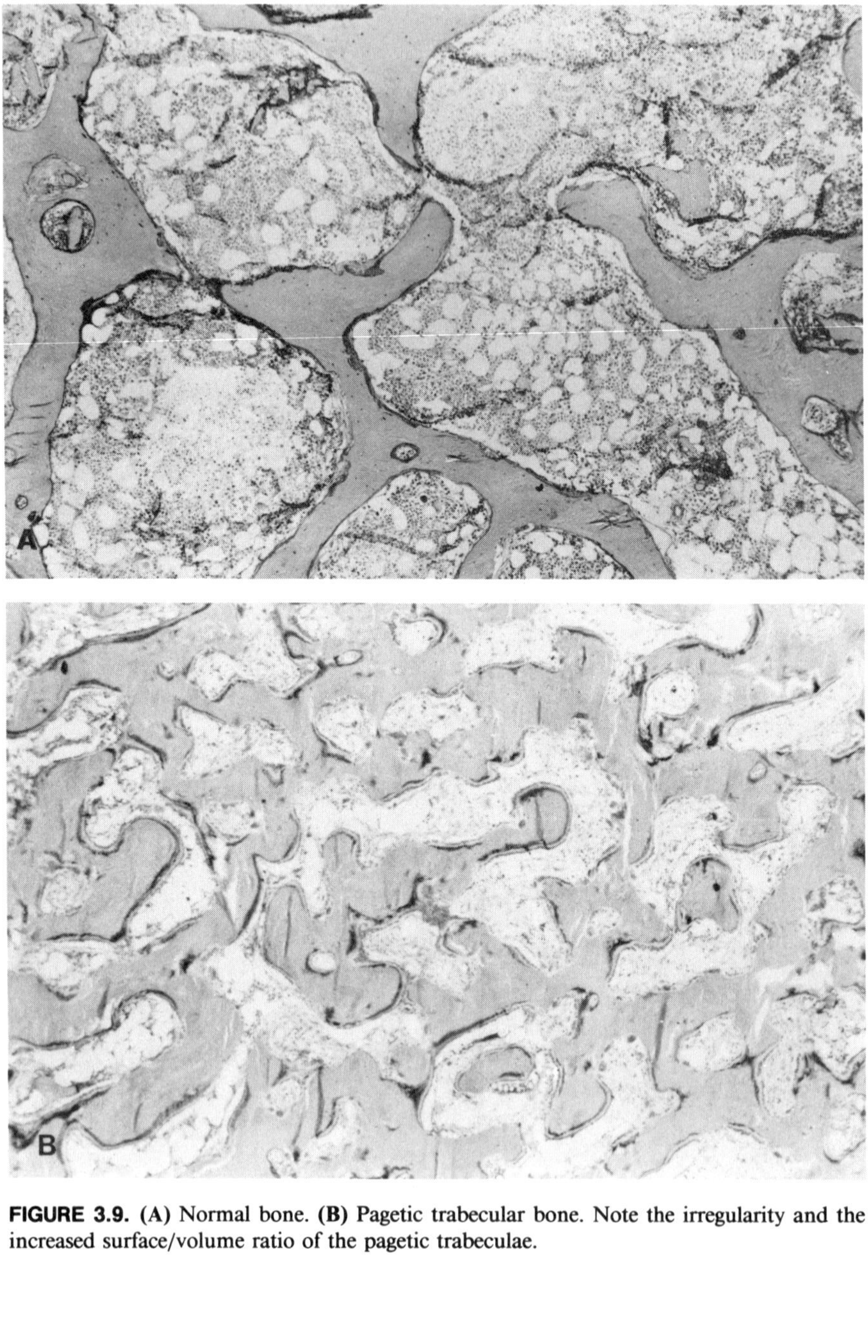

FIGURE 3.9. **(A)** Normal bone. **(B)** Pagetic trabecular bone. Note the irregularity and the increased surface/volume ratio of the pagetic trabeculae.

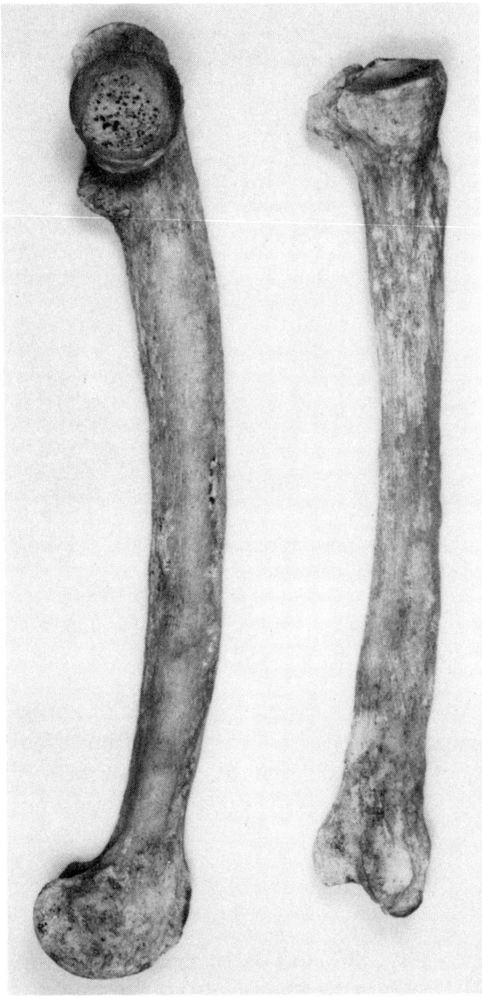

FIGURE 3.10. Femur and tibia of a pagetic patient. Note the femoral bowing and the irregular surface of the tibia.

pagetic lesion generally rests on identification of pathognomonic osteoclasts.

Recent years have seen the development of agents such as calcitonin[19] and the bisphosphonates,[20] which are effective in the treatment of Paget's disease. As both agents directly target osteoclasts and inhibit their activity,[21,22] they block the initial stage of the pagetic lesion and thus the abnormal remodeling that characterizes the disorder. These changes are evidenced histologically by a decrease in parameters of both bone formation and resorption after treatment.[19] The fact that lytic pagetic lesions

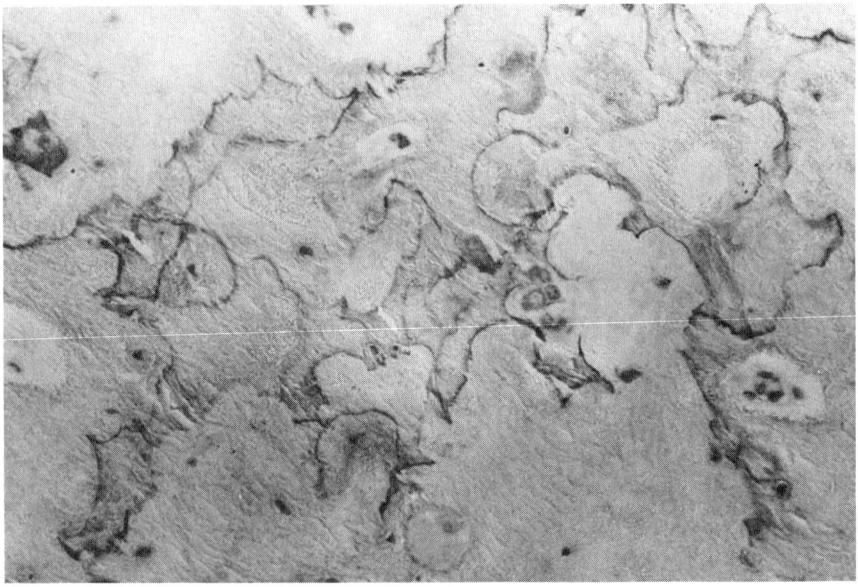

FIGURE 3.11. Mosaic pattern of Paget's disease. The irregular cement lines reflect the rapid and abnormal remodeling that preceded the inactive phase

may heal with treatment indicates that the net effect of these agents favors bone formation.[23]

Paget's disease is also associated with an increased incidence of malignant bone tumors. They arise in pagetic lesions and are most often osteosarcomas, although the incidence of other sarcomas is also enhanced.[24] These tumors tend to be anaplastic, and the prognosis of pagetic sarcomas is generally dismal.[25]

REFERENCES

1. Schmorl G: Ueber osteitis deformans Paget. *Virchows Arch (Pathol Anat)* 1932;283:694.
2. Meunier PJ, Coindre JM, Edouard CM, et al: Bone histomorphometry in Paget's disease: Quantitative and dynamic analysis of pagetic and nonpagetic bone tissue. *Arthritis Rheum* 1980;23:1095.
3. Williams CP, Meachim G, Taylor WH: Effect of calcitonin treatment on osteoclast counts in Paget's disease of bone. *J Clin Pathol* 1978;31:1212.
4. Matthews JL, Martin JH: Intracellular transport of calcium and its relationship to homeostasis and mineralization. *Am J Med* 1971;50:589.
5. Talmage RV, Grubb SA: A laboratory model demonstrating osteocyte-osteoblast control of calcium concentrations. *Clin Orthop* 1977;22:299.
6. Fallon MD, Teitelbaum SL: The interpretation of fluorescent tetracycline markers in the diagnosis of metabolic bone diseases. *Hum Pathol* 1982;13:416.

7. Coccia PF, Krivit W, Cervenka J, et al: Successful bone marrow transplantation for infantile malignant osteopetrosis. *N Engl J Med* 1980;302:701.
8. Alvarez JI, Teitelbaum SL, Menton D, Blair HC: Osteoclast generation from avian marrow monocytic precursors *in vitro*: Characterization by isoenzymes, ultrastructure, and bone resorption showing identity with freshly isolated osteoclasts. *J Bone Mineral Res* 1989;4:S265.
9. Blair HC, Kahn AJ, Crouch EC, et al: Isolated osteoclasts resorb the organic and inorganic components of bone. *J Cell Biol* 1986;102:1164.
10. Blair HC, Teitelbaum SL, Ghiselli R, Gluck S: Osteoclasts bone resorption by a polarized vacuolar proton pump. *Science* 1989;245:855.
11. Frost HM: Tetracycline-based histological analysis of bone remodeling. *Calcif Tissue Res* 1969;3:211.
12. Parfitt AM: The coupling of bone formation to bone resorption: A critical analysis of the concept and of its relevance to the pathogenesis of osteoporosis. *Metab Bone Dis* 1982;4:1.
13. Rebel A, Malkani K, Basle M, Bregeon C: Osteoclast ultrastructure in Paget's disease. *Clin Orthop* 1987;217:4.
14. Mills BG, Singer FR, Weiner LP, et al: Evidence for both respiratory syncytial virus and measles virus antigens in the osteoclasts of patients with Paget's disease of bone. *Clin Orthop* 1984;183:303.
15. Mills BG, Singer FR: Critical evaluation of viral antigen data in Paget's disease of bone. *Clin Orthop* 1987;217:16.
16. Basle MF, Fournier JG, Rosenblatt S, et al: Measles virus RNA detected in Paget's disease of bone tissue by in situ hybridization. *J Gen Virol* 1986;67:907.
17. Lai MC, Wang Y-J, Mills B, and Singer F: Molecular cloning and characterization of a paramyxovirus RNA: Sequences in Paget's disease of bone. *J Bone Mineral Res* 1989;4:198.
18. Friedenstein AJ: Precursor cells of mechanocytes. *Int Rev Cytol* 1976;47:327.
19. Fallon MD, Schwamm HA: Paget's disease of bone: An update on the pathogenesis, pathophysiology, and treatment of osteitis deformans. *Pathol Annu* 1989;24:115.
20. Altman RD, Johnston CC, Khairi MR, et al: Influence of disodium etidronate on clinical and laboratory manifestations of Paget's disease of bone (osteitis deformans). *N Engl J Med* 1973;289:1379.
21. Chambers TJ, Moore A: The sensitivity of isolated osteoclasts to morphological transformation by calcitonin. *J Clin Endocrinol Metab* 1983;57:819.
22. Carano A, Teitelbaum SL, Konsek JD, et al: Bisphosphonates directly inhibit the bone resorption activity of isolated avian osteoclasts in vitro. *J Clin Invest* 1990;85:456.
23. Murphy WA, Whyte MP, Haddad JG Jr: Paget bone disease: Radiologic documentation of healing with human calcium therapy. *Radiology* 1980;136:1.
24. Huvos AG, Butler A, Bretsky SS: Osteogenic sarcoma associated with Paget's disease of bone: A clinicopathologic study of 65 patients. *Cancer* 1983;52:1489.
25. Haibach H, Farrell C, Dittrich FJ: Neoplasms arising in Paget's disease of bone: A study of 82 cases. *Am J Clin Pathol* 1985;83:594.

CHAPTER 4

Indications for Medical Treatment of Paget's Disease of Bone

Ethel S. Siris

INTRODUCTION

Paget's disease of bone was first described in 1876,[1] but efficacious and safe medical treatments did not become widely available until nearly 100 years later. To some degree, this delay reflected ignorance of the intrinsic abnormality that produces the characteristic changes in bone. With the emergence of a better understanding of the pathophysiology of Paget's disease, logical approaches to therapy have become possible. Today, after nearly 20 years of experience with specific antipagetic medications, we have acquired some knowledge of what medical treatments can accomplish, but we are still developing guidelines regarding when, whom, and why to treat.

In this chapter, the intent is to consider the indications for medical treatment of Paget's disease. In order to achieve this, it is necessary to review the clinical aspects of this disorder, the principles of medical treatment, and the goals of such treatment in a variety of clinical settings.

CLINICAL PRESENTATION OF PAGET'S DISEASE

Paget's disease is a localized disorder of bone remodeling in which abnormal osteoclasts at affected skeletal sites produce an increase in the rate and extent of bone resorption. A secondary increase in osteoblastic new bone formation follows the increase in bone resorption with the creation of bone that is structurally chaotic, less compact, more vascular, and prone to deformity and fracture. Depending on the specific bones that are affected and the level of activity of the ongoing remodeling abnormality, there may be no obvious signs and symptoms, as may occur in a majority of patients, or there may be a spectrum of abnormal physical findings and related complaints that range from minimally troublesome to severely disabling.

Involvement of the skeleton may be monostotic, with only one skeletal site involved, or polyostotic, with structural changes in several different areas of the skeleton. Common sites of Paget's disease include the pelvis, femur, spine, skull, tibia, and humerus. Less commonly involved are bones of the forearm, clavicles, scapulae, and ribs. Isolated involvement of a patella, metacarpal, or metatarsal is occasionally seen. The presentation of this disorder may vary from patient to patient as a result of its localized nature; for example, one patient may have pagetic changes in the skull and two noncontiguous vertebral bodies, and another may have the disease in half the pelvis, the proximal femur on one side, and the contralateral tibia.

Table 4.1 lists sites of involvement in a series of 864 patients from across the United States who were studied in an epidemiologic survey performed by our group.[2] Of these patients 25% had monostotic disease, and the rest polyostotic. As can be inferred from this diverse listing of sites, the symptoms of Paget's disease, when present, may be quite variable. Table 4.2 lists the reported symptoms in this population, who clearly represent the symptomatic end of the spectrum, at the time they were first diagnosed, at a mean age of 58 years, and since diagnosis, a mean of 13 years later, when completing our survey.

The most frequent complaints involved bone pain, a symptom that can be very difficult for the clinician to interpret. Bone pain in Paget's disease can be a dull, nonspecific aching in the bone itself. Sharper, more localized pain may result from microfractures that may or may not be visible on radiographs. When there is pagetic involvement adjacent to a

TABLE 4.1 Sites of Paget's Disease

Site	Patients, %
Pelvis/hip	63
Femur	41
Spine	34
Tibia	33
Skull	31
Humerus	23
Forearm	12

TABLE 4.2 Paget's Disease Symptoms*

Symptom	Patients with Symptom at Diagnosis (%)	Patients with Symptom Since Diagnosis (Mean = 13 years) (%)
Bone pain with movement	53	73
Joint pain	44	65
Bone pain at rest	43	68
Heat over bone	29	42
Bowing deformity	22	35
Radicular pain	17	24
Skull enlargement	12	18
Hearing loss	9	18
Headache	9	14
Fracture through pagetic bone	7	12
Asymptomatic	32	25

*In 864 patients who completed a questionnaire.

major joint in weight-bearing bones (such as the hip, knee, or ankle), pain due to a secondary osteoarthritis may arise and is a common source of discomfort and potential disability. Headache or a bandlike tightening across the forehead can occur with skull involvement. Paget's disease of the vertebral bodies may cause localized back pain as well as pain from various neurologic compression syndromes. Encroachment of enlarged pagetic vertebrae on nerve roots, particularly in the lumbar area, may produce pain from radiculopathy. This may occasionally occur in the setting of a compression fracture of a vertebral body but typically occurs without fracture. Lumbar involvement may lead to spinal stenosis with pain in the back or lower extremities.

It is important to emphasize that patients with Paget's disease often have significant degenerative disease at nonpagetic sites; thigh pain attributed to a narrowed pagetic hip joint might actually be the result of nonpagetic lumbar disk disease. Thus, just as it is incorrect to ascribe pagetic pain to arthritis or "old age" (as apparently is often done), it is also wrong to label all pain as pagetic, when some is originating in a nonpagetic area. Not only are these considerations important in diagnosis but they are also critical in assessing the effectiveness of antipagetic therapy in the relief of symptoms.

As shown in Table 4.2, bone deformity may occur in Paget's disease. A bowing deformity or simply an asymmetric enlargement of an extremity, acetabular protrusion of the hip or other pelvic deformity, frontal bossing or enlargement or ridging of the skull, and various degrees of kyphosis or scoliosis are examples of this. Bone deformity may lead to clinical problems. A bowed femur or tibia is typically associated with some shortening of the affected leg, which may produce limping or a more serious gait disturbance. Abnormal mechanical forces may then predispose the patient to the development of a secondary, so-called Paget's arthritis (osteoarthritis) of the hip, knee, or ankle in the region of the bowing or perhaps promote arthritis on the contralateral side, if the gait disturbance is severe. Acetabular protrusion may also be the source of severe hip joint dysfunction.

Pagetic bone is associated with increased vascularity when the abnormal bone turnover is markedly increased, manifested by moderate elevations in the serum alkaline phosphatase (reflecting the secondary increase in bone formation) and urinary hydroxyproline (a marker of the initiating lesion, the increase in bone resorption). When such bone is adjacent to neural structures, the combination of expanded bone size and vascular engorgement may produce neurologic complications. When extensive skull involvement is complicated by basilar invagination, patients may occasionally develop hydrocephalus, due to obstruction of cerebral spinal fluid flow, or frank brain stem compression.[3] This may lead to a variety of slowly progressive neurologic problems including ataxia, dementia, and cranial nerve abnormalities. Less severe and more common neurologic sequelae of extensive skull overgrowth may include progressive hearing loss, usually due to contributions of both sensorineural—including 8th nerve damage—and bone-related problems.[4] Other cranial nerve palsies (such as Bell's palsy) are sometimes observed. As mentioned previously, radiculopathy can occur particularly with lumbar spine involvement. A more serious but infrequent complication in patients with thoracic vertebral body involvement is spinal cord compression accompanied by paraparesis or paraplegia.[3]

In some cases of metabolically active Paget's disease these neurologic conditions may reflect either pressure on neural structures by enlarged and highly vascular pagetic bone or a "steal syndrome" in which blood is directed away from neural structures toward pagetic tissue.[5] Aggressive medical management to decrease pagetic bone turnover may often produce substantial benefit. Orthopedic or neurosurgical intervention may also be needed when the problem is the result of a more direct bone impingement on nerve tissue.

The hypervascularity of pagetic bone may be associated with an increase in blood flow to adjacent soft tissue and skin leading to an increase in skin temperature, most easily appreciated in the tibia or skull. This may be an annoying symptom for some patients. Occasionally it is mistaken for a sign of inflammation or infection, and it has led to the incorrect prescription of antibiotics or even to an unwarranted biopsy.

Fracture of pagetic bone may include traumatic or pathologic fracture of an extremity, compression fracture of a vertebra, or small, partial fissure fractures along the convex cortical surfaces of weight-bearing bones. These small fissure fractures are often asymptomatic and long-standing; occasional medial extension of such a small fracture requires careful observation, especially if it becomes painful, as this may be a sign of impending complete fracture at the site.

An infrequent but often mentioned nonskeletal complication of metabolically active Paget's disease is high-output cardiac failure. Although an increase in cardiac output may be measured in some patients with very active and extensive Paget's disease,[6] our experience indicates that most patients who have frank congestive heart failure usually have underlying cardiac disease as well, very possibly exacerbated by the increased skeletal blood flow demands from the vascular pagetic bone.

Neoplastic changes in pagetic bone are extremely rare. It is believed that less than 1% of patients experience malignant degeneration with the develop of osteogenic sarcoma, fibrosarcoma, or chondrosarcoma at pagetic sites.[7] Benign giant cell tumors (sometimes called reparative granulomas rather than true neoplasms) occur rarely as well.[8] It is unclear whether the recent availability of medications that suppress pagetic bone turnover will affect the development of these neoplastic complications.

Paget's disease may sometimes be associated with alterations in calcium and uric acid metabolism.[9] Uric acid levels are often slightly elevated for reasons not understood, and occasionally acute gout at typical sites of involvement may occur.[10] Uric acid–containing kidney stones may develop in some patients with hyperuricemia. It is uncertain whether suppression of pagetic bone turnover will decrease the incidence of hyperuricemia or its complications.

Urinary calcium may sometimes be elevated in patients with active Paget's disease, presumably as a result of the markedly increased bone resorption, and calcium-containing kidney stones may form. In our survey of 864 patients with Paget's disease and 500 age- and gender-matched controls, we found that 14% of men and 7% of women with pagetic disease had experienced gout, but this was not significantly different from the experiences of male and female controls. Similarly, 5% of women patients and 3% of female controls reported having had kidney stones, a difference that was not significant. However, a history of kidney stones in men was significantly higher in patients (13%) than in controls (7%; $P < 0.05$).[11]

Serum calcium level is typically normal in Paget's disease, presumably because of normal renal function and, more importantly, a relatively close coupling of bone resorption—tending to release calcium from bone—and new bone formation, serving presumably to reuse calcium during bone accretion. However, hypercalcemia can occur in association with Paget's disease in some individuals. Several authors have noted a possible increase in the frequency of primary hyperparathyroidism occurring in Paget's disease patients[12]; in our survey,[11] a history of primary hyperparathyroidism was obtained from 5% of the pagetic subjects, but from only 1% of the controls ($P < 0.001$). Another type of calcium problem, immobilization hypercalcemia, is sometimes seen in patients with markedly increased bone turnover who are put to bed for a period of time for a concurrent illness. With the loss of weight bearing and a subsequent decrease in bone formation, ongoing bone resorption may present increased calcium to the extracellular fluid and hypercalcemia may ensue.

MEDICAL TREATMENT OF PAGET'S DISEASE

In the United States today there are four medications available to the practicing physician for use in Paget's disease. The first two of these are salmon calcitonin (Calcimar [Rhone-Poulene-Rorer]) and human calcitonin (Cibacalcin [Ciba-Geigy]). Only parenteral formulations can be obtained at present, necessitating a subcutaneous or intramuscular mode of administration. The cost per year for full daily doses is in the range of $3,500 at this writing. Most patients can tolerate dose reductions, however, after the first months of treatment. A nasal spray form of calcitonin is being investigated at this time but will probably become available in the near future. The calcitonins are discussed in detail elsewhere in this volume.

The bisphosphonate (diphosphonate) etidronate disodium (Didronel [Norwich Eaton]) is an oral agent, generally taken for courses of 6 months followed by at least 6 months of no therapy. Cost of one course of this drug at the usual dosage is approximately $400 to $500. An intravenous formulation of etidronate, approved for use in hypercalcemia, is also available, but this mode of administration has had limited study in Paget's disease. Several other promising bisphosphonates are currently being investigated and may become available in the next 3 to 4 years. This class of compounds is also discussed extensively in this volume.

Plicamycin, previously termed mithramycin (Mithracin [Miles]), is used on occasion for Paget's disease. Although this agent is approved in the United States only for the management of hypercalcemia, it has been administered successfully to patients with Paget's disease and is discussed in Chapter 13.

Gallium nitrate is another agent under active investigation in the United States for its effectiveness in Paget's disease. It has been approved for use in hypercalcemia, but there is as yet a very limited experience with the agent in pagetic subjects.[13]

INDICATIONS FOR TREATMENT OF PAGET'S DISEASE

With the review of the localized nature of Paget's disease and the description of the breadth and variety of the signs and symptoms that may result in some patients, the indications for treatment with antipagetic therapy can be considered. It should be reiterated that most patients with Paget's disease are asymptomatic. Thus, the first questions to ask when treatment decisions are weighed are: What is the disease doing to the patient, and what will treatment do to the disease process? Current therapies are directed at suppression of pagetic activity; the calcitonins, bisphosphonates, plicamycin, and gallium all appear to work primarily through a suppression of the increased osteoclastic bone resorption that initiates the abnormal remodeling process. Each of these agents promotes a decrease in pagetic bone turnover. In situations where suppression of increased bone turnover is likely to be associated with either some relief of symptoms or a slowing or arrest of localized disease progression, use of antipagetic therapy is logical. Conversely, when symptoms or problems are primarily due to mechanical changes produced by past pagetic activity and long-standing structural change in bone, these agents may be less effective in producing symptomatic benefit.

Indications for therapy are shown in Table 4.3. The presence of treatable symptoms is the first of these. Symptoms such as pain in an extremity, headache, or back pain (assuming the source of the pain is a site of Paget's disease), and increased warmth over bone often respond well to a decrease in pagetic bone turnover. Some neurologic compression syndromes may also respond, particularly when there is very active disease and the impairment may be due to vascular engorgement of the pagetic

TABLE 4.3 Indications for Treatment with Antipagetic Therapy

Symptoms likely to benefit from a decrease in pagetic bone turnover
Prevention of local progression and future complications
Planned surgery at a pagetic site
Prolonged immobilization and risk of hypercalcemia

bone and soft tissue; with a reduction in bone turnover, hypervascularity may decrease and relieve the compression. Even with severe secondary arthritic changes, some back, hip, or knee pain may decrease substantially with treatment, particularly if there is active bone turnover (as determined by the biochemical markers), but this may be difficult to predict. Conversely, hearing loss is unlikely to improve (although it may progress less quickly),[14] a bowed limb will remain bowed (and may continue to bow, for mechanical reasons), and a misshapen hip or knee joint may remain mechanically dysfunctional.

It should be noted that treatment of symptomatic patients can also include other modalities, such as analgesic and nonsteroidal antiinflammatory drugs, canes, shoe lifts, and hearing aids.

Controversy exists with respect to the use of antipagetic medication in the absence of symptoms. However, an understanding of the pathophysiology of this disorder and the mechanisms of action of the currently available drugs suggests that treatment may be appropriate when there is active disease (that is, serum alkaline phosphatase greater than three to four times normal level) at sites where there is a risk of future complications and the development of symptoms if disease progresses. As shown in Table 4.4, treatment is recommended even in asymptomatic patients if there is ongoing active disease involving the extremities (especially weight-bearing bones), where a future bowing deformity might occur; with vertebral body involvement, where late fracture or development of spinal nerve or cord compression could arise; with extensive skull involvement, where future hearing loss, headache, or basilar invagination and risk of neurologic compression exists; and for Paget's disease involving the acetabular region of the pelvis or a long bone in an area adjacent to a major joint (such as the hip, knee, ankle, or shoulder), where future osteoarthritis might emerge as a consequence of structural changes in bone at the site. It is probably impossible to predict the natural evolution of an area of Paget's disease in a particular patient; nonetheless, as shown in Figure 4.1 (A through C) progressive changes can occur over time. Similarly, as shown in Table 4.2, increased numbers of patients developed symptoms as time passed after initial diagnosis. Whether these problems can be prevented by treatment

TABLE 4.4 Sites to Consider Treating in Asymptomatic Patients

Long bones (especially weight bearing)
Vertebral bodies
Skull
Areas adjacent to major joints

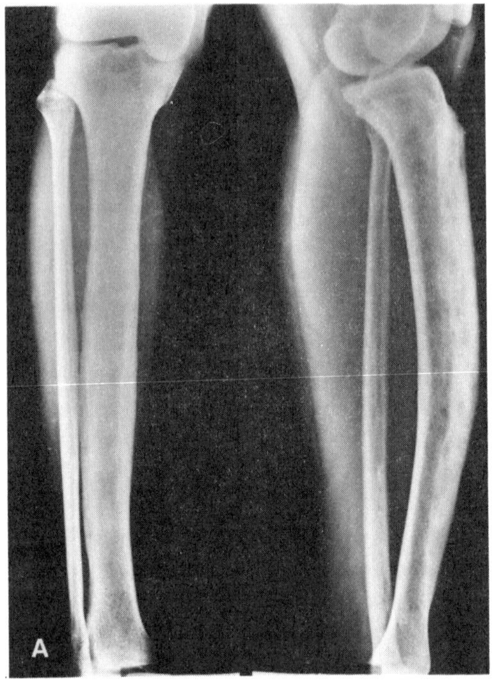

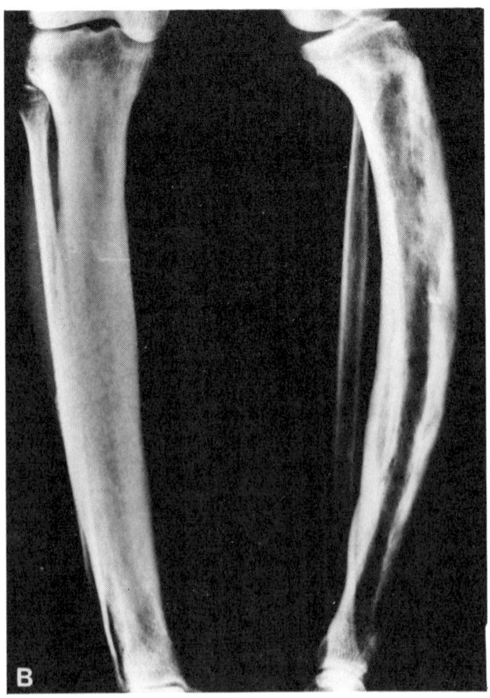

FIGURE 4.1. Progression of tibial Paget's disease in an untreated patient is shown in these radiographs. **(A)** Anteroposterior and lateral views of the right tibia 2 years after the initial diagnosis. Cortical thickening and expansion of bone, with anterior and early lateral bowing, are present. **(B)** and **(C)** Radiographs of the same leg taken 7 and 20 years later, respectively. Progressively increasing deformity has occurred, with extension of disease distally exhibited in the second radiograph and marked increases in both the lateral and anterior bowing over the 20-year period. Using the normal fibula and distal femur as landmarks, the shortening and transverse expansion of the tibia can be readily appreciated.

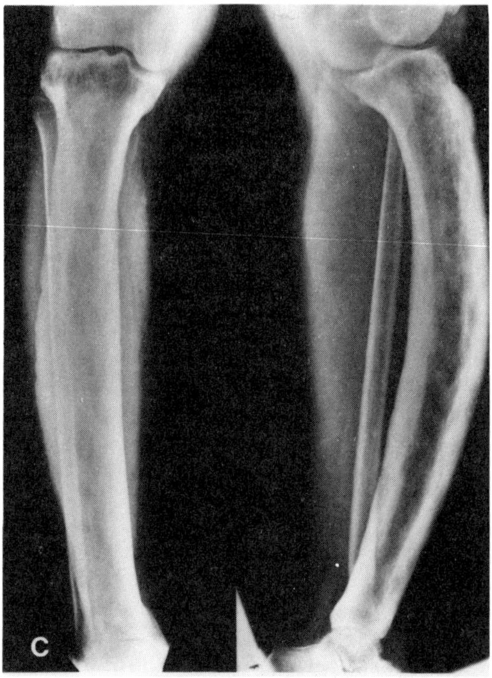

remains unknown, but studies describing the reduction in osteoclast number and the restoration of more normal bone architecture after treatment[15] support the view that arrest or slowing of progression with medication may truly occur.

A third indication for treatment arises in the setting of elective surgery planned at a site of Paget's disease. Three to 6 months of administration of a calcitonin or bisphosphonate before surgery may successfully decrease hypervascularity and make the surgeon's task easier by reducing blood loss. This concept is based primarily on clinical experience and seems to be valid. In my own experience, pretreatment is not needed if the serum alkaline phosphatase is only mildly elevated (for example, less than two times normal) but may be warranted for activity greater than this.

Finally, prolonged immobilization of a patient with active, polyostotic Paget's disease is sometimes associated with hypercalcemia, as discussed previously. Suppression of the bone resorption should lower the calcium level in this setting, and antipagetic therapy may be of value when initiated promptly in such a patient.

Table 4.5 lists several other issues regarding treatment that should be addressed, as these involve common clinical questions. The first concerns

TABLE 4.5 Controversial Treatment Issues

Patient age
Level of elevation of biochemical indices
Cardiovascular disease
Recent fracture or orthopedic surgery

patient age. It is my impression that many practicing physicians tend to avoid treatment in elderly patients. Conversely, many medical specialists in the field believe that patient age should not impede therapeutic intervention if that treatment is likely to offer relief of symptoms. Although some have suggested that preventive treatment in elderly people makes little sense, I take care of a number of otherwise healthy patients in their early 80s, whose potential life span is not easily predicted; to my mind, indications for therapy as previously described continue to apply. At the other end of the age spectrum, it is extremely important to review carefully the situation of younger patients, such as those in their 40s or 50s, in whom early therapeutic intervention may be of long-term benefit. The patient whose tibia is shown in Figure 4.1 was 42 years old and asymptomatic when her "mild" lesion was first discovered; today many specialists would try to suppress activity aggressively in such an individual, in the hope of preventing the severe bone deformity that eventually emerged.

Another commonly asked clinical question concerns the level of elevation of the biochemical markers at which to treat. I believe that the level of alkaline phosphatase (the simpler of the two markers to obtain routinely) should be viewed in terms of the sites of involvement, radiographic appearance, and symptoms. A test result of less than twice the upper limit of normal, in association with extensive changes at many sites, may reflect a late "burned-out" phase of Paget's disease, and in general, I might observe such a patient for a period of time without treating. If the patient with the same mild elevation in the test has minor changes in the pelvis not involving the acetabulum or has a patch of lytic disease or sclerosis in one area of the skull, I would probably observe the individual without treatment. The same test result in a patient with early changes in a weight-bearing bone, however, would worry me more; asymptomatic femoral or tibial involvement, particularly with a lytic "blade of grass" lesion, deserves treatment, in my view, even if the alkaline phosphatase is only mildly elevated, as such bone changes are likely to progress. Finally, in the presence of symptoms, as described earlier, I would probably treat if I believed that the symptoms reflected the abnormal—although low—level of increased bone turnover. Although I generally do not treat patients with radiographic evidence of Paget's disease but presently normal values for serum alkaline phosphatase and urinary hydroxyproline, localized lytic disease in a weight-bearing area or vertebra would lead me to choose treatment.

Many patients are quite concerned about their specific levels of serum alkaline phosphatase, becoming alarmed by changes of 10% to 20%. It is worth noting that serial measurements of this enzyme in a single day, over several days, or over several months in an untreated patient can show variations of 5% to 15%. It is also a point of clinical interest that the very highest levels of alkaline phosphatase often occur in patients with skull involvement. In our hospital a normal serum alkaline phosphatase level is 30 to 100 IU/L; it is not unusual for someone with Paget's disease of only the skull to have a value greater than 1,000 IU/L, when another patient with extensive pelvis and spine involvement might have a result of 500 to 600 IU/L. It is my clinical impression that lower values are preferable to higher, but we must always remember that we are attempting to treat the affected skeleton, not the alkaline phosphatase level per se.

As discussed, the vascular nature of pagetic bone can result in an increase in cardiac output when there is extensive polyostotic disease undergoing high levels of bone turnover, as reflected by the biochemical indices. In older patients who also have underlying heart disease, this may lead to cardiac decompensation. I have treated a few patients in this category, with initial serum alkaline phosphatase levels above 2,000 IU/L, in whom symptoms of angina or congestive heart failure improved after the Paget's activity was successfully reduced. However, congestive heart failure arising in the setting of milder Paget's disease is much less likely to be affected by improvement of the pagetic process.

Orthopedic surgeons often ask whether antipagetic therapy is appropriate after fracture or elective surgery, when normal bone healing must occur. There are virtually no data from human studies to indicate whether bone healing will be impaired by a suppression of pagetic bone turnover in this type of patient; limited animal data suggest that healing after fracture may be enhanced by calcitonin. From the experience of a number of my colleagues, there seems to be no hesitation in administering a calcitonin to such a patient if it is otherwise indicated. There is some theoretical concern about the use of etidronate in this setting, based on the fact that high doses of this agent for prolonged periods can result in an impairment of mineralization. Although the recommended lower doses given for no longer than 6 months at a time would be unlikely to cause a problem, prudence dictates that a calcitonin is a better choice in this situation.

In summary, there are several antipagetic medications available in the United States today (and additional agents are in use in Europe, as described elsewhere) that may afford benefit to a substantial number of patients. Although moderately expensive, these treatments appear to be well tolerated and free of serious adverse effects in a great majority of patients. As newer safe, efficacious, and easily administered therapies emerge, even more aggressive approaches to management may develop. Physicians should be cognizant of the pharmacologic principles through which these agents have effects on bone. Pagetic patients may manifest a wide range of signs and symptoms; as practitioners consider offering these medications, the probability of benefit in each individual patient must always be taken into account.

REFERENCES

1. Paget J: On a form of chronic inflammation of bones. *Med Chir Trans* 1877:60:37–63.
2. Siris E, Kelsey J, Flaster E, et al: Paget's disease in the United States: A survey of 700 patients. *J Bone Mineral Res* 1988;3(suppl 1):S93.
3. Schmidek HH: Neurologic and neurosurgical sequelae of Paget's disease of bone. *Clin Orthop* 1977;127:70–77.
4. Nager GT: Paget's disease of the temporal bone. *Ann Otol Rhinol Laryngol* 1975; 84(suppl 22):1–32.
5. Herzberg L, Bayliss E: Spinal-cord syndrome due to noncompressive Paget's disease of bone: A spinal-artery steal phenomenon reversible with calcitonin. *Lancet* 1980;2:13–15.
6. Howarth S: Cardiac output in osteitis deformans. *Clin Sci* 1953;12:271–275.
7. Poretta CA, Dahlin DC, Janes JM: Sarcoma in Paget's disease of bone. *J Bone Joint Surg [Am]* 1957;39:1313–1329.
8. Jacobs TP, Michelsen J, Polay J, et al: Giant cell tumor in Paget's disease of bone. *Cancer* 1979;44:742–747.
9. Singer FR: *Paget's Disease of Bone.* New York, Plenum, Medical Book 1977, pp 113–114.
10. Franck WA, Bress NM, Singer FR, Krane SM: Rheumatic manifestations of Paget's disease of bone. *Am J Med* 1974;56:592–603.
11. Siris E, Kelsey J, Flaster E, et al: Environmental exposures and medical histories in Paget's disease. *J Bone Mineral Res* 1988;3(suppl 1):S93.
12. Posen S, Bligh PC, Wilkinson M: Paget's disease of bone and hyperparathyroidism: Coincidence or causal relationship? *Calcif Tissue Res* 1978;26:107–109.
13. Matkovic V, Apseloff G, Sheppard DR, Gerber N: Use of gallium to treat Paget's disease of bone: A pilot study. *Lancet* 1990;1:72–75.
14. ElSammaa M, Linthicum FH Jr, House HP, House JW: Calcitonin as a treatment for hearing loss in Paget's disease. *Am J Otol* 1986;7:241–243.
15. Meunier PJ, Chapuy MC, Delmas P, et al: Intravenous disodium etidronate therapy in Paget's disease of bone and hypercalcemia of malignancy: Effects on biochemical parameters and bone histomorphometry. *Am J Med* 1987;82(suppl 2A):71–78.

CHAPTER 5

Experiences with Porcine and Salmon Calcitonin in the Treatment of Paget's Disease

Stanley Wallach

INTRODUCTION

The development of calcitonin (CT) as the first effective therapeutic agent for Paget's disease is not just of historic significance but also of current interest as the most effective treatment for Paget's disease available in the United States. Calcitonin, in fact, has provoked the reawakening of interest in Paget's disease during the past two decades, 100 years after Sir James Paget's description in the late 1800s. Agents used in the 1940–1960 era, such as corticosteroids, sodium fluoride, estrogens, and aspirin, have not stood the test of time since none produced the spectacular effects that were so evident with CT. The rapidity, within a decade, with which the discovery of CT was translated into effective treatment by collaboration among basic researchers, clinical investigators, and industrial research and development groups is awesome.

Harold Copp deserves the credit for the discovery of CT in the early 1960s when he conducted a variety of unusual experiments in which he was able to set up a perfusion system that controlled the calcium concentration of the blood flowing through the thyroid-parathyroid axis independent of the systemic circulation but also allowed resulting hormonal effluents from the thyroid-parathyroid axis to reach the periphery to affect the skeleton and therefore, the systemic calcium concentration.[1] In experiments in which he perfused first high-calcium blood and then low-calcium blood through the thyroid-parathyroid axis,[1] the expected inverse effects on the systemic calcium concentration occurred. The high-calcium blood was presumed to have "turned off" the parathyroids and consequently decreased systemic blood calcium concentration, whereas the low-calcium blood treated with edetate (EDTA) to complex the ionic calcium caused a reversal of this process. However, Copp carried the experiment a step further by excising the thyroid-parathyroid axis after exposure to low-calcium blood. To his surprise, the systemic blood calcium concentration, which should have then decreased, continued to rise. This effect could not be explained on the basis of sole parathyroid control of calcium metabolism acting through enhanced bone resorption. Copp's most graphic experiment was one in which he compared the ability of perfusion of high-calcium blood to lower the systemic blood calcium concentration by "turning off" the parathyroids with that of surgical removal of the thyroid-parathyroid axis. Contrary to prediction, the decrease in the systemic blood calcium concentration was more rapid with high-calcium perfusion, indicating that there was not only cessation of parathyroid secretion during high-calcium perfusion but another factor operative in assisting in the decrease in the systemic blood calcium concentration. He named that putative factor, which he did not identify, CT and theorized that the factor was secreted somewhere within the thyroid-parathyroid axis independently of parathyroid hormone.

It was left to Hirsch and Foster and their associates in 1964[2,3] to show that a principle in the mammalian thyroid, not the parathyroid, was capable of lowering the blood calcium level. Subsequent work identified that principle as authentic CT produced by the parafollicular (C) cells, which are distinct from the thyroid follicular cells that produce thyroxine and triiodothyronine. The C cells do not abut the thyroid colloid but are within the basement membrane of the thyroid follicles, having migrated to the thyroid anlage from the neural crest during embryonic life, after temporary residence in the ultimobranchial bodies of the neck.

Porcine CT (PCT) was the first to be recognized, characterized, and synthesized. All the CTs have an amino acid length of 32 and a molecular weight of approximately 3,000 kD. Essential to biologic activity is a seven-member aminoterminal ring connected through a disulfide bond. However, the CTs of various species differ from one another in molecular structure because of amino acid substitutions that influence their biologic properties. Eight CTs have been characterized and synthesized thus far: pig, rat, cow, sheep, chicken, salmon, eel, and human. Four CTs are now in use in the treatment of human disease. PCT was the first to be used, and Bijvoet takes the credit for demonstrating its biologic activity in Paget's disease.[4] PCT underwent extensive clinical trials in both Europe and the United States and is still in use in some parts of the world, although it was never licensed in the United States. The two CTs that are in regular use in the United States for the treatment of Paget's disease are salmon CT (SCT) and human CT (HCT). Modified eel CT is also available[5] and is the treatment of choice in Japan, where it was first developed.

Calcitonins have a large number of biologic activities in both hard and soft tissues, but their most prominent action is to decrease bone resorption by inhibition of osteoclast activity. There is also evidence of a capacity to increase bone formation and a number of effects on the kidney, the gastrointestinal (GI) tract, the liver, and the pancreas. In the central nervous system, CT may have an analgesic effect, as well as cause satiety. Some of the peripheral effects may be due to central nervous system influence since small doses injected intraventricularly mimic some of the effects of GI instillation and of systemic administration. It is probable that many actions of CT are related to altered calcium transport in soft and hard tissues. In addition, certain breast tumors have CT receptors, and it has been shown recently that cellular zinc transport is also influenced by CT, specifically in Leydig's cells and certain types of lymphocytes.[6] Whether any of these other actions of CT can be used in human therapy remains to be determined.

Next we will consider the major action of CT on bone to decrease bone resorption by osteoclast inhibition, since this is the major basis for its ability to treat Paget's disease. The observations that demonstrate beneficial effects of CT on Paget's disease can be divided into three groups; biochemical and metabolic studies, physiologic and histologic alterations, and clinical effects. As shown in Figure 5.1, PCT has a dramatic effect in decreasing the serum alkaline phosphatase, and some patients return to the normal range after several months of treatment. The group of patients in Figure 5.1 was then switched to SCT with a further small effect.[7] In this same group, urinary total hydroxyproline excretion showed a similar pattern but with a major difference: an "escape" and return to baseline levels by the end of treatment with PCT. With a switch to SCT, the inhibitory effect resumed.

This is one example of the curious dissociation phenomenon associated with CT and other treatments of Paget's disease. In many patients there is good concordance between the declines in the various parameters of disease activity, such as alkaline phosphatase and urinary hydroxyproline, but in other patients the parameters are dissociated. It is possible that antibodies develop against the PCT, but this does not explain the dissociation phenomenon.

The return to baseline of hydroxyproline excretion during PCT treatment was a major reason why it was not licensed in the United States, whereas the more potent SCT was licensed. Figure 5.2 portrays a group of 28 patients who were treated with SCT alone for 1 to 2 years. A pattern similar to the previous pattern was observed, as the alkaline phosphatase

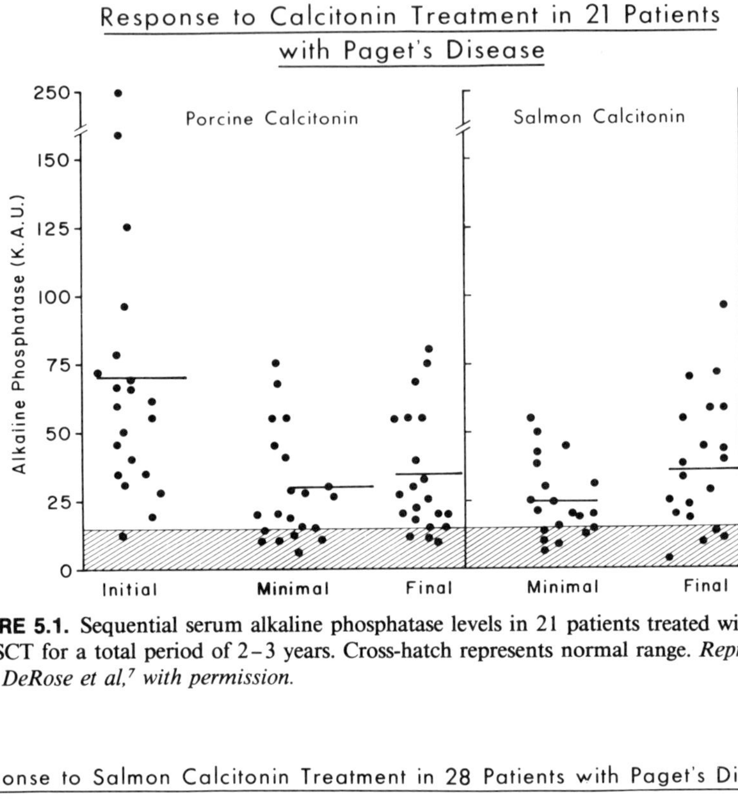

FIGURE 5.1. Sequential serum alkaline phosphatase levels in 21 patients treated with PCT and SCT for a total period of 2–3 years. Cross-hatch represents normal range. *Reproduced from DeRose et al,[7] with permission.*

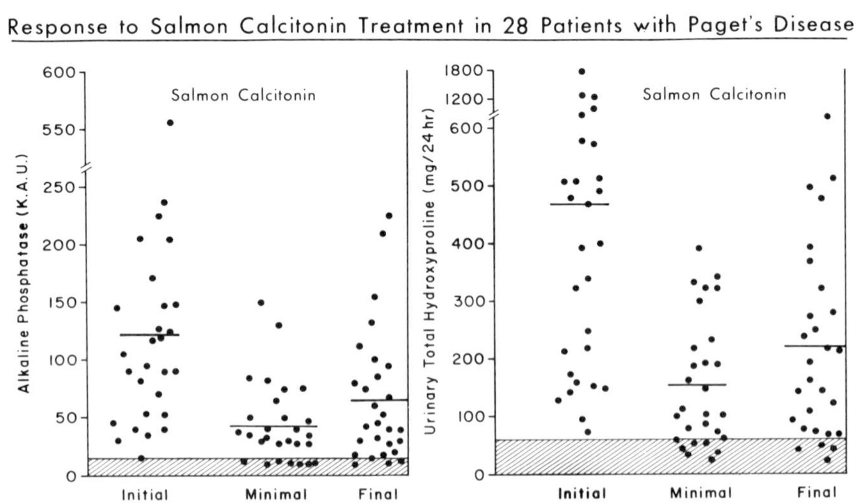

FIGURE 5.2. Sequential serum alkaline phosphatase and total urinary hydroxyproline levels in 28 patients treated with SCT for 1–2 years. Cross-hatch represents normal range. *Reproduced from DeRose et al,[7] with permission.*

level declined approximately 50%, with a slight rebound by the end of treatment. Hydroxyproline excretion responded similarly, but with more scatter and a greater degree of rebound by the end of treatment, again demonstrating dissociation of the responses of the two parameters. The correlation coefficient of the decrease in the two parameters was 0.65 (Figure 5.3).

Among the physiologic effects of CT, a marked decrease in radiocalcium turnover, reflecting decreased skeletal turnover, is prominent. Compartmental analysis to yield skeletal calcium flux rates indicates a significant decrease in skeletal turnover as a result of CT treatment (Table 5.1). The effect of CT in decreasing skeletal calcium turnover is generally maximal after 12 to 18 months of treatment, whereas the effect noted after 1 to 2 months of treatment is generally smaller. In three cases a paradoxical increase in turnover was recorded after 1 month of CT administration. In approximately half the patients studied, there was a later waning of the inhibitory effect on calcium turnover, and this could occur as soon as 1 year of CT treatment.

Figures 5.4 and 5.5 compare the results of CT treatment on bone turnover (F_{34}) with concurrent changes in alkaline phosphatase levels and urinary hydroxyproline excretion. Again, marked concordance between

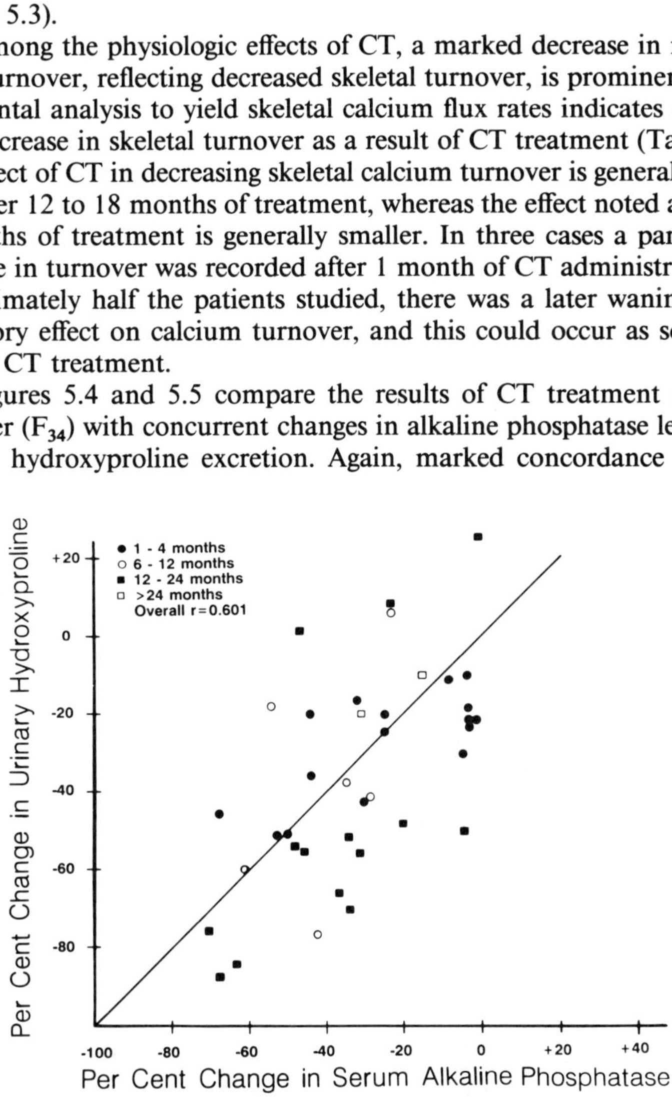

FIGURE 5.3. Correlation of individual percentage changes in serum alkaline phosphatase and urinary hydroxyproline during calcitonin treatment. $R = 0.601$. *Reproduced from Wallach et al,[9] with permission.*

TABLE 5.1 Effect of Calcitonin on Radiocalcium Turnover in Paget's Disease

Patient	Treatment, months*	Change in Skeletal Calcium Uptake, %
A.W. (I)	PCT 8 IU/kg qd (1)	−24
(II)	PCT 200 IU qd (1)	−24
M.B.	PCT 8 IU/kg qd (1)	−27
	PCT 200 IU qd (3)	−27
	PCT 200 IU qd (11)	−8
	SCT 100 IU qd (5)	+31
	SCT 100 IU qd (20)	+37
A.V.	PCT 8 IU/kg qd (2)	−34
	SCT 100 IU qd (11)	−49
C.E.L	PCT 8 IU /kg qd (1)	−12
F.J.C	PCT 8 IU/kg qd (1)	−6
	PCT 200 IU qd (6)	−6
	SCT 100 IU qd (11)	−31
	SCT 50 IU tiw (26)	+2
P.K.	PCT 8 IU/kg qd (1)	−13
	SCT 100 IU qd (7)	+7
M.M.	SCT 100 IU qd (1)	−69
	SCT 50 IU tiw (17)	−27
S.D.	SCT 100 IU tiw (1)	+1
	SCT 50 IU tiw (12)	−17
	SCT 50 IU tiw (24)	−15
E.F.	SCT 50 IU tiw (1)	+35
	SCT 50 IU tiw (17)	−46
D.A.	SCT 50 IU tiw (1)	−18
	SCT 50 IU tiw (12)	−71
K.F.	SCT 100 IU qd (1)	−12
	SCT 50 IU tiw (17)	−33
P.T.	SCT 100 IU qd (1)	−2
	SCT 50 IU qd (16)	−91
P.G.	SCT 100 IU qd (1)	−15
	SCT 50 IU tiw (13)	−42
	SCT 50 IU tiw (22)	−10
P.R.	SCT 50 IU tiw (2)	−5
	SCT 50 IU tiw (11)	−26
	SCT 50 IU tiw (22)	−44
D.K.	SCT 100 IU tiw (1)	−42
	SCT 50 IU tiw (13)	−25
M.C.	SCT 50 IU tiw (1)	−6
	SCT 50 IU tiw (10)	−51
J.D.	SCT 50 IU tiw (4)	−44
	SCT 50 IU tiw (16)	−17
B.H.	SCT 50 IU tiw (1)	+240
E.F.	SCT 50 IU tiw (1)	+33

*PCT, porcine calcitonin; SCT, salmon calcitonin; qd, daily; tiw, three times a week.

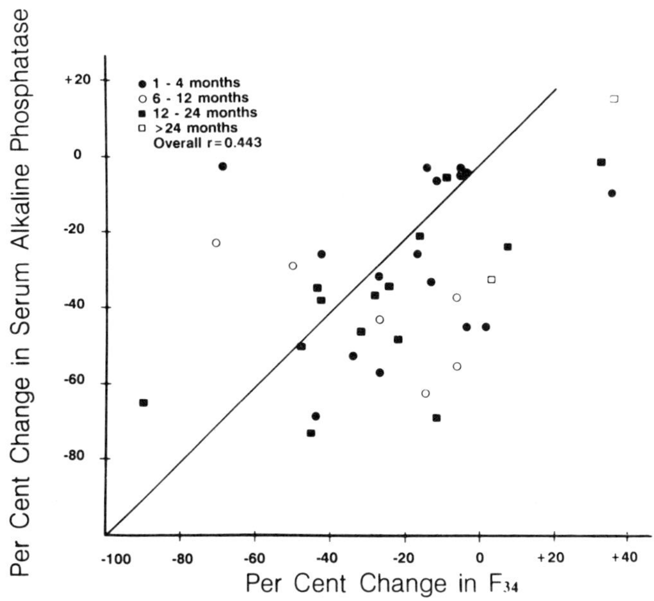

FIGURE 5.4. Correlation of individual percentage changes in serum alkaline phosphatase and skeletal calcium turnover (F_{34}) during calcitonin treatment. R = 0.443. *Reproduced from Wallach et al,[9] with permission.*

the parameters was present in some patients and unexplained dissociation in others. The correlation coefficients for F_{34} and the two biochemical parameters were between 0.4 and 0.5, indicating significant dissociation. There was also a lesser decline in skeletal turnover than in the static biochemical parameters. These dissociations have not as yet been adequately explained and have also been noted when other agents were used in treatment.

Calcium balance during CT treatment becomes positive during the first 4 to 6 weeks. As shown in Table 5.2, in seven of ten studies using SCT, there was an increase in calcium balance exceeding 10% of the dietary intake, which is explained by the effect of CT on inhibition of bone resorption.[8] The positive calcium balance is temporary since a coupled inhibition of bone formation occurs later. Total body calcium measurements indicate that the average pagetic patient has 22% more body calcium than predicted at baseline with a decrease of approximately 4% with long-term treatment.[9] These findings correlate very well with the change toward normality of the histologic pattern of the pagetic bone. Another physiologic effect of CT is to reverse the increased bone blood flow characteristic of this disorder. Normalization of bone blood flow, and of the corresponding increase in cardiac output, usually occurs within 2 weeks of CT treatment.

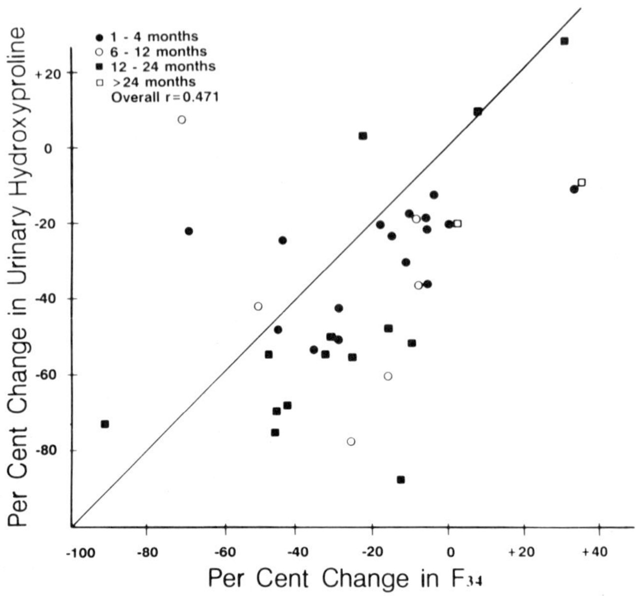

FIGURE 5.5. Correlation of individual percentage changes in urinary total hydroxyproline and skeletal calcium turnover (F_{34}) during calcitonin treatment. $R = 0.471$. *Reproduced from Wallach et al,[9] with permission.*

Normal bone is affected in pagetic patients when CT is given, as shown by Toh et al.,[10] who measured forearm bone mineral density of the uninvolved radius. Calcitonin-treated patients showed no decrease in bone mineral density over a 3-year period, whereas a control group followed without treatment had a measurable decrease in bone mineral density over this same period.

TABLE 5.2 Effect of Calcitonin on Short-Term Calcium Balance in Paget's Disease

Patient	Calcium Intake, mg/day	Change in Calcium Balance, mg/day
P.G.	580	+169
P.T.	572	+190
K.F.	662	+113
M.M.	665	−3
S.D.	572	+217
D.K.	588	+100
B.H.	694	−1
E.F.	717	+327
M.C.	774	+142
D.A.	826	+35

The clinical effects of CT treatment are best discussed in the context of the indications for treatment. Pain is the predominant disabling symptom for which most patients seek treatment. Although pagetic pain can sometimes be relieved effectively by nonsteroidal antiinflammatory agents and other analgesics, when it cannot, CT relieves the pain or causes it to be markedly ameliorated in more than 80% of patients. This is not to gainsay the use of nonsteroidal antiinflammatory agents since these can be used alone in mild cases or together with CT in patients who have an arthritic component to their Paget's disease. Progressive skeletal involvement, that is, complications such as fracture, platybasia, vertebral compression, acetabular protrusion, and progressing deformity, is a strong indication for CT treatment since it is possible to arrest such complications. Unfortunately, supporting research in this area is incomplete because of the difficulty in making serial quantitative measurements. Many of these progressive skeletal complications occur in patients who also have an extensive bone resorption component of the disease, for example, osteoporosis circumscripta, resorptive fronts, lenticular shaped areas of resorption, and fissure fractures. Calcitonin is effective in reducing the excessive bone resorption component.

Neurologic deficits, with the exception of nonprogressive deafness, are always an indication for CT treatment, since it is possible to achieve moderate to near-complete relief of neurologic deficits in many cases.[11,12] Patients being prepared for orthopedic surgery should also be treated with CT since there is ample evidence that bleeding from bone is greatly decreased by prior treatment, making orthopedic procedures simpler.[13] Calcitonin is also of value in prolonged immobilization, not so much to prevent immobilization-related hypercalcemia, which is rare, as to prevent the increased bone resorption and bone loss that occur in pagetic limbs after they fracture and are immobilized. Calcitonin reduces osteoclastic activity in this situation and eliminates the areas of excessive pagetic bone resorption that may have originally led to the fractures. Cardiovascular complications that are secondary to increased cardiac output, which are fortunately rare, are also well treated with CT. In my opinion it is also justifiable to treat extreme elevations of the biochemical parameters in the absence of any of these indications.

Many graphic examples of the therapeutic effects of CT are available. Osteoporosis circumscripta of the skull, resorptive fronts, lenticular-shaped areas of bone rarefaction, fissure fractures, and so on, have all been demonstrated to remodel toward more normal architecture with 1 to 2 years of CT treatment.[7] Even when the Paget's disease is in a sclerotic phase, it is possible to alter bony architecture so that thickened pagetic bone is reduced in diameter, including that of pagetic vertebral bone encasing the spinal canal and causing impaired spinal reserve capacity.[14] It is now possible to measure this very accurately by computerized axial tomography (CAT) scanning and to follow CT treatment of such neurologic complications.[14]

The earliest report of the relief of spinal block with CT treatment was made in 1974. The index patient had complete paraplegia, sphincter loss, and a sensory level at the T-9 level. After 2 years of CT treatment, the patient had lost her paraplegia and sensory level, had regained sphincter control, and was living independently. A repeat myelogram showed that the dye was able to flow through the previous area of block, indicating relief of spinal block by medical therapy.[11]

The logistics of CT treatment of Paget's disease relate to the dose, duration, and other technical aspects of treatment. Several years ago, data were presented to show that 50 IU three times a week was as effective as 100 IU/d (Table 5.3), and for the average patient this is still true. At 6 months of treatment, however, the data suggested that 50 IU three times a week was less effective. In recent years, some patients in whom the therapeutic response was slower than expected with 50 IU three times a week have been encountered, and it is now advisable to increase the dose in selected patients with severe disease in whom a sluggish response to a lower dose occurs.

With regard to administering less than 50 IU of CT three times a week or administering it less often, a study conducted several years ago in which patients were treated with 50 IU once a week showed that the alkaline phosphatase decreased, but not as much as with more intensive treatment.[15] Also, only half the patients had relief of symptoms. For these reasons, it is probably suboptimal to treat less than three times a week.

The side effects of SCT treatment are negligible in terms of serious organ toxicity. Persistent side effects sufficiently severe to force discontinuation of treatment are rare. In my experience approximately 1% of pa-

TABLE 5.3 Effects of Different SCT Doses on Biochemical Parameters

	Mean Percentage Decrease from Baseline*		
	100 IU qd	**100 IU tiw**	**50 IU tiw**
Alkaline phosphatase			
6 months	51 (8)	60 (8)	33 (10)
Urinary hydroxyproline			
4 weeks	19 (4)	22(2)	20 (4)
6 months	54 (8)	56 (8)	33 (10)

*Parentheses indicate number of patients; qd, daily; tiw, three times a week.

tients develop urticaria some time during the first 2 months of treatment, and this indicates that SCT cannot be used. Unfortunately, such a response cannot be predicted in advance by skin testing. Approximately 10% of patients develop one or more gastrointestinal symptoms, 10% have flushing of the face and ears, and 10% have a nonspecific rash either at the site of injections or more generally. In most cases, these side effects are mild to moderate, ameliorate over a 2- to 3-month period of continued treatment, and do not require discontinuation of treatment. A rare patient may not be able to tolerate these side effects.

The optimal duration of CT treatment is an unanswered question. In a group of patients treated for approximately 2 years in whom treatment was then discontinued, the alkaline phosphatase increased gradually over a period of 6 months post treatment and returned nearly to baseline, whereas urinary hydroxyproline excretion took much longer and at the end of 1 year was still 50% lower than baseline. Ten of 13 patients continued to have a clinical remission of Paget's symptoms for a year after treatment was stopped.[16] These data differ from those of O'Donoghue and Hosking,[17] who gave only 6 months of CT treatment. After their treatment was stopped, all the patients were back to baseline levels for both alkaline phosphatase and hydroxyproline excretion within 6 months. These comparisons suggest that the proper duration of CT treatment is nearer to 2 years than 6 months. A reasonable policy at present is to give 18 months of treatment before making a decision as to whether to continue or stop and observe. It is difficult to advise continuous treatment extending over several years, since anecdotal experience with patients treated for 5 to 12 years indicates that the effects of the treatment largely disappear. Therefore, CT is better given in courses than as long-term continuous treatment.

Even when CT is administered in courses, it is not uncommon to find patients in whom the results of treatment after a second, third, or fourth course are not as complete as after the first course. This raises the question of resistance to CT, which is discussed in greater detail in Chapter 7. Figure 5.6 gives an example of secondary resistance in a patient whose baseline alkaline phosphatase level was 1,300 IU. He had a marked clinical and biochemical effect with treatment, with a small biochemical rebound but continued clinical improvement. Calcitonin was discontinued after 8 months. The patient's symptoms returned, and retreatment begun when the alkaline phosphatase reached 1,000 IU did not result in a decline in the alkaline phosphatase or relief of the patient's symptoms.

It is commonly accepted that secondary resistance is related to neutralizing antibody formation in some cases but not others.[7] In a group of 28 patients who received SCT alone, approximately half maintained their nadirs in alkaline phosphatase and urinary hydroxyproline levels and half

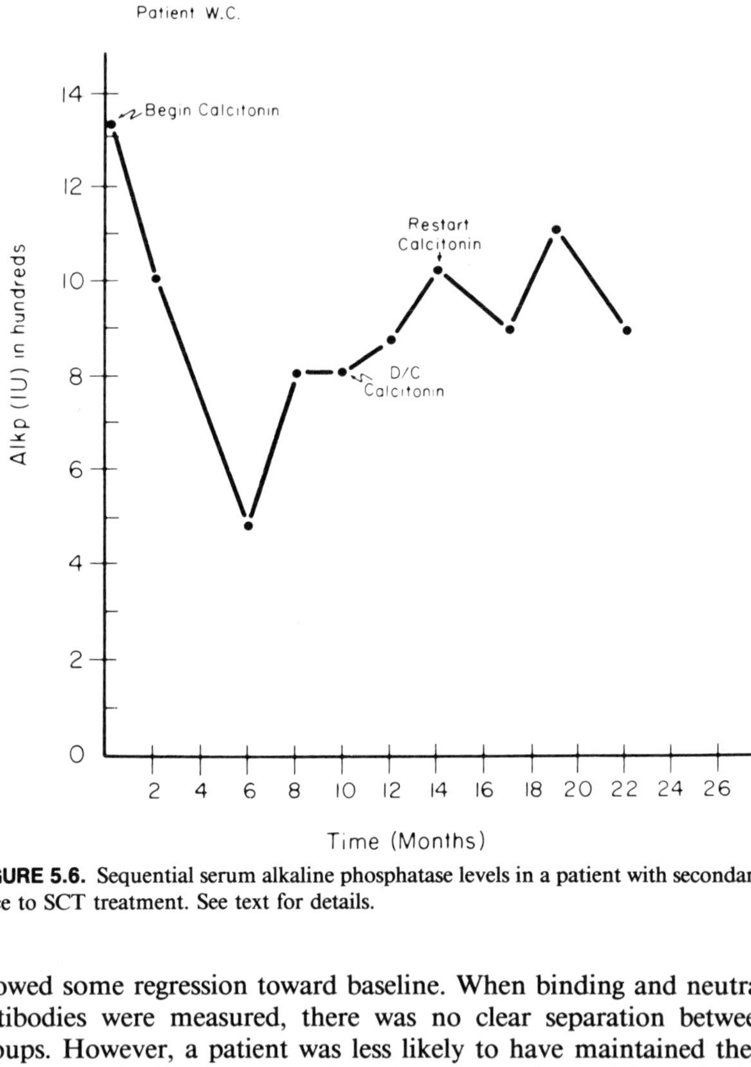

FIGURE 5.6. Sequential serum alkaline phosphatase levels in a patient with secondary resistance to SCT treatment. See text for details.

showed some regression toward baseline. When binding and neutralizing antibodies were measured, there was no clear separation between the groups. However, a patient was less likely to have maintained the nadir when an antibody was present than when it was absent. These binding and neutralizing antibody studies did not use the sophisticated methods that now exist, and a better correlation between resistance and antibody formation will probably be found as more studies are made.

The exact degree to which patients on SCT develop antibodies is still unclear. Resistance is only an occasional problem during the first 2 years of treatment, but as patients are retreated, an increasing number show secondary resistance to CT treatment. Calcitonin is nevertheless the most physiologic form of therapy available at present and is the mainstay of

Paget's disease treatment in the United States. As is discussed in Chapter 11 intranasal CT can be nearly as effective as parenteral CT in Paget's disease when a sufficient dose is administered and is nearing the approval process for general use in the United States.[18,19]

REFERENCES

1. Copp DH: Calcitonin comes of age: A quarter century in perspective, in Pecile A (ed): *Calcitonin: Chemistry, Physiology, Pharmacology and Clinical Aspects.* Amsterdam, Elsevier Science Publishing, 1985; pp 3–9.
2. Hirsch PF, Munson PL: Thyrocalcitonin. *Physiol Rev* 1969;49:548–622.
3. Foster GV, Baghdiantz A, Kumar MA, et al: Thyroid origin of calcitonin. *Nature* 1964;202:1303–1305.
4. Bijvoet OLM, van der Sluys Veer J, Jansen AP: Effects of calcitonin on patients with Paget's disease, thyrotoxicosis, or hypercalcemia. *Lancet* 1986;1:876–881.
5. Caniggia A, Nuti R, Galli M, et al: Effect of a long-term treatment with the aminosuberic analog of eel calcitonin on osteocalcin in Paget's disease. *Panminerva Med* 1987;29:1–5.
6. Chausmer AB, Chavez C, Wain RM, Dakka Y: Calcitonin, zinc and testicular function. *Metabolism* 1989;38:714–717.
7. DeRose J, Singer FR, Avramides A, et al: Response of Paget's disease to porcine and salmon calcitonins. *Am J Med* 1974;56:858–866.
8. Shai F, Baker RK, Wallach S: The clinical and metabolic effects of porcine calcitonin on Paget's disease of bone. *J Clin Invest* 1971;50:1927–1939.
9. Wallach S, Avramides A, Flores A, et al: Skeletal turnover and total body elemental composition during extended calcitonin treatment of Paget's disease. *Metabolism* 1975;24:745–753.
10. Toh SH, Claunch BC, Brown PH: Effect of calcitonin treatment on the natural course of bone demineralization in Paget's disease. *J Clin Endocrinol Metab* 1983;56:405–409.
11. Chen JR, Rhee RSC, Wallach S, et al: Neurologic disturbances in Paget disease of bone: Response to calcitonin. *Neurology* 1979;29:448–457.
12. El Samma M, Linthicum FH Jr, House HP, House JW: Calcitonin as treatment for hearing loss in Paget's disease. *Am J Otol* 1986;7:241–243.
13. Meyers M, Singer FR: Osteotomy for tibia vera in Paget's disease under cover of calcitonin. *J Bone Joint Surg* 1978;60(A):810–814.
14. Weisz GM: Lumbar canal stenosis in Paget's disease: The staging of the clinical syndrome, its diagnosis, and treatment. *Clin Orthop* 1986;206:223–227.
15. Avramides A, Flores A, DeRose J, Wallach S: Treatment of Paget's disease of bone with once a week injections of salmon calcitonin. *Br Med J* 1975;3:632.
16. Avramides A, Flores A, DeRose J, Wallach S: Paget's disease of the bone: Observations after cessation of long-term synthetic salmon calcitonin treatment. *J Clin Endocrinol Metab* 1976;42:459–463.
17. O'Donoghue DJ, Hosking DJ: Biochemical response to combination of disodium etidronate with calcitonin in Paget's disease. *Bone* 1987;8:219–225.
18. Reginster JY, Jeugmans-Huynen AM, Albert A, et al: One year's treatment of Paget's disease of bone by synthetic salmon calcitonin as a nasal spray. *J Bone Mineral Res* 1988;3:249–252.
19. Gagel RF, Logan C, Mallette LE: Treatment of Paget's disease of bone with salmon calcitonin nasal spray. *J Am Geriatr Soc* 1988;36:1011–1014.

CHAPTER 6

Experiences with Human Calcitonin in the Treatment of Paget's Disease of Bone

John G. Haddad

INTRODUCTION

With the discovery of the hormone calcitonin 28 years ago, increasing interest was centered on its composition, secretion, and mechanisms of action.[1-5] Eventually, the porcine, human, and salmon calcitonins were sequenced and synthesized,[2,3,6] and growing enthusiasm for their anti-bone resorption effect led to many clinical investigations of their influences on disorders of mineral and skeletal homeostasis. The hormone's physiologic role is still not clearly understood. However, its interference with some portions of osteolytic mechanisms has been repeatedly observed to lead to beneficial effects on bone turnover and skeletal remodeling. Since this interference is most rapidly and clearly seen in conditions of accelerated bone turnover, many of the hormone's convincing effects have been appreciated in patients with Paget's bone disease.[7-10]

HUMAN CALCITONIN

Very shortly after the identification and sequencing of the porcine-derived peptide, the human calcitonin peptide was isolated and sequenced.[2] As with other calcitonins, human calcitonin (HCT) is a 32-amino-acid peptide with a disulfide bond between cysteine residues at positions 1 and 7 and a proline amide at position 32. All of the peptide appears to be required for its hypocalcemic activity, and biologic activity is altered by opening the disulfide ring or producing modifications or shortening of the peptide.[5]

By 1969, a long-term trial of the therapeutic efficacy of HCT in Paget's bone disease had started at the Hammersmith Hospital in London, and promising results led to additional clinical trials elsewhere, including the United States. Although the results were excellent, marketing decisions delayed the appearance of HCT on the prescription formulary in the United States until much later.

CLINICAL STUDIES

Initially, HCT was available for the treatment of 41 patients with Paget's disease studied by the Hammersmith group.[7] In general, the human peptide caused effects not unlike those seen with the porcine, salmon, and eel calcitonins.[8-16]

Most of the reported studies characterize the extent and severity of the disease by providing biochemical indexes of bone turnover and radiographic and bone scan data. In addition, symptoms of the disease and side effects of the therapy are often cited. In some instances, very careful radiographic follow-up has led to a recognition of an influence of HCT on skeletal morphology.[17-19]

Pain relief during HCT treatment has been reported to occur in 82% of patients (Table 6.1). This is in accord with results reported for salmon calcitonin in several studies. Significant reductions in biochemical parameters of skeletal turnover are also observed during HCT treatment. Reduction of the serum total alkaline phosphatase and the urine total hydroxyproline is well recognized. As indicated in Table 6.2, decreases in these parameters are regularly seen in spite of varied dosage schedules and study durations.

TABLE 6.1 Pain Relief During HCT Treatment of Paget's Disease

Reference	Patients Experiencing Pain Relief, %	Patients Studied, No.
8	80	13
13	95	12
15	90	17
9	80	16
7	40–100*	33

*Categorized by skeletal regions, with best results at tibia, spine, and pelvis.

TABLE 6.2 Responses of Serum Alkaline Phosphatase and Urine Hydroxyproline to HCT Treatment of Paget's Disease

Reference	No. of Patients Studied	Weekly Dosage, mg	Alkaline Phosphatase, % of Baseline	Hydroxyproline, % of Baseline	Duration of Therapy, months
7	33	7.0	60	62	12
8	13	2.5–3.5	67	57	5–20
18	6	4.5	45	41	6
11	7	1.75–3.0	50	—	2–30
9	17	7.0	50	50	6

As emphasized earlier,[20] the serum and urine test results can indicate that a quantitative influence on bone remodeling has been achieved, but other information is required in order to be able to estimate the quality of the skeletal change. For these purposes, careful radiologic examination of affected bones has uniformly indicated a beneficial effect of HCT on focal bone balance. Not all lesions are easily estimated, and lytic areas such as advancing fronts or "blade of grass" lesions in the appendicular skeleton are particularly easy to follow.[17–20] In addition, expansile lytic areas, cortical and endosteal surfaces, and trabecular density have been studied. In some studies, the improvement associated with HCT treatment has been the arrest of the progression of a lytic front and/or the remineralization of lytic foci. When HCT therapy is withheld, the lesions often become lytic again. On reintroduction of HCT treatment the lesions again improve. Overall, the influence of HCT is dramatic in osteolytic Paget's disease, but the effect must be considered a suppression of disease activity. Most observers consider daily doses of HCT of 50 to 100 IU (0.25 to 0.5 mg) to be those most often associated in radiographic findings with improvement[7,18] although lower doses (on a weight basis) of salmon calcitonin have been reported to have similar effects.[20]

OTHER CONSIDERATIONS

Side effects of calcitonin therapy are similar in nature, regardless of the calcitonin used. Flushing sensations, anorexia, nausea, other gastrointestinal (GI) symptoms, increased urinary frequency, and altered taste sensations are sometimes reported. Most clinicians advise a presleep injection schedule in order that their patients who are susceptible to nausea can avoid it. Most of the side effects last for only a few minutes or 1 to 2 hours. Many observers believe that GI effects are most frequent with HCT.

Can the calcitonins prevent the development of deformity? This is not a clear issue, for the natural history of the disorder indicates that deformation is a chronic process. Certainly, the use of calcitonin for 2 to 3 months before surgery on affected areas reduces the vascularity of the lesions. Also, this is not associated with an impairment of fracture healing or the recovery from bone surgery. Some reports of improved neurologic function (deafness, nerve compressions) have appeared, but such responses are clearly not the uniform general experience.

A clear-cut need for HCT has been shown in patients who have developed immunologic resistance after repeated exposure to animal-derived calcitonin therapy.[12,14,16,21,22] In such instances, therapy with HCT results in the responses seen with the animal-derived calcitonins before the development of resistance.

Comparative studies of the calcitonins are few, but comparable effects have been observed.[23]

SUMMARY

The availability of HCT provides an additional suppressive agent for treating Paget's disease of bone. The original isolation and characterization of this peptide occurred at about the same time as other calcitonins were investigated. Similarly, clinical trials with HCT and other calcitonins occurred contemporaneously. The overall results with HCT in Paget's bone disease are similar to those observed during treatment with the porcine, salmon, and eel peptides. Since immunologic resistance to HCT is rarely encountered,[24] it is an important agent in the treatment of this disease.

REFERENCES

1. Rittel W, Brugger M, Kamber B, et al: Thyrocalcitonins: III. Synthesis des alpha-thyrocalcitonins. *Helv Chim Acta* 1968;51:924–928.
2. Neher R, Riniker B, Rittel W, Zuber H: Menschliches Calcitonin: III. Struktur von Calcitonin M and D. *Helv Chim Acta* 1968;51:1900–1905.
3. Niall HD, Keutmann HT, Copp DH, Potts JT Jr: Amino acid sequence of salmon ultimo-branchial calcitonin. *Proc Natl Acad Sci USA* 1969;64:771–775.
4. Martin TJ: Actions of calcitonin and mithramycin. *Arthritis Rheum* 1980; 23:1131–1138.
5. MacIntyre I, Evans IMA, Hobitz HHG, et al: Chemistry, physiology and therapeutic applications of calcitonin. *Arthritis Rheum* 1980;23:1139–1147.

6. Kahnt FW, Riniker B, MacIntyre I, Weher R: Thyrocalcitonin: 1. Isolierung und charakterisierung wirksamer peptide aus schwineschilddrusen. *Helv Chim Acta* 1968; 51:214–219.
7. Evans IMA: Human calcitonin in the treatment of Paget's disease: Long-term trials, in MacIntyre I (ed): *Human Calcitonin and Paget's Disease.* Bern, Stuttgart, Vienna, Hans Huber Publishers, 1977, pp 111–123.
8. Burckhardt P, Ducommun J, Hessler C: Treatment of Paget's disease with human calcitonin, in MacIntyre (ed): *Human Calcitonin and Paget's Disease.* Bern, Stuttgart, Vienna, Hans Huber Publishers, 1977, pp 155–166.
9. Ziegler R, Holz G, Rave F, et al: Therapeutic studies with human calcitonin, in MacIntyre (ed): *Human Calcitonin and Paget's Disease.* Bern, Stuttgart, Vienna, Hans Huber Publishers, 1977, pp 167–178.
10. Nagant de Deuxchaisnes C: Calcitonin in the treatment of Paget's disease. *Triangle* 1983;22:103–128.
11. Singer FR, Rude RK, Mills BG: Studies of the treatment and etiology of Paget's disease of bone, in MacIntyre I (ed): *Human Calcitonin and Paget's Disease.* Bern, Stuttgart, Vienna, Hans Huber Publishers, 1977, pp 93–110.
12. Haddad JG: Effective human calcitonin therapy following immunological resistance to salmon calcitonin therapy in Paget's bone disease, in MacIntyre (ed): *Human Calcitonin and Paget's Disease.* Bern, Stuttgart, Vienna, Hans Huber Publishers, 1977, pp 195–206.
13. Lang R, Milkman M, Jensen PS, Vignery AMC: Chronic treatment of Paget's disease of bone with synthetic human calcitonin. *Yale J Biol* 1981;54:355–365.
14. Rojanasathit S, Rosenberg E, Haddad JG: Paget's bone disease: Response to human calcitonin in patients resistant to salmon calcitonin. *Lancet* 1974;2:1412–1415.
15. Nuti R, Vattimo A: Synthetisches human-calcitonin hei osteodistrophia deformans (Paget) und osteoporose. *Dtsch Med Wochenschr* 1981;106:149–152.
16. Altman RD, Collins-Yudiskas B: Synthetic human calcitonin in refractory Paget's disease of bone. *Arch Intern Med* 1987;147:1305–1308.
17. Doyle RH, Pennock J, Greenberg P, et al: Radiological evidence of a dose-related response to long-term treatment of Paget's disease with human calcitonin. *Br J Radiol* 1974;47:1–8.
18. Murphy WA, Whyte MP, Haddad JG: Paget's bone disease: Radiological documentation of healing with human calcitonin therapy. *Radiology* 1980;136:1–4.
19. Woodhouse NJY, MacIntyre L, Joplin GF, Doyle FH: Radiological regression in Paget's disease treated by human calcitonin. *Lancet* 1972;2:992–994.
20. Nagant de Deuxchaisnes C, Maldague B, Malghem J, et al: The action of the main therapeutic regimes on Paget's disease of bone, with a note on the effect of vitamin D deficiency. *Arthritis Rheum* 1980;23:1215–1234.
21. Haddad JG, Caldwell JG: Calcitonin resistance: Clinical and immunological studies in subjects with Paget's disease of bone treated with porcine and salmon calcitonin. *J Clin Invest* 1972;51:3133–3341.
22. Singer FR, Fredericks RS, Minkin C: Salmon calcitonin therapy for Paget's disease of bone: The problem of acquired clinical resistance. *Arthritis Rheum* 1980;23:1148–1154.
23. Nagant de Deuxchaisnes C: Calcitonin in the treatment of Paget's disease. *Triangle* 1983;22:103–128.
24. Dietrich FM, Fischer JA, Bijvoet OLM: Formation of antibodies to synthetic human calcitonin during treatment of Paget's disease. *Acta Endocrinol* 1979;92:468–476.

CHAPTER 7

Resistance to Calcitonin

Frederick R. Singer and Karla Ginger

For more than 20 years, calcitonin has been used in the treatment of Paget's disease. With long-term administration of the hormone, two main patterns of biochemical response have been observed.[1] In most patients, serum alkaline phosphatase activity and urinary hydroxyproline excretion fall over a period of months and reach a plateau at an average reduction of about 50% below pretreatment levels. Biochemical indexes may remain suppressed to this degree for more than 10 years as treatment continues (Figure 7.1). In a smaller group of patients after an initial period of typical biochemical suppression, the indices gradually rise, and with continuing treatment they reach pretreatment or even higher levels (Figure 7.2). This latter pattern of acquired clinical resistance appears to occur most commonly when salmon or porcine calcitonin is administered, but a similar clinical course has been observed in a few patients on human calcitonin therapy. Primary clinical resistance may occur but appears to be unusual.

ACQUIRED CLINICAL RESISTANCE: ANTIBODY MEDIATED

In early studies of patients treated with salmon or porcine calcitonin it was generally found that about 50% or more developed specific antibodies to these hormones in serum or plasma.[2-9] This was not unexpected in view of the considerable difference in amino acid sequences of the salmon or porcine hormone when compared to that of human calcitonin.[10]

Patients who developed particularly high titers of calcitonin antibodies

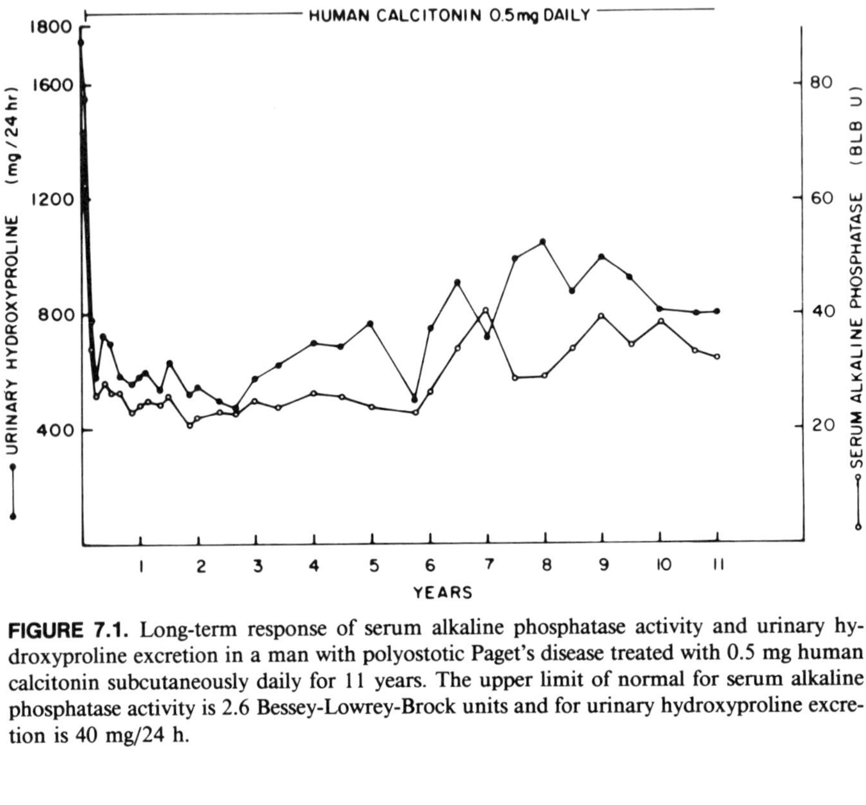

FIGURE 7.1. Long-term response of serum alkaline phosphatase activity and urinary hydroxyproline excretion in a man with polyostotic Paget's disease treated with 0.5 mg human calcitonin subcutaneously daily for 11 years. The upper limit of normal for serum alkaline phosphatase activity is 2.6 Bessey-Lowrey-Brock units and for urinary hydroxyproline excretion is 40 mg/24 h.

in the circulation were likely to become resistant to the hormone with chronic treatment. The course of the first patient reported to exhibit this phenomenon is illustrated in Figure 7.2.[2] The initial fall in urinary hydroxyproline excretion and serum alkaline phosphatase activity was not sustained during the 11.5 months of daily therapy with 100 MRC units of salmon calcitonin. Stored plasma obtained during the course of treatment was later evaluated and found to bind increasing amounts of radiolabeled salmon calcitonin as treatment continued. By using radioimmunoelectrophoresis immunoglobulin G was identified as the source of the plasma binding. A variety of other studies in this patient proved highly instructive and helped to define the syndrome of antibody-mediated clinical resistance to calcitonin. In Figure 7.3, the acute plasma calcium responses to calcitonin during the course of treatment are illustrated. The patient initially had an acute decrease in plasma calcium of 1 mg/dL after 20 MRC units of salmon calcitonin was administered intravenously (Figure 7.3A). After 7 months of treatment, when the antibody titer was quite high, 100 MRC units administered intravenously failed to alter the plasma calcium con-

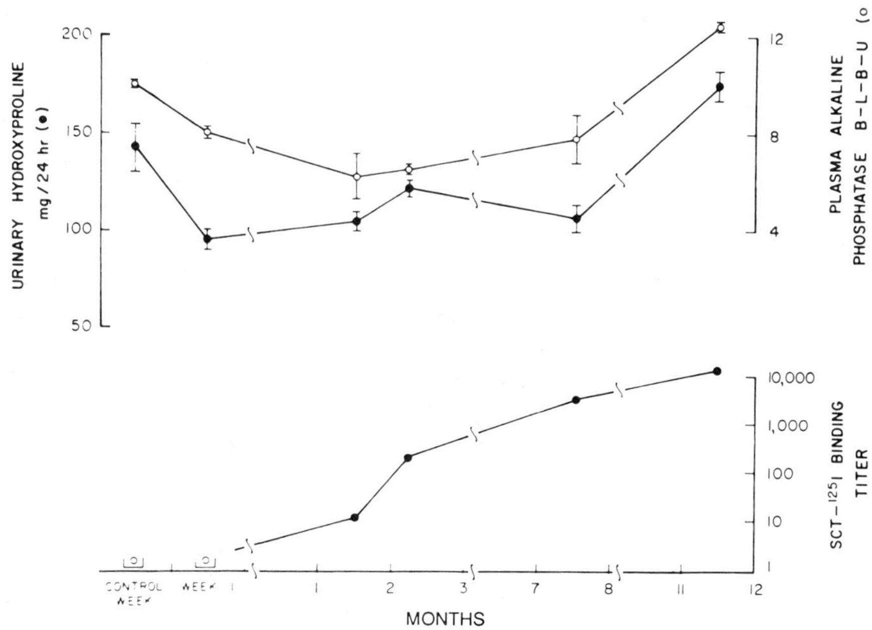

FIGURE 7.2. Plasma alkaline phosphatase activity, urinary hydroxyproline excretion, and salmon calcitonin-^{125}I binding titer in serum before and during treatment of a 51-year-old man with Paget's disease. He received 100 MRC units of salmon calcitonin subcutaneously daily for 11.5 months. The hydroxyproline data points represent the mean ± SEM of at least five 24-hour urine collections during a 1-week period. The alkaline phosphatase data points represent the mean ± SEM of at least three blood samples taken during the week. The binding titer is plotted on a logarithmic scale. SEM, standard error of the mean. *(Reproduced from Singer et al,[2] p. 2333, with permission.)*

centration (Figure 7.3B). At the twelfth month of therapy 1,000 MRC units given intravenously was shown to produce hypocalcemia (Figure 7.3C) but at 15 months the same dose given subcutaneously failed to reproduce the effect of the intravenous dose (Figure 7.3D). These plasma calcium profiles were interpreted to reflect the effect of high titers of specific anti–salmon calcitonin antibodies in the circulation. Before treatment, a small dose of hormone inhibited bone resorption and produced hypocalcemia. When high antibody titers were present, the hormone binding capacity of the extracellular fluid was sufficient to block the biologic activity of injected calcitonin. Only by administering a rapid intravenous injection of 1,000 MRC units of hormone could the hormone-binding capacity be overcome, allowing free hormone to reach the calcitonin receptors on osteoclasts and thus initiate the inhibition of bone resorption. This neutralization of the biologic effect of calcitonin was again demonstrable when the patient's plasma was incubated with salmon calcitonin and injected into rats.[2]

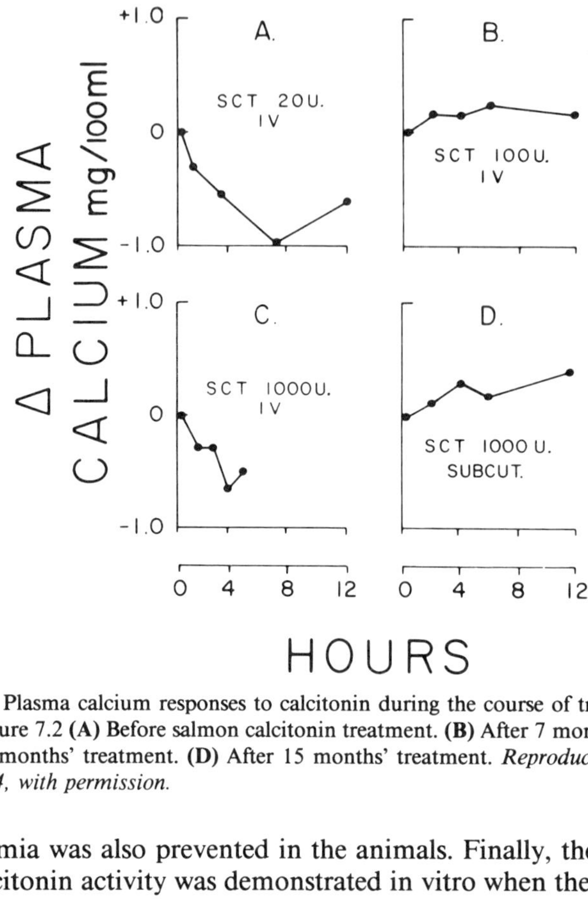

FIGURE 7.3. Plasma calcium responses to calcitonin during the course of treatment of the patient in Figure 7.2 **(A)** Before salmon calcitonin treatment. **(B)** After 7 months' treatment. **(C)** After 12 months' treatment. **(D)** After 15 months' treatment. *Reproduced from Singer et al,[2] p. 2334, with permission.*

Hypocalcemia was also prevented in the animals. Finally, the neutralization of calcitonin activity was demonstrated in vitro when the plasma was preincubated with salmon calcitonin before addition to mouse bone organ cultures. The plasma prevented the inhibitory effect of calcitonin on the release of ^{45}Ca from the cultured bones.[8] Neutralizing antibodies to salmon calcitonin associated with calcitonin resistance have also been found in patients treated with intranasal hormone.[11,12] Previous treatment with parenteral salmon calcitonin is a common feature in patients treated with intranasal salmon calcitonin who become resistant to intranasal therapy and exhibit an increase in antibody titers.[11-15] The earlier exposure of the immune system to salmon calcitonin appears to prime the antibody-producing cells for a more vigorous response on reexposure to the hormone.

The antibodies generated in patients treated with parenteral salmon calcitonin have not shown a significant affinity for human calcitonin. This has allowed successful control of Paget's disease with human calcitonin in patients who become resistant to parenteral salmon calcitonin as a result of antibody formation.[2,16,17] (Figures 7.4 and 7.5). Most recently, the effective use of intranasal human calcitonin has been reported in patients who became resistant to treatment with intranasal salmon calcitonin.[18] Similar success with human calcitonin therapy also has been reported in patients resistant to porcine calcitonin who have anti-porcine calcitonin antibodies in the circulation.[19] In this study, there was no significant binding of human calcitonin by antibodies to porcine calcitonin, thus accounting for the excellent result achieved with human calcitonin therapy.

In the largest series of patients reported on parenteral salmon calcitonin therapy, 22 of 85 patients (26%) became resistant to continuing treatment after an initial response.[17] In 19 of these patients, the antibody titer was 1 : 1,500 or greater. The remaining three patients had undetectable antibodies (< 1 : 5 titer); they are discussed later. Overall, 56 of 85 patients (66%) had detectable antibodies in the circulation during treatment, but all the patients with detectable antibody titers less than 1 : 1,500 remained response to therapy. Much lower antibody titers have been associated with resistance in some patients treated with intranasal salmon calcitonin.[12,13,15] This may be due to a lower peak level of calcitonin in the circulation produced by intranasal therapy. Therefore, lower antibody titers could inhibit the responsiveness of these patients.

In our experience of patients treated for 6 months or longer, antibody-

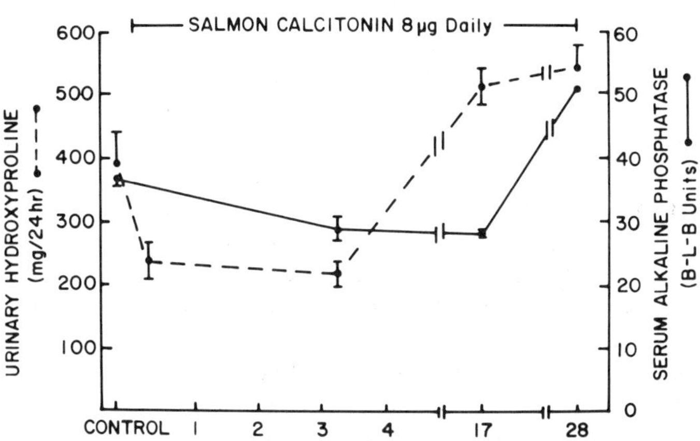

FIGURE 7.4. Response of a 62-year-old woman treated for 28 months with salmon calcitonin. After an initial decrease in the biochemical indexes, the patient became resistant to continuing treatment. Antibodies to salmon calcitonin were present in her serum at a titer of 1:8,000 at 28 months. *Reproduced from Singer et al,[26] with permission.*

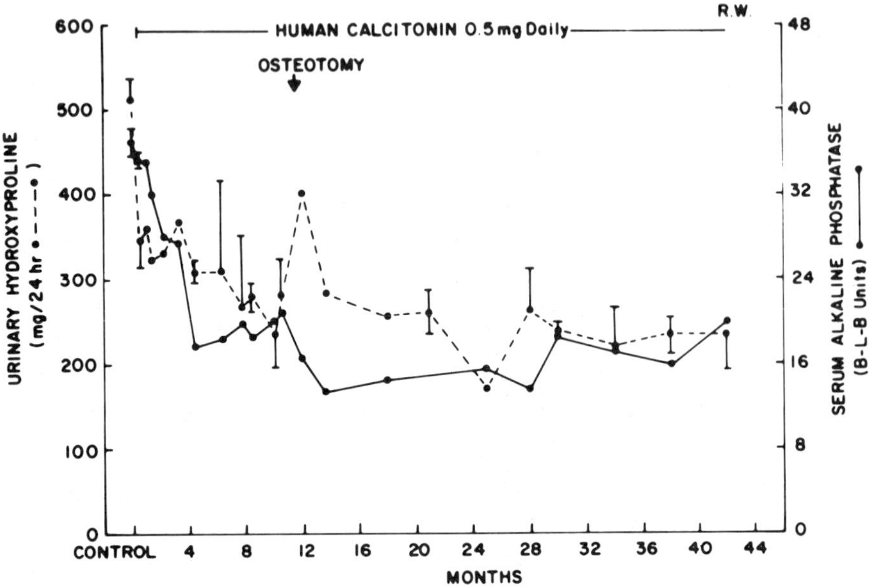

FIGURE 7.5. Results of human calcitonin treatment of the patient with resistance to salmon calcitonin illustrated in Figure 7.4. Note the continuing response to treatment after 44 months.

mediated clinical resistance is not unusual. However, some investigators have expressed the opinion that this event is rare[7–9,20] or may not even occur.[21] It is not entirely clear why there is a difference of opinion in respect to the occurrence of antibody-mediated calcitonin resistance. One major factor appears to be the relatively short-term treatment courses reported in studies in which antibodies were interpreted as not playing a significant role in the clinical course. For example, Reginster and colleagues[21] treated patients for only 3 months before concluding that antibodies were of no significance. Since the pharmacologic effects of calcitonin may persist for many months after cessation of calcitonin therapy in responsive patients,[22] it is inappropriate to draw conclusions as to the role of calcitonin antibodies in patients treated for relatively short periods.

Although we have invariably found that high titers of antibodies to salmon calcitonin are associated with clinical resistance in patients treated for 6 months or more, there are a few examples in the literature where this is not the case. Martin describes two patients treated with parenteral salmon calcitonin with continued biochemical responsiveness over several years despite very high titers of antibodies.[20] A reasonable explanation for this phenomenon is that, in some cases, the antibodies do not bind the hormone at a site on the molecule that prevents interaction of calcitonin with its receptor on the osteoclast plasma membrane. Recently, new in vitro methods for assessing the neutralization properties of calcitonin antibodies have been developed,[11,12] but more studies need to be made before the question of the relevance of nonneutralizing antibodies can be answered.

Definitive criteria for defining the presence of antibody-mediated calcitonin resistance are the following:

1. Demonstration of an early phase of biochemical suppression followed by return to pretreatment biochemical levels despite continuing treatment
2. Demonstration of specific antibodies to calcitonin in the circulation
3. Successful biochemical suppression achieved by treatment with human calcitonin

The last criterion is mandatory in respect to validating the clinical significance of the antibodies. We have administered human calcitonin to 14 patients with antibody titers greater than 1 : 1,000 and acquired clinical resistance to salmon calcitonin. In each patient, good biochemical response was noted. There are at least 23 additional cases in the literature with high antibody titers in whom human calcitonin has been used after development of resistance to salmon (12 cases) or porcine calcitonin (11 cases).[12,15,16,18,19] In 22/23 patients, human calcitonin was effective, although in 1 patient, a second course of therapy was not effective.[19] Thus, in 35/37 patients judged to have antibody-mediated calcitonin resistance, human calcitonin has been an effective therapeutic agent. Antibodies to human calcitonin (in a low titer) have been reported in only one patient treated with this species of calcitonin.[23] Since as yet antibodies to salmon or porcine calcitonin have not bound human calcitonin, it would be expected that human calcitonin should be initially effective in any patient with antibody-mediated resistance to salmon or porcine calcitonin.

ACQUIRED CLINICAL RESISTANCE: ABSENT ANTIBODIES

Although most of the attention has been focused on the role of antibodies in the pathogenesis of acquired clinical resistance to calcitonin, a few patients who had no detectable antibodies in the circulation have been described. We have previously reported three patients treated with salmon calcitonin who became unresponsive despite continuous treatment.[17,24] They had no detectable antibodies and differed from most of our patients with antibody-mediated resistance in that they continued to have a significant acute hypocalcemic response after salmon calcitonin injections. Martin has also reported one antibody-negative patient who had a decrease in urinary hydroxyproline excretion greater than 50% after 7 months of treatment with salmon calcitonin and then had a return of hydroxyproline to pretreatment levels by 12 months.[20] More recently, we have followed a fourth patient treated with salmon calcitonin who had excellent control of her serum alkaline phosphatase activity for 10 years but gradually lost responsiveness over the next 3 years (Figure 7.6). She had barely detectable antibodies in multiple serum specimens and was unresponsive to a 9-month course of subcutaneous human calcitonin 0.5 mg daily. Six months after receiving three intravenous infusions of 30 mg pamidronate on consecutive days, her serum alkaline phosphatase activity decreased by 83%.

Resistance to human calcitonin has also been observed during long-term treatment.[25] This is an unusual event and has not been associated with antibodies to calcitonin. We have observed one excellent example of this clinical course in a man treated for 5 years with 0.5 mg human calcitonin daily (Figure 7.7). After decreases of 60% and 79% of urinary hydroxyproline excretion and serum alkaline phosphatase activity, respectively, these biochemical indexes rose to pretreatment levels or above

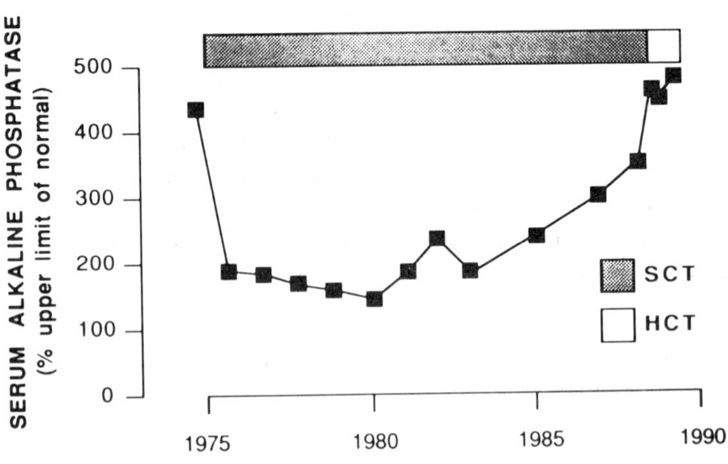

FIGURE 7.6. Serum alkaline phosphatase activity expressed as a percentage of the upper limit of normal in a woman treated with subcutaneous salmon calcitonin then human calcitonin over a 13-year period (age 34–47). During the first 1½ years she received 50 IU salmon calcitonin twice weekly, during the next year 100 IU daily, and then 100 IU twice daily until 1989. She received 0.5 mg human calcitonin for 9 months.

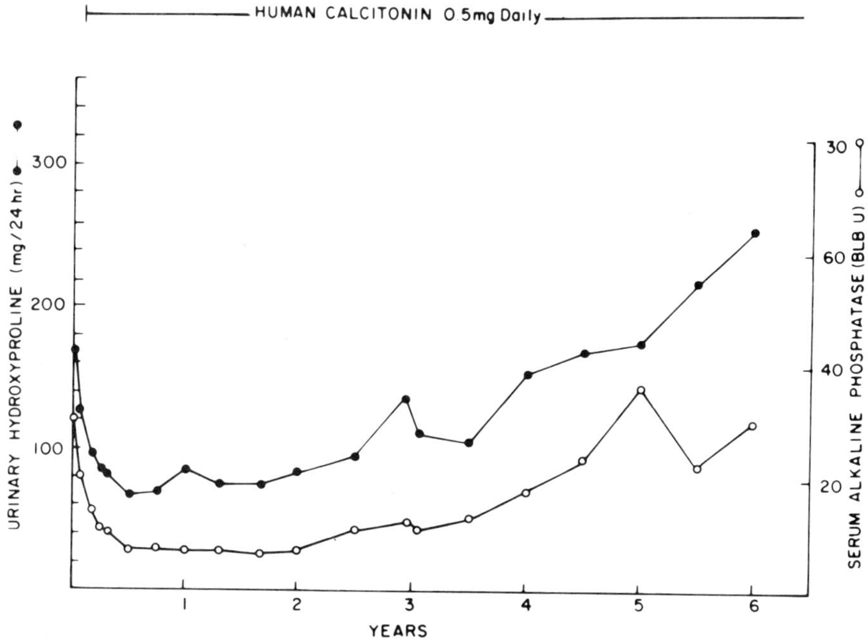

FIGURE 7.7. Long-term response of serum alkaline phosphatase activity and urinary hydroxyproline excretion in a man with polyostatic Paget's disease treated with 0.5 mg human calcitonin subcutaneously daily for 6 years. An example of acquired clinical resistance to human calcitonin.

despite continuing therapy. Subsequently, he has been treated with residronate and has responded well.

The explanation for calcitonin resistance in the absence of antibodies is not known. There is no evidence that secondary hyperparathyroidism can account for this. It has not been possible, for technical reasons, to study receptor down regulation in these patients. Since most hypercalcemic patients treated with calcitonin quickly become unresponsive, receptor down regulation would be a plausible explanation. However, the unusual occurrence of clinical resistance in Paget's disease as well as the long-time course of development make this particular explanation less appealing. Another interesting proposal (S. M. Krane, personal communication) is that with chronic exposure to calcitonin, there is a diminution in the number of calcitonin-sensitive osteoclasts. Over a period of months or years, clones of calcitonin-insensitive osteoclasts may come to dominate the pagetic lesions. Absent or low concentrations of calcitonin receptors might account for the lack of response to calcitonin. As has been demonstrated, agents other than calcitonin would be effective in this setting. Proof of this hypothesis will require better methods of studying pagetic osteoclasts and definitive characterization of the calcitonin receptor.

One other mechanism may be responsible for calcitonin resistance in the absence of antibodies in patients treated with intranasal calcitonin.[14] It is possible that chronic irritation of the nasal mucosa could result in relative mucosal impermeability. This could be tested by measuring hormone concentrations in serum at the start of the treatment course and at the time a resistant state becomes apparent.

SUMMARY

Loss of effectiveness of salmon and porcine calcitonin in the long-term treatment of patients with Paget's disease is a relatively common event (up to 26%). In most patients this is associated with high titers of antibodies to calcitonin in the circulation. These patients almost always respond to treatment with human calcitonin. However, in a small number of cases, the resistant state develops in patients treated with salmon or human calcitonin who have no detectable antibodies. The explanation for this remains to be established.

REFERENCES

1. Singer FR, Keutman HT, Neer RM, et al: Pharmacological effects of salmon calcitonin in man, in Talmage RV, Munson PL (eds): *Calcium, Parathyroid Hormone and the Calcitonins.* Amsterdam, Excerpta Medica Foundation, 1972, pp 89–96.
2. Singer FR, Aldred JP, Neer RM, et al: An evaluation of antibodies and clinical resistance to salmon calcitonin. *J Clin Invest* 1972;51:2331–2338.
3. Haddad JG Jr, Caldwell JG: Calcitonin resistance: Clinical and immunologic studies in subjects with Paget's disease of bone treated with porcine and salmon calcitonins. *J Clin Invest* 1972;51:3133–3141.
4. Dube WJ, Goldsmith RS, Arnaud SB, et al: Development of antibodies to porcine calcitonin during treatment of Paget's disease of bone. *Mayo Clin Proc* 1973;48:43–46.
5. DeRose J, Singer FR, Avramides A, et al: Response of Paget's disease to porcine and salmon calcitonins. *Am J Med* 1974;56:858–866.
6. Plehwe WE, Hudson J, Clifton-Bligh P, et al: Porcine calcitonin in the treatment of Paget's disease of bone. *Med J Aust* 1977;1:577–581.
7. Woodhouse NJY, Mohamedally SM, Saed-Nejad F, et al: Development and significance of antibodies to salmon calcitonin in patients with Paget's disease in long-term treatment. *Br Med J* 1977;9:927–929.
8. Martin TJ, Jerums G, Melick RA, et al: Clinical, biochemical and histological observations on the effect of porcine calcitonin in Paget's disease of bone. *Aust NZ J Med* 1977;7:36–43.
9. Hosking DJ, Denton LB, Cadge B, et al: Functional significance of antibody formation after long-term salmon calcitonin therapy. *Clin Endocrinol* 1979;10:243–252.

10. Azria M: The calcitonins. In *Physiology and Pharmacology.* Basel, Karger, 1989.
11. Levy F, Muff R, Dotti-Sigrist S, et al: Formation of neutralizing antibodies during intranasal synthetic salmon calcitonin treatment of Paget's disease. *J Clin Endocrinol Metab* 1988;67:541–545.
12. Grauer A, Friedhelm R, Schneider H, et al: In vitro detection of neutralizing antibodies after treatment of Paget's disease of bone with nasal salmon calcitonin. *J Bone Mineral Res* 1990;5:387–391.
13. D'Agostino HR, Barnett CA, Zielinski XJ, et al: Intranasal salmon calcitonin treatment of Paget's disease of bone. *Clin Orthop* 230:223–228.
14. Singer FR, Villanueva R, Ginger K: Acquired resistance to salmon and human calcitonin during treatment of Paget's disease of bone. *Calcif Tissue Int* 1989;44(suppl):S87.
15. Nagant de Deuxchaisnes C, Devogelaer JP: Alternative modes of administration of salmon calcitonin as assessed in Paget's disease of bone. In Singer FR, Wallach S (eds): *Paget's Disease of Bone: Clinical Assessment, Present and Future Therapy.* New York, Elsevier Science Publishing Co, 1991, pp 135–165.
16. Rojanasathit S, Rosenberg E, Haddad JG Jr: Paget's bone disease: Response to human calcitonin in patients resistant to salmon calcitonin. *Lancet* 1974;2:1412–1415.
17. Singer FR, Fredericks RS, Minkin C: Salmon calcitonin therapy for Paget's disease of bone: The problem of acquired clinical resistance. *Arthritis Rheum* 1980;23:1148–1154.
18. Muff R, Dambacher MA, Perrenoud A, et al: Efficacy of intranasal human calcitonin in patients with Paget's disease refractory to salmon calcitonin. *Am J Med* 1990; 89:181–184.
19. Lo Cascio V, Adami S, Galvanini G, et al: Response of Paget's disease to human calcitonin in patients resistant to porcine calcitonin. *J Endocrinol Invest* 1984;7:85–88.
20. Martin TJ: Treatment of Paget's disease with calcitonins. *Aust NZ J Med* 1979;9:36–43.
21. Reginster JY, Gennari C, Mautalen C, et al: Influence of specific anti–salmon calcitonin antibodies on biological effectiveness of nasal salmon calcitonin in Paget's disease of bone. *Scand J Rheumatol* 1990;19:83–86.
22. Avramides A, Flores A, DeRose J, et al: Paget's disease of the bone: Observations after cessation of long-term synthetic salmon calcitonin treatment. *J Clin Endocrinol Metab* 1976;42:459–463.
23. Dietrich FM, Fischer JA, Bijvoet OLM: Formation of antibodies to synthetic human calcitonin during treatment of Paget's disease. *Acta Endocrinol* 1979;92:468–476.
24. Singer FR, Ahrne-Collier I: Salmon calcitonin therapy: Antibodies and clinical resistance in patients with Paget's disease of bone. In MacIntyre I, Szelke M (eds): *Molecular Endocrinology.* Amsterdam, Elsevier/North Holland Biomedical Press, 1977, pp 207–212.
25. MacIntyre I, Evans IMA, Hobitz HG, et al: Chemistry, physiologic and therapeutic applications of calcitonin. *Arthritis Rheum* 1980;23:1139–1147.
26. Singer FR, Rude RK, Mills BG: Studies in the treatment and etiology of Paget's disease of bone, in MacIntyre I (ed): *International Symposium on Human Calcitonin and Paget's Disease.* Bern, Stuttgart, Vienna, Hans Huber Publishers, 1977, p. 93.

CHAPTER 8

Treatment of Paget's Disease with Etidronate Disodium

Pierre J. Meunier and Alain Ravault

Eighty-eight patients with Paget's disease were treated with etidronate disodium at an oral dose of 5 mg/kg/d and followed up for an average of 5.2 years. Each course of treatment lasted 6 months and was repeated once or several times. Of the symptomatic patients 75% showed improvement at the end of the follow-up period, whereas 85% of the asymptomatic patients developed no complications that might have been expected if preventive treatment had not been undertaken. Overall, there was clinical deterioration in 28% of the patients during the study. Despite the generally beneficial results, cranial symptoms were not always decreased, and hypoacusis appeared or worsened in some patients. Twenty-three fractures occurred, including eight in pagetic bone, but fracture risk was not increased by etidronate disodium. Extraskeletal side effects were rare. However, there was a delayed exacerbation of bone pain in approximately 12% of patients. This side effect resolved when etidronate disodium was stopped except in one case in which a fracture ensued. Of the patient population 25% were resistant to etidronate disodium; resistance generally appeared between the second and third courses of etidronate disodium treatment. In summary, when etidronate disodium is prescribed over a prolonged period at a dose of 5 mg/kg/d in 6-month courses, the drug improves or stabilizes the condition of three quarters of the patients with Paget's disease, both clinically and biochemically.

INTRODUCTION

Treatment for Paget's disease of bone generally uses the antiosteoclastic properties of calcitonin and the bisphosphonates. The first bisphosphonate to be used was etidronate disodium or ethane-hydroxy-1,1-diphosphonate (EHDP [Didronel]). The effectiveness of this drug on the clinical and biochemical symptoms of Paget's disease has been demonstrated by many studies,[1-16] most of which have addressed the short-term and intermediate-term effects of etidronate disodium treatment. Skeletal side effects, secondary to an induced mineralization defect, are observed when etidronate disodium is used at high doses (>10 mg/kg/d) or when it is administered continually.[4,11] Therefore, a therapeutic scheme has been widely adopted in which the course of treatment is 6 months at a dose of 5 mg/kg/d (approximately 400 mg/d) in an attempt to prevent this side effect. The antiosteoclastic activity of etidronate disodium does not cure the disease but results in prolonged remissions. Remissions are often followed by relapses that necessitate further treatment. The effect of reintroducing the drug is variable, since some patients develop resistance. The aim of this study is to analyze the results of long-term follow-up in 88 pagetic patients treated with etidronate disodium in courses of 5 mg/kg/d, each course lasting 6 months. The mean follow-up time was 5.2 years.

MATERIALS AND METHODS

Patients

This study was carried out in patients recruited between 1972 and 1983 by the Department of Rheumatology and Metabolic Bone Diseases at the Edouard Herriot Hospital in Lyon, France. The patients had never previously been treated with bisphosphonates, but nine patients had previously been given calcitonin. All previous treatment was discontinued at least 2 months before etidronate disodium was started. Follow-up was for a period of 3 to 10 years. All patients had biochemical studies, a bone scan, and radiographs of pagetic sites at the beginning of the study. These examinations were repeated during the follow-up period and at the end of the study. The serum alkaline phosphatase (AP) and 24-hour urine hydroxyproline (OHPU) findings were sometimes normal when the disease involved a small amount of skeleton. All patients had normal renal function (serum creatinine less than 130 μmol/L) and were free of hepatodigestive disorders and other bone diseases. None was receiving cortisone, fluoride, or estrogens.

Therapy and Follow-Up

Etidronate disodium was prescribed orally at 5 mg/kg/d for 6 months. Treatment was repeated once or several times when clinical and/or biochemical relapse occurred, with intervals between courses of therapy of approximately 6 months. Patients without symptoms but with pagetic involvement in the skull; cervical, thoracic, or lumbar spine; sacrum; hip joint; or long bones were treated to prevent possible complications. Clinical and biochemical evaluations were made at the beginning and end of each course of treatment.

Patients with symptoms were assigned to the following categories on the basis of their overall course from the beginning to the end of the study: (1) improved, (2) unchanged, or (3) worse. When possible, the cause of their pain was categorized as bone, articular, or mixed (bone and articular). The progress of the disease was evaluated independently of whether symptoms were present or not and was judged as (a) favorable, when complications (deafness, arthropathy, deformity, and so on) did not appear or if present, lessened, or remained unchanged or (b) unfavorable, when complications appeared or worsened, or there were other indications that the disease had progressed.

Resistance to a course of treatment was defined as absence of any clinical effect on bone pain, as well as absence of a significant biochemical effect, with both serum alkaline phosphatase and OHPU levels at the end of a course still at 70% of their values before treatment. Resistance was considered mild when both serum alkaline phosphatase and OHPU levels at the beginning and end of treatment were less than 1.5 times the upper limit of normal (ULN). Long-term resistance was defined as a lack of both clinical and biochemical effects from the beginning to the end of the study.

On the basis of the assessments of symptoms, disease progress, and resistance discussed, patients were classified into three groups as follows: (1) sensitive: good response throughout all courses of treatment; (2) resistant: long-term resistance to all courses of treatment; (3) intermediate response: resistance to only a single course of treatment or long-term resistance of mild degree.

The extent of disease (IE) was calculated from radiographic data and was expressed as a percentage of the total skeleton.[17]

Phosphatemia was measured by the method of Misson (normal = 34 ± 4.8 mg/L) and 24-hour OHPU by the method of Prockop (normal = 30 ± 15 mg/24 h). Several methods were used to measure serum alkaline phosphatase levels, and for each method, the ratio of the value obtained to the upper limit of normal was determined (x/ULN). Variations in AP and OHPU values were expressed as percentages of initial values.

The chi-square test was used for qualitative variables, the test of least squares for comparisons of two means, the Student *t* test for quantitative variables in paired series, and the analysis of variance for comparisons of two or more means. The results were expressed as means ± standard deviation.

RESULTS

The characteristics of the treated patients are shown in Table 8.1. Men had a greater extent of disease (IE) and higher mean OHPU at baseline than women. The 20 asymptomatic patients differed significantly from those with symptoms (Table 8.2) in their IE and baseline alkaline phosphatase and OHPU values. Seventeen of 20 asymptomatic patients remained so and had a favorable course of etidronate disodium treatment used as a preventive drug against the risk of osteoarthritis of the hip, spinal cord

TABLE 8.1 Characteristics of Population Studied

Number	88
Age, years	63.6 ± 11.4 (24–83)*
Sex M/F	43/45
Extent of disease (IE), %	
Men	14.1 ± 12.5 (2–48)
Women	9.1 ± 8.2† (1–4)
Initial mean AP value, *x*/ULN	4.1 ± 5.8 (0.5–42)
Initial mean OHPU value, mg/24 h	
Men	149 ± 177 (27–1,073)
Women	88 ± 62† (30–353)
Duration of follow-up, years	5.2 ± 1.6 (3–10)
Number of patient-years	458
Number of treatment-years	155
Number of courses of treatment/patient	3.0 ± 1.5 (1–6)
Number of courses of treatment/patient/year	0.6 ± 0.3 (0.2–1.2)
Duration of first remission, years	2.0 ± 1.4 (0.2–7.4)

*Parentheses indicate ranges.
†$P < 0.05$.

TABLE 8.2 Comparison of Asymptomatic and Symptomatic Patients

	Asymptomatic, $n = 20$	Symptomatic, $n = 68$	
Age, years	63.6 ± 10	63.7 ± 12.0	NS*
Sex M/F	13/7	30.38	NS
Extent of disease (IE), %	6.7 ± 4.0	13.0 ± 11.8	$P < 0.001$
Initial mean AP, x/ULN	2.4 ± 2.8	4.6 ± 6.3	$P < 0.01$
Initial mean OHPU, mg/24 h	74 ± 46	132 ± 149	$P < 0.01$
Duration of follow-up, years	4.7 ± 1.4	5.4 ± 1.6	NS
Number of courses of treatment/ patient	3.0 ± 1.5	2.9 ± 1.5	NS
Duration of first remission, years	1.6 ± 1.0	2.2 ± 1.5	NS
Progress favorable/ unfavorable	15/5	48/20	NS

*NS = not significant.

dysfunction, and other complications. The three unfavorable outcomes among the 20 initially asymptomatic patients consisted of one case of a loosened total hip prosthesis and two cases of fracture (femur, humerus).

Among the patients with symptoms, 76% (52/68) were improved at the end of the follow-up period. Twenty-two percent (22%) of the cases (15/68) were unchanged, and 2% (1/68) were worse. At baseline, 35 patients had bone pain, 4 patients had articular pain, and 21 had a mixture. Bone and mixed pain were relieved more often than articular pain ($P < 0.01$).

Changes in alkaline phosphatase and OHPU values during successive courses of treatment are shown in Table 8.3. Changes in OHPU induced

TABLE 8.3 Mean Values of Alkaline Phosphatase and OHPU for Successive Courses of Etidronate Disodium Treatment

Course No.	AP (xULN) Before	AP (xULN) After	ΔAP, %	OHPU, mg/24 h Before	OHPU, mg/24 h After	ΔOHPU, %
1	4.1 ± 5.8 $n = 88$	2.1 ± 2.9 $n = 85$	41 ± 81 $n = 85$	119 ± 135 $n = 88$	77 ± 84 $n = 86$	25 ± 41 $n = 85$
2	4.0 ± 6.5 $n = 70$	3.4 ± 4.9 $n = 71$	7 ± 37 $n = 68$	95 ± 127 $n = 68$	82 ± 75 $n = 70$	17 ± 38 $n = 68$
3	5.2 ± 7.0 $n = 48$	4.0 ± 6.2 $n = 43$	15 ± 30 $n = 44$	120 ± 128 $n = 48$	85 ± 68 $n = 43$	11 ± 39 $n = 44$
4	5.4 ± 7.9 $n = 34$	5.0 ± 6.8 $n = 33$	2 ± 31 $n = 31$	177 ± 271 $n = 33$	129 ± 188 $n = 32$	21 ± 31 $n = 31$
5	4.4 ± 2.6 $n = 12$	4.1 ± 2.2 $n = 12$	−1 ± 21 $n = 9$	120 ± 61 $n = 11$	96 ± 40 $n = 11$	21 ± 35 $n = 9$

by etidronate disodium for successive courses were similar. However, treatment-induced changes in alkaline phosphatase were progressively attenuated with successive courses of treatment. For the total population at the end of follow-up, the mean alkaline phosphatase was 3.5 ± 4.6 ULN and the mean OHPU value was 104 ± 143 mg/24 h. These values were not significantly different from the AP and OHPU values recorded at the beginning of the study.

The progression of the disease was judged favorable in 63 patients (72%), with a similar outcome in both sexes. As expected, patients who had an improvement in symptoms had a favorable outcome more often than those in whom symptoms persisted (41 versus 8; $P < 0.05$). Disease progression was unfavorable in 25 patients (28%). In 13 patients, this was due to resistance to treatment, as in the following three examples:

Example 1. A 68-year-old woman, with involvement of the entire pelvis, both femurs, the skull, the spine (T-8 to L-5), and one tibia (IE = 16%), had osteoarthritis of the hip. Despite five courses of treatment, deformity of the hip progressed, accompanied by an osteolytic resorptive front of the tibia. Bilateral hypoacusis with Meniere's disease also appeared.

Example 2. A 75-year-old woman with an IE of 41% was followed for 7.7 years and given four courses of etidronate disodium. Despite this treatment, osteoarthritis of both hips and a 1.5-cm increase in cranial perimeter, accompanied by increased bilateral deafness, occurred.

Example 3. A 29-year-old man with an IE of 48% was followed for 7 years and despite four courses of treatment with etidronate disodium, developed radiologic extension of the pagetic process in six long bones with the appearance of deformation of both femurs, the pelvis, and one humerus. He also lost 10 cm in height with compression of the seventh cervical vertebra and the second through fifth lumbar vertebrae. Pagetic fractures of the clavicle and a humerus occurred. The cranial perimeter increased 2 cm, with deafness and symptoms of basilar impression. Initially, his alkaline phosphatase value was 15 × ULN and OHPU 590 mg/24 h. At the end of study, the alkaline phosphatase value had increased to 32 × ULN and OHPU to 1,232 mg/24 h.

Other resistant patients manifested the onset of or an increase in deafness, increased cranial perimeter, osteoarthritis of the hip, and progression of osteolytic resorption fronts in the skull or long bones. In one case, a dissociation of the clinical response occurred in that spastic paraparesis caused by pagetic thoracic involvement was markedly improved during five courses of etidronate disodium over a 6-year period, but radiologically demonstrable extension of lesions of the distal femur and the skull occurred at the same time.

Five patients with Paget's disease of the thoracic spine had myelopathic involvement, usually in the lower half of the thoracic spine. In one patient, paraplegia was relieved by laminectomy before treatment began and there was no relapse during two courses of treatment with etidronate disodium over a 4-year period. Four patients with progressive spastic paraparesis had etidronate disodium prescribed orally for 6 months at 5 to 10 mg/kg/d. In one patient, salmon calcitonin (SCT), 50 IU/d, was also given for the first 6 weeks. Treatment produced complete remission of symptoms in all four cases, but relapse also occurred 6 months to 2 years after treatment. Fortunately, the patients responded to reintroduction of etidronate disodium, and three patients had a complete remission of their neurologic complications. The fourth patient had a 75% remission. In all, two to five courses of treatment were given during a 3- to 8-year period.

Hypoacusis, unilateral or bilateral, was present in 55% (16/29) of the patients with skull involvement and did not improve with treatment. Skull parameters remained stable in 13 of these patients and increased in 3 patients by 1.5 to 3 cm. These patients had extensive disease (IE = 40, AP > 10 ULN, OHPU > 150 mg/24 h) and were generally more resistant to etidronate disodium, with an unfavorable outcome.

There were 23 complete fractures distributed among 16 patients. Eight fractures occurred in pagetic bone and 15 in nonpagetic bone. The overall frequency of fractures was 26%, pagetic bone fractures constituted 9%. The fracture rate was 5/100 patient-years for all fractures and 1.7 for pagetic fractures. Fractures of the femoral diaphysis occurred only in pagetic bone, whereas femoral neck, rib, and vertebra fractures generally occurred in nonpagetic bone. Eight patients had fissure fractures, either single or multiple. Three of these appeared during treatment with etidronate disodium and were accompanied by renewed episodes of pain, necessitating the discontinuance of etidronate disodium and the introduction of SCT.

Side Effects

Side effects of etidronate disodium were observed mainly in the skeletal system. Minor digestive disturbances (gastralgia, nausea, diarrhea, constipation) were observed in eight instances, pruritus twice, and dizziness once. These problems did not require stopping treatment. Transitory hyperphosphatemia greater than 5.0 mg/dL was present at the end of 9 of 218 courses of treatment. A renewed outbreak of pain in pagetic bone during the third month of treatment or later was experienced by 11 patients (12.5%), representing a rate of 7/100 treatment-years. The pain was localized to the tibia (6/11), the femur (2/11), the astragalus (1/11), or multiple sites (2/11). The painful areas were invariably sites of preexisting osteolytic foci in the subperiosteum associated with cortical thinning (7/11) or fissure fractures (5/11). Improvement occurred 1 to 3 months after etidronate disodium was stopped, except in one case, in which a fissure fracture of a pagetic femur progressed to a complete fracture.

Resistance

As noted in Table 8.4, 31% of the patients retained sensitivity throughout, 45% had an intermediate response, and 24% were resistant to etidronate disodium. The patients in the resistant group had a lower mean age, a greater number of courses of treatment, and a shorter first remission than the other two groups. Many of the patients in the sensitive group received only a single course of treatment, which usually resulted in a prolonged remission lasting on average 3.6 years. These patients tended to have less severe disease (IE = 7.6%; AP = 2.4 ULN; OHPU = 94 mg/24 h). There were no significant differences among the three groups classified by degree of resistance in baseline values of AP and OHPU at the end of either the first or the second course of treatment.

Patients showed improvement in symptoms proportional to their degree of resistance: sensitive: 85%; intermediate: 55%; resistant: 33% ($P < 0.02$). Similarly, there was a favorable overall outcome in 85% of sensitive patients, 70% in intermediate patients, and only 57% in resistant patients. However, more than half the resistant group had a favorable outcome despite resistance. Resistance appeared most often between the second and third courses of treatment.[1,3] Some resistant patients were retreated with etidronate disodium by using a more aggressive therapeutic scheme (5 mg/kg/d intravenously for 7 days or 20 mg/kg/d orally for 1 month), and this maneuver was effective in 7 of 14 patients. Substitution of SCT was effective in 7 of 10 patients.

DISCUSSION

During this study of etidronate disodium at a dose of 5 mg/kg/d orally, approximately 100 other patients having extensive Paget's disease were treated more aggressively with clodronate or with etidronate disodium at a dose of 20 mg/kg/d orally or 5 mg/kg/d intravenously. Thus this study is not representative of severe Paget's disease but is illustrative of the results of etidronate disodium treatment in moderate Paget's disease.

The data support the finding that etidronate disodium has a preventive and beneficial action since 85% of the group had a favorable outcome. The use of etidronate disodium may also be justified when there is localized disease and alkaline phosphatase and OHPU values are normal, if the sites of the Paget's disease or its character presage future complications.

TABLE 8.4 Characteristics of the Sensitive (S), Intermediate (I), and Resistant (R) Groups

Patients, no. (%)	Sex M/F	Age, years	Extent of disease, %	Duration of follow-up, years	Duration of first remission, years	AP		OHPU	
						Beginning	End	Beginning	End
S 27 (31%)	17/10	67.4 ± 7.6	13.5 ± 11.6	5.0 ± 1.8	2.8 ± 1.4	5.1 ± 8.3	2.3 ± 2.5*	160 ± 197	74 ± 58*
I 40 (45%)	16/24	65.4 ± 10.4	10.5 ± 10.4	5.2 ± 1.5	2.0 ± 1.4*	3.2 ± 3.9	3.1 ± 2.6	96 ± 74	86 ± 72
R 21 (24%)	10/11	55.5 ± 13.4*	11.7 ± 10.7	5.5 ± 1.4	1.2 ± 0.8*	4.6 ± 4.7	5.7 ± 6.8	107 ± 119	176 ± 257

*P 0.01–0.05.

The percentage of patients with improvement in this series is similar to that found in other long-term studies.[10,18,19] The greater effectiveness of etidronate disodium in relieving bone pain than articular pain has also been noted by Khairi et al.[10] and by Alexandre et al.[2]

The degree of decrease in alkaline phosphatase and OHPU values at the end of the first course of treatment, 41% and 25%, respectively, is lower than the 40% to 50% generally reported[2-4,20] because several patients had initial values close to normal. The lesser biochemical efficacy in reducing alkaline phosphatase values of etidronate disodium during the second course of treatment has not been previously reported and may represent an uncoupling of its effects on bone resorption and bone formation resulting from the preponderantly antiosteoclastic activity of etidronate disodium.[21] Khairi et al.[10] have noted that alkaline phosphatase values relapse earlier than OHPU values after treatment with etidronate disodium and have speculated that there is a greater decrease in the number of osteoclasts than of osteoblasts with etidronate disodium treatment.

The effectiveness of bisphosphonates for spinal dysfunction in Paget's disease has been noted previously.[1,22-24] In these earlier studies, consisting of eight patients treated with etidronate disodium successfully, only two were treated with the low dose used here. It is therefore important to note the restorative effect of the 5 mg/kg dose of etidronate disodium administered orally in four cases of myelopathic involvement with spastic paraparesis. Although myelopathic relapses occurred after a variable period of time, the patients remained susceptible to retreatment and the long-term outcomes were favorable. Efficacy is even greater when the myelogram result is normal, suggesting that spinal ischemia caused by the "stealing" of blood flow from the spinal cord to the adjacent pagetic vertebrae is at fault.

The frequency of hypoacusis in the patients with pagetic skull involvement (55%) is in accord with that found by Nager of 30% to 50%.[25] Nager also noted an absence of improvement with treatment, and in such patients the outcome of the disease may be unfavorable.

Analysis of fractures in pagetic patients treated with etidronate disodium poses a problem because fracture rates, as claimed with high doses of etidronate disodium (10 to 20 mg/kg/d)[4,6,8,10,26] in either pagetic or nonpagetic bone,[27] must be compared with the frequency of fractures in patients not treated with etidronate disodium, and the latter is not known with certainty. In nonpagetic bone, fracture frequencies of 9% to 28% have been reported[6,24,28,30,31] compared to 9% in the present series. Also, the rate of fracture in pagetic bone of 1.7/100 patient-years in the present study compares well with rates of 0.8 to 1.6 reported in three other series of untreated patients.[6,28,30] In previous studies of treatment with calcitonin[32-45] totaling 431 patients and 427 patient-years of treatment, no non-traumatic fractures of a pagetic femur were observed. In four other series,[46-49] one traumatic fracture of a pagetic femur was observed in 497 patients (0.2%). Although it is possible that calcitonin diminishes the risk of fracture in Paget's disease, this also cannot be confirmed without a controlled study. The present observations indicate that etidronate disodium at 5 mg/kg/d does not increase the risk of fracture in patients with Paget's disease.

Delayed pain as a side effect of etidronate disodium is well known to occur with doses of 20 mg/kg/d[4,6,10,50] but has been reported in the literature less frequently in patients treated with 5 mg/kg/d.[51-53] A delayed exacerbation of pain occurred in eight patients who nevertheless had a favorable outcome with one exception. The mechanism of the exacerbation of pain is not known, but in certain reports,[27,51,52] it has been associated with histologic abnormalities in mineralization. The time of onset is variable,[4,54,55] and it is independent of vitamin D status.[56]

The emergence of resistance to etidronate disodium at 5 mg/kg/d in approximately a quarter of the patients after an average of 2.5 courses of treatment was noted previously only by Siris et al.,[15] and neither Khairi et al.[10] nor Altman[18] reported such resistance. The absence of a significant difference in disease extent or in biochemical abnormalities in the resistant patients compared to sensitive patients is at variance with the results of Altman[18] and of Siris et al.[15] It is possible that resistance to etidronate disodium depends not only on the extent of disease but also on factors not measured by the biochemical parameters. The amelioration of symptoms and the favorable objective outcome observed in many patients in the resistant group provide evidence that etidronate disodium may have a degree of effectiveness even when the biochemical parameters do not so indicate. These findings suggest that etidronate disodium should not necessarily be abandoned early in a patient who appears resistant on the basis of biochemical data but has otherwise progressed favorably from the clinical point of view.

In conclusion, this study, which has limitations because of its retrospective nature, shows that etidronate disodium, prescribed in discontinuous courses of treatment of 6-months' duration at a dose of 5 mg/kg/d, results in improvement and a stabilization in three quarters of patients with Paget's disease. In the remaining cases, alternative therapy, such as calcitonin and second-generation bisphosphonates, should be considered.

REFERENCES

1. Alexandre C, Chapuy MC, Bressot C, et al: Traitement de la maladie osseuse de Paget par l'éthanc-1-hydroxy-1, diphosphonate à faible posologic. *Nouv Presse Méd* 1980;9:3429–3433.

2. Alexandre C,Chapuy MC, Vignon E, et al: Treatment of Paget's disease of bone with ethane-1-hydroxy-1, 1-diphosphonate (EHDP) at a low dosage (5 mg/kg/day). *Clin Orthop* 1983;174:193–205.
3. Altman RD, Johnston CC, Khairi MRA, et al: Influence of disodium etidronate on clinical and laboratory manifestations of Paget's disease of bone (osteitis deformans). *N Engl J Med* 1973;189:1379–1384.
4. Canfield RE, Rosner W, Skinner J, et al: Diphosphonate therapy of Paget's disease of bone. *J Clin Endocrinol Metab* 1977;44:96–106.
5. Devries HR, Bijvoet OLM: Results of prolonged therapy with EHDP in Paget's disease. *Neth J Med* 1974;17:281–298.
6. Finerman GA, Gonick HC, Smith RK, Mayfiel JM: Diphosphonate treatment of Paget's disease. *Clin Orthop* 1976;120:115–124.
7. Guncaga J, Lauffenburger T, Lentner C, et al: Diphosphonate treatment of Paget's disease of bone: A correlated metabolic calcium kinetic and morphometric study. *Horm Metab Res* 1974;6:62–69.
8. Kantrowitz FG, Byrne MH, Schiller AL, Krane SM: Clinical and biochemical effects of diphosphonates in Paget's disease of bone, abstracted. *Arthritis Rheum* 1975;18:407.
9. Khairi MRA, Johnston CC, Altman RD, et al: Treatment of Paget's disease of bone (osteitis deformans): results of a one year study with sodium etidronate. *JAMA* 1974;230:562–267.
10. Khairi MRA, Altman RD, De Rosa GP, et al: Sodium etidronate in the treatment of Paget's disease of bone: A study of long-term results. *Ann Intern Med* 1977;87:656–663.
11. Khairi MRA, Johnston CC: Treatment of Paget's disease of bone (osteitis deformans) with sodium etidronate. *Clin Orthop* 977;127:94–105.
12. Rampon S, Bussière JL: Coxopathies pagétiques, In: *La Maladie Osseuse de Paget.* Premier Colloque de pathologie locomotrice, Montpellier, 1974. Paris, Galliena, 1975 pp 29–34.
13. Renier JC, Bontoux-Carre E, Bontoux L, et al: Le traitement de la maladie de Paget par l'éthane-hydroxy-1, 1-diphosphonate (EHDP). *Rev Rhum* 1982;49:87–92.
14. Ravault A: Maladie osseuse de Paget. Suivi à long terme de 88 patients traites à l'etidronate disodique en discontinu à faible dose (5 mg/kg/j). Thesis. Lyon I University, 1986.
15. Siris ES, Canfield RE, Jacobs TP, et al: Clinical and biochemical effects of EHDP in Paget's disease of bone: Pattern of response to initial treatment and to long-term therapy. *Metab Bone Dis* 1981;4–5:301–308.
16. Smith R: *Paget's Disease of Bone: Biochemical Disorders of the Skeleton.* London, Butterworth Publishers, 1979.
17. Meunier PJ, Salson C, Mathieu L, et al: Skeletal distribution and biochemical parameters of Paget's disease. *Clin Orthop* 1987;217:37–44.
18. Altman RD: Long-term follow-up of therapy with intermittent etidronate disodium in Paget's disease of bone. *Am J Med* 1985;79:583–590.
19. Siris ES, Canfield RE, Jacobs TP, Baquiran DC: Long-term therapy of Paget's disease of bone with EHDP. *Arthritis Rheum* 1980;23:1177–1184.
20. Johnston CC, Khairi MRA, Meunier PJ: Use of etidronate (EHDP) in Paget's disease of bone. *Arthritis Rheum* 1980;23:172–176.
21. Basle MF, Rebel A, Renier JC, et al: Bone tissue in Paget's disease treated by ethane-1-hydroxy-1, 1-diphosphonate (EHDP): Structure, ultrastructure and immunocytology. *Clin Orthop* 1984;184:281–288.
22. Charhon S, Chapuy MC, Valentin-Opran A, Meunier PJ: Intravenous etidronate for spinal cord dysfunction due to Paget's disease. *Lancet* 1982;1:391–392.
23. Douglas DL, Duckworth T, Kanis JA, et al: Spinal cord dysfunction in Paget's disease of bone and its treatment: Has medical treatment a vascular basis? *J Bone Joint Surg* 1981;63B:495–503.

24. Douglas DL, Kanis JA, Duckworth T, et al: Paget's disease: Improvement of spinal cord dysfunction with diphosphonates and calcitonin. *Metab Bone Dis* 1981;3:327–336.
25. Nager GT: Paget's disease of the temporal bone. *Ann Otol Rhinol Laryngol* 1975;84(suppl 22):1–32.
26. Ibbertson HK, Henley JW, Fraser TR, et al: Paget's disease of bone-clinical evaluation and treatment with diphosphonate. *Aust NZ J Med* 1979;9:31–35.
27. Mautalen G, Gonzales D, Blumenfeld E, et al: Spontaneous fractures of uninvolved bones in patients with Paget's disease during unduly prolonged treatment with disodium etidronate (EHDP). *Clin Orthop* 1986;207:150–155.
28. Altman RD, Collins B: Musculoskeletal manifestations of Paget's disease of bone. *Arthritis Rheum* 1980;23:1121–1127.
29. Dickson DD, Camp JD, Ghormley RK: Osteitis deformans: Paget's disease of the bone. *Radiology* 1945;44:449–455.
30. Nagant de Deuxchaisnes C, Dufour JP, Devogelaer JP, et al: Etidronate and the risk of fractures. *Lancet* 1985;1:610–611.
31. Traver CA: The association of fractures and Paget's disease (osteitis deformans). *N Y State J Med* 1936;36:242–246.
32. Bouvet JP: Traitement de la maladie de Paget par la thyrocalcitonine de saumon: Etude coopérative en double insu. *Nouv Presse Med* 1977;6:1447–1450.
33. Burckhardt P, Ducommun J, Hessler C: Treatment of Paget's disease of bone with human calcitonin, in McIntyre I (ed): *Human Calcitonin and Paget's Disease* Bern, Hans Huber, 1977, pp 155–160.
34. De Rose J, Singer FR, Avramides A, et al: Response of Paget's disease to porcine and salmon calcitonin. *Am J Med* 1974;56:858–866.
35. Grunstein HS, Clifton-Bligh P, Posen S: Paget's disease of bone: Experience with 100 patients treated with salmon calcitonin. *Med J Aust* 1981;2:278–280.
36. Hamilton CR: Effects of synthetic salmon calcitonin in patients with Paget's disease of bone. *Am J Med* 1974;56:315–322.
37. Jaeger P, Bischof F, Delaloye A, Burckhardt P: Le traitement combiné de la maladie de Paget de l'os par la calcitonine et le diphosphonate EHDS, *Schweiz Med Wochenschr* 1981;111:1893–897.
38. Kanis JA, Horn DB, Scott RDM, Strong JA: Treatment of Paget's disease of bone with synthetic salmon calcitonin. *Br Med J* 1974;3:727–731.
39. Kuhlencordt F, Ringe JD, Kruse HP: Behandlung der Ostendystrophia deformans Paget mit Lachs-Calcitonin. *Dtsch Med Wochenschr* 1981;106:1620–1623.
40. Lang R, Milkman M, Jensen PS, Vignery AMC: Chronic treatment of Paget's disease of bone with synthetic human calcitonin. *Yale J Biol Med* 1981;54:355–365.
41. Martin TJ, Jerums G, Melick RA, et al: Clinical, biochemical and histological observations on the effect of porcine calcitonin in Paget's disease of bone. *Aust NZ J Med* 1977;7:36–43.
42. Nuti R, Vattimo A: Synthetisches human-calcitonin bei osteodystrophic deformans (Paget) und osteoporose. *Dtsch Med Wochensch* 1981;106:149–152.
43. Plehwe WE, Hudson J, Clifton-Bligh P, Posen S: Porcine calcitonin in the treatment of Paget's disease of bone: Experience with 32 patients. *Med J Aust* 1977;1:577–581.
44. Sturtridge WC, Harrison JE, Wilson DR: Long-term treatment of Paget's disease of bone with salmon calcitonin. *Can Med Assoc J* 1977;117:1031–1034.
45. Ziegler R, Holz G, Raue F, et al: Therapeutic studies with human calcitonin, in McIntyre I. (ed): *Human Calcitonin and Paget's Disease*. Proceedings of the International Workshop). Bern, Hans Huber, 1977, p. 167.
46. Evans IMA: Human calcitonin in the treatment of Paget's disease of bone: Long term trials, in McIntyre I (ed): *Human Calcitonin and Paget's Disease*. Bern, Hans Huber, 1977, pp 111–123.

47. Fornasier VL, Stapleton K, Williams CC: Histological changes in Paget's disease treated with calcitonin. *Hum Pathol* 1978;9:455–461.
48. Singer FR, Rude RK, Mius BG: Studies of the treatment and aetiology of Paget's disease of bone, in McIntyre I (ed): *Human Calcitonin and Paget's Disease.* Bern, Hans Huber, 1977, pp 93–110.
49. Woodhouse NJY, Chalmers AH, Wells IP, et al: Paget's disease: Radiological changes occurring in untreated patients and those on therapy with salmon calcitonin during two years observation. *Br J Radiol* 1977;50:699–705.
50. Fromm G, Schajowicz F, Casco C, et al: The treatment of Paget's bone disease with sodium etidronate. *Am J Med Sci* 1979;277:29–37.
51. Boyce BF, Fogelman I, Ralston S, et al: Focal osteomalacia due to low-dose diphosphonate therapy in Paget's disease of bone. *Lancet* 1984;1:821–824.
52. Evans RA, Dunstan CR, Holls E, Wong SYP: Pathologic fracture due to severe osteomalacia following low-dose diphosphonate treatment of Paget's disease of bone. *Aust NZ J Med* 1983;13:277–279.
53. Nagant de Deuxchaisnes C, Rombouts-Lindemans C, Huaux JP: Roentgenologic evaluation of the action of the diphosphonate EHDP and of combined therapy (EHDP and calcitonin) In Paget's disease of bone, in McIntyre I. Szelke M (eds): *Molecular Endocrinology.* Proceedings of Endocrinology 79. Amsterdam, Elsevier North Holland Biomedical Press, 1979, pp 405–433.
54. Alexandre C, Meunier PJ, Edouard C, et al: Effects of ethane-1-hydroxy-1, 1-diphosphonate (5 mg/day/dose) on quantitative bone histology in Paget's disease of bone. *Metab Bone Dis* 1981;3:309–316.
55. Russell RGG, Smith R, Preston C, et al: Diphosphonates in Paget's disease. *Lancet* 1974;1:894–898.
56. Nagant de Deuxchaisnes C, Maldague B, Malghem J, et al: The action of the main therapeutic regimens on Paget's disease of bone with a note of the effect of vitamine D deficiency. *Arthritis Rheum* 1980;23:1215–1234.

CHAPTER 9

Disodium Pamidronate Therapy of Paget's Disease

Olav L. M. Bijvoet

INTRODUCTION

Several bisphosphonate analogues are currently in use for the treatment of bone disorders, with the best known being etidronate disodium, disodium clodronate (Cl_2 MDP), and disodium pamidronate, also known as disodium APD.[1] APD is chemically disodium (3-amino-1-hydroxy-propylidene)-1, 1-bisphosphonate. The inhibitory action of the bisphosphonates on bone resorption requires prior chemisorption to the calcified bone matrix,[2-4] which is achieved through two phosphonate groups connected by a central carbon atom, the P-C-P bond, which all the bisphosphonates have in common. The two phosphonates form complexes with calcium salts and with the hydroxyapatite crystals embedded in bone matrix.[1] Their presence on crystal surfaces changes the energy distribution on these surfaces and the chemical composition of the mineral, according to the nature of the nonbisphosphonate groups of the bisphosphonate, so that some of them make crystals grow more slowly and also dissolve more slowly. In addition, several bisphosphonates alter biologic processes taking place at the surface of bone crystals. Some may inhibit bone resorption by direct inhibition of bone-resorbing cells, others by impairing accession to bone of these cells. The high affinity of bisphosphonates for bone mineral is exploited in scintigraphy, in which bisphosphonates bound to radioactive tracers localize to bony areas having increased turnover. Phosphonate bonds are not hydrolyzable by alkaline phosphatases or pyrophosphatases. This, together with their strong chemisorption to bone mineral, is responsible for a long half-life once deposited there.

The two valence positions of the central carbon atom not connected to the phosphonate groups are occupied by chlorine atoms in clodronate. Both etidronate and APD, on the other hand, have a hydroxyl group satisfying one of these valence positions that assists in the chemisorption process to bone mineral. The fourth valence position is again occupied by different residues in various bisphosphonates, and this fourth residue is as important in determining the biologic properties of the analogue as the P-C-P bond itself.[3,5] When one adds different bisphosphonates to cell cultures, their biologic effects may vary enormously.[5] Yet when these bisphosphonates are given to animals, they all cause the serum calcium concentration to decrease. Histologic and radiologic studies, combined with metabolic balance studies, indicate this is due primarily to inhibition of bone resorption.[1,6,7] Not only do the bisphosphonates differ in molar potency, but in vivo and in vitro studies have also uncovered significant qualitative differences in their mechanisms of action. There is evidence that clodronate is cytotoxic for the osteoclasts that ingest it while resorbing bone mineral. APD, on the other hand, seems to act by preventing recognition of the bone matrix by both osteoclast precursors and mature osteoclasts.[2-4] Etidronate, the first-generation bisphosphonate in which the inhibitory action of the bisphosphonates on bone resorption was first established, also produces a significant inhibitory effect on the mineralization of newly formed bone matrix. APD and clodronate do not share this latter property.

The evidence that APD seems to act by preventing recognition of the bone matrix by both osteoclast precursors and mature osteoclasts may in part explain the paradox that soon after inhibition of bone resorption, when there is also a secondary rise in serum parathyroid hormone levels, the number of multinucleate osteoclastlike cells is increased, rather than decreased, although these cells are not contiguous to bone.[6] In vitro, when osteoclast precursors are permitted to migrate into bone containing APD, the precursors become multinucleate but are unable to resorb bone. The resulting cells have different staining characteristics and other properties than osteoclasts and are not authentic osteoclasts.

Relative to etidronate and clodronate, APD has not only a different mechanism of action but a greater quantitative potency to inhibit bone resorption. Analogues of APD with longer side chains have also been produced, such as the aminobutane and aminohexane derivatives, and these have properties similar to those of APD. The aminobutane derivative is more potent on a weight base but has no essential advantage. The aminohexane compound, on the other hand, is much less active. The clinical data on these newer compounds are, however, scarce.[5-11] The properties of the aminobisphosphonates can be further improved by retaining the nitrogen atom in the fourth residue but replacing its hydrogen atoms with carbon atoms. The simplest of these third-generation bisphosphonates, Me_2APD (3-dimethylamino-hydroxypropylidene-bisphosponate), is almost completely nontoxic in in vitro cell cultures, and its antiresorption potency and inhibitory effect on bone recognition by osteoclasts are increased.[2]

CLINICAL ASPECTS

The second-generation bisphosphonates, APD and clodronate, represent a significant advance over the first-generation bisphosphonate, etidronate, because of their potency and lack of an inhibitory effect on mineralization in the doses used. Clodronate has a potency against bone resorption roughly equivalent to that of etidronate, whereas APD has a tenfold higher antiresorptive potency and achieves its effect in a quite different manner. In animals, APD has been shown to impair mineralization only at doses higher than those needed to obtain the antiosteoclastic effect.[6]

The second-generation bisphosphonates have been investigated in Paget's disease for almost two decades. With APD, when administered in the appropriate dose and according to an appropriate treatment schedule, it is possible to achieve a complete biochemical and clinical response in approximately 90% of patients, together with full suppression of disease activity (Figure 9.1).[8,10,12] This response is associated with a disappearance of hyperemia and edema in and around the bony lesions within weeks, and with a gradual loss of bone pain. If secondary arthritis is present, it is not usually benefited. These results can be obtained with APD courses of short duration.[13] As a result, with adequate monitoring on an outpatient basis, patients can be freed of the necessity for prolonged treatment. As noted, these effects are obtained without disturbing bone mineralization and with improvement of bone structure, as documented by histologic and radiologic observations.

The improvement of clinical results obtained with this bisphosphonate has a profound effect on the indications for treatment and the associated diagnostic measures as well as the long-term prognosis for patients with Paget's disease. There is insufficient space to summarize this here, but for the benefit of patients and treating physicians, the author has given a detailed account in a recently published review, "Clinical Disorders of Bone and Mineral Metabolism."[14]

Bone biopsies after APD treatment have documented a normalization of the cellularity of pagetic bone and a reduction, rather than an increase, in the amount of osteoid.[8,15] The improvement in bone structure can be quite evident in radiographs (Figure 9.2) and is there similar to those

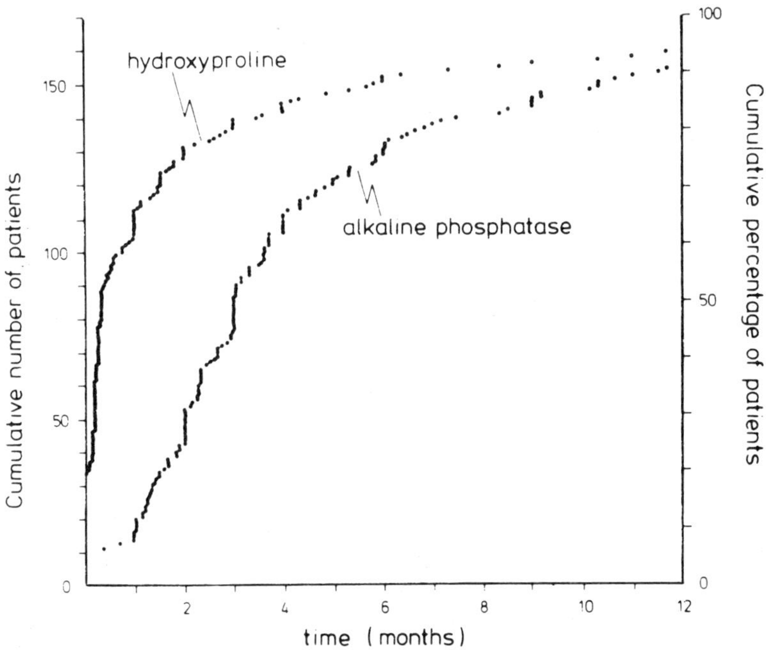

FIGURE 9.1. Cumulative number and percentage of patients (100% = 170 patients) with normal values of OHP and AP with time after initiation of APD treatment. *Reproduced from Harinck et al,[8] with permission.*

obtained with calcitonin, especially in lytic lesions, and no histologic deterioration occurs, as it sometimes does with etidronate. In contrast to that with calcitonin, the improvement with APD is *sustained* after treatment is stopped.[12,16–18] The early suppression of bone resorption, without suppression of mineralization, causes bone balance to change to a positive value of as much as 400 mg/d, roughly equal to the amount of calcium absorbed from the gut.[15] This effect of APD is associated with a decrease in serum and urinary calcium levels and a rise in serum concentrations of parathyroid hormone and 1,25-dihydroxyvitamin D.[19,20] These effects of APD are either absent or less evident when etidronate is given intravenously in doses high enough to mimic the effects of the second-generation bisphosphonates on bone resorption.[10] The reason may be that the impairment of mineralization associated with administration of such high doses of etidronate may reduce the uptake of calcium in newly formed bone mineral to the same extent as it reduces the calcium release through resorption inhibition.

Caution should be exerted against infusing patients with doses of APD

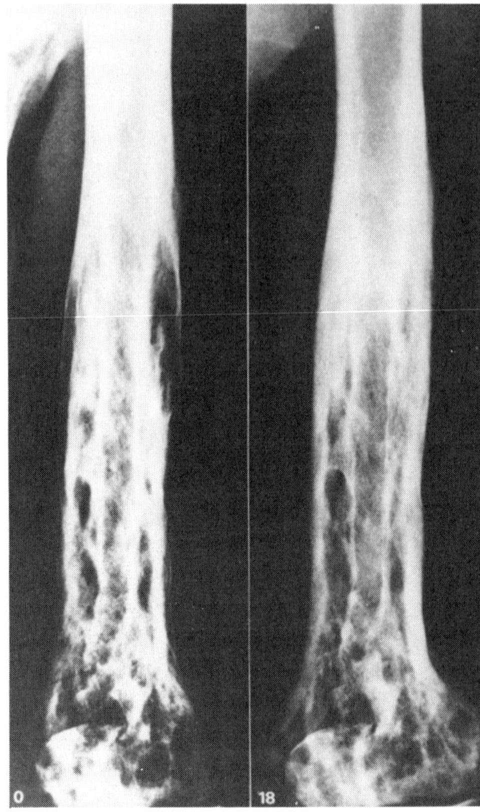

FIGURE 9.2. Radiologic improvement in the humerus during APD therapy (remineralization and remodeling). Eighteen months after the start of treatment the humerus had assumed a more slender and normal shape, the unmineralized bone regained its normal density, the osteolytic clefts were filled, and the proximal border of the lesion had faded away. *Reproduced from Vellenga CJLR, Mulder JD, Bijvoet OLM: Radiological demonstration of healing in Paget's disease of bone treated with APD. Br J Radiol 1985;58(693):834, with permission.*

of 30 mg or higher every 6 hours. With an intravenous dose of 30 mg every 6 hours, the decrease in urinary calcium is less precipitous than the decrease in urinary hydroxyproline. In addition, the usual decrease in serum phosphate seen with parathyroid stimulation is sometimes replaced by an increase in serum phosphate. These signs are evident within 48 hours, are similar to effects of intravenous etidronate, and may reflect an impairment of mineralization.[10] I have not investigated this phenomenon further since doses of 30 mg or more may have a damaging action on bone and are not necessary. In patients with hypercalcemia of malignancy in whom the rate of bone formation is not so greatly increased, this phenomenon is less likely to be evident at higher APD doses.

With APD, the definition of a remission in Paget's disease activity is different from that used for the calcitonins or etidronate. Remission with APD means a complete absence of biochemical disease activity, together with an arrest of radiologic progression, after cessation of therapy. The end of remission is defined as any sustained increase in the serum alkaline phosphatase activity or urinary hydroxyproline excretion, even of small degree. Actuarial analysis has shown that 50% of APD-treated patients are still in complete remission 18 months after treatment, (Figure 9.3) and in 30% the remission lasts 4 years or more.[8,13] Recurrence is always slow and can be monitored by yearly or twice-yearly determinations of the serum alkaline phosphatase level. Recurrence is sometimes first noted by the patient when pain begins to recur. The duration of remission is related to the degree of suppression of the urinary hydroxyproline excretion that was achieved after the end of the initial treatment phase, and monitoring during treatment to achieve a maximal beneficial effect pays later dividends.[8,13] The urinary hydroxyproline excretion is therefore preferred to the serum alkaline phosphatase activity for monitoring early efficacy of treatment.

Reitsma et al.[6] have shown in animal studies, and Frijlinck et al. in humans that the earliest biochemical event after inhibition of bone resorption is a decrease in urinary hydroxyproline excretion, whereas the serum alkaline phosphatase activity remains unchanged during the early treatment period. Normalization of bone formation occurs later, and it takes 3 to 6 months for equilibrium between bone formation and resorption to be

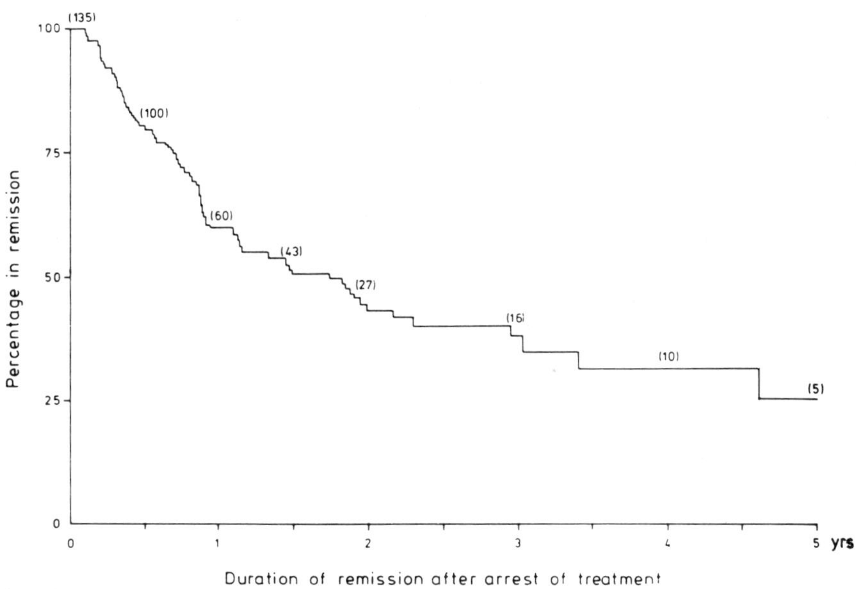

FIGURE 9.3. Duration of remission after arrest of treatment. Actuarial analysis of the duration of remission after arrest of APD treatment in 135 patients with Paget's disease of bone. *Reproduced from Harinck et al,[8] with permission.*

reestablished at a lower, now normal rate. This normalization of bone resorption should be distinguished from impairment of mineralization and is probably due to regulatory mechanisms proper to the bone tissue that tend to maintain equilibrium between activity of osteoblasts and osteoclasts. In the intervening period before adaptive reduction in bone formation rate is fully achieved, bone balance is positive. This causes a drain of calcium from the circulation to the skeleton, with secondary elevations of serum parathyroid hormone and 1,25-dihydroxyvitamin D levels, thereby mediating an increased calcium absorption from the gut.[19,20] As a result, symptomatic hypocalcemia is extremely rare. We have found that parathyroid hormone (PTH) may partially reverse the effect of APD on osteoclasts,[4] and this may also partially account for the rarity of hypocalcemia.

Scintigraphy can register the beneficial effects of treatment, but comparative repeat evaluations should be applied since effective treatment is not associated with a complete disappearance of excessive radioisotope uptake into pagetic lesions. On the average, about 20% of the initial excess uptake persists, possibly as a result of structural abnormalities in the calcified matrix.[21] If the scintigraphy is not quantitated but only visually assessed and the initial tracer uptake into bone is high, the 80% reduction in activity is likely to remain unnoticed; the remaining 20% of excess uptake may be sufficient to cause confusion between activity and remission!

The inhibitory effect of APD on osteoclastic bone resorption is the only one needed for therapeutic efficacy. It has been demonstrated that the short- and long-term effects of treatment are not different, whether treatment is continued for months until the serum alkaline phosphatase activity has normalized or given only for the few weeks needed for the urinary hydroxyproline excretion to decrease into the midnormal range.[8,13] Monitoring the degree of suppression of urinary hydroxyproline excretion allows an early assessment of the efficacy of treatment and prevents many months of superfluous drug administration.

APD SIDE EFFECTS

Still unexplained are complex immunologic phenomena that appear and disappear during the first treatment week with amino bisphosphonates such as APD.[8,12,13] These occur only during the first episode of treatment and never with retreatment. Half the patients have a transient increase in body temperature exceeding 0.5°C. The fever is associated with mild influenzalike symptoms and with transient hematologic changes. There are a rise in granulocyte count at 24 hours and a decrease in lymphocyte count to a minimum of 65% of initial value at 72 hours. All changes revert to baseline by 9 days. This complex of changes is similar in nature and time course to a complex of changes noted after administration of various interleukins and has there been termed "acute phase reaction." Since APD interferes with the accession of osteoclast precursors in bone and the immune system has an important role in the modulation of cell-cell interactions in bone, these symptoms of initial APD exposure may represent trapping of lymphocytes in bone with stimulation of interleukin production.[2,3,12,22] This entire phenomenon, which is likely to be a typical acute-phase reaction, requires further investigation. A paradoxical increase in osteoclasts or osteoclastlike cells may also be seen during the early phase of bisphosphonate treatment, and this may also be a local effect; it seems too early to represent a response to the secondary increase in PTH secretion.

Side effects of oral APD on the gastrointestinal mucosa are frequent at doses higher than 300 mg daily are due to irritation of the gastric mucosa, and may prevent effective use of oral APD preparations as the sole treatment in many patients. This problem indicates that intravenous APD therapy should be the treatment of choice at least for the initial phase of treatment.[8]

RESISTANCE

Primary and secondary resistance to second-generation bisphosphonates, although rare, has been reported. Among the 5% of nonresponders in our experience,[8] most have partial resistance. We have noted only two patients with complete resistance to APD. After relapse in initially responsive patients, there is usually a new response to retreatment with APD, although the rate of decrease of urinary hydroxyproline excretion is occasionally slowed.

DOSE SCHEDULES

Intravenous APD has been used in doses ranging from 5 to 200 mg daily. The extant data, however, suggest that single intravenous infusions should not exceed 15 to 20 mg/d, since 1 mg every 6 hours is the lowest effective dose and the short-term effects of APD do not increase significantly at higher rates greater than 15 to 20 mg/d. Theoretical reasons for not exceeding 15 to 20 mg/d were indicated earlier in this chapter. A large proportion of administered APD is retained on the bone, and efficacious treatment appears to require a total of approximately 200 mg administered parenterally and within 6 weeks, according to whatever schedule. The standard treatment schedule is a 10-day infusion course of 20 mg/d. One modification that has been proposed is to give serial weekly APD infusions at doses higher than 20 mg, using doses as high as 120 mg weekly. There are practical advantages to such an approach, although the total time needed to monitor therapy is increased. There is also concern that very high rates may damage bone structure through the induction of osteomalacia. Data supporting efficacy of this weekly treatment approach equal to that of the standard treatment schedule have yet to be generated. A third and more practical schedule is to administer a dose of 180 mg through six biweekly infusions of 30 mg, with each infusion lasting 4 hours. If, after 6 weeks, the urine hydroxyproline/creatinine ratio has not normalized, further infusions are given until the ratio has normalized. Additional infusions are likely to be necessary in more severely afflicted patients in whom the initial level of serum alkaline phosphatase activity and/or fasting urinary hydroxyproline/creatinine ratio exceeds 3.5 times the upper limit of normal.

The reason that bisphosphonate infusions are generally given slowly lies in the ability of the bisphosphonate to form insoluble complexes with calcium, if the combined calcium and bisphosphonate concentrations become too high. This may cause renal damage and has been observed with etidronate, but not as yet with the other bisphosphonates. A second reason is that damage to osteoblasts resulting in a disturbance of mineralization and eventual toxicity to other cells could be the result of an excessive circulating bisphosphonate concentration, rather than an excessive concentration on the bone surface. One tends, therefore, to administer the bisphosphonate in such a manner that a sufficiently high bone surface coverage is achieved at the cost of minimal elevation of the circulating bisphosphonate concentration.

Oral absorption of APD is approximately 1% and this means that a dose of 500 mg orally is equivalent to 5 mg intravenously.[8] Unfortunately, high oral doses are not well tolerated because of gastrointestinal side effects. However, our studies have demonstrated that following initial intravenous treatment courses with oral doses of 150 to 600 mg daily, in those patients in whom the initial treatment did not achieve normalization of hydroxyproline, eventually induces remission in the large majority of patients. Maximal results are achieved in 6 to 12 months.

Oral APD as the sole treatment should not be recommended mainly because of the necessary long duration of treatment and monitoring and the likelihood of gastrointestinal side effects if higher doses are to be used. In the past, studies with oral treatment have, however, produced interesting results in that they established that normalization of hydroxyproline, even in the absence of normalization of alkaline phosphatase, is sufficient to achieve complete remission at a later stage, even when the treatment is discontinued at the moment urine hydroxyproline excretion is normal. In one report, three different regimens were tested: (1) 600 mg APD daily orally until 6 months after the serum alkaline phosphatase level returned to normal, (2) 600 mg APD daily orally until the urinary hydroxyproline excretion returned to normal and alkaline phosphatase had only partially normalized, and (3) 20 mg as daily intravenous infusions for 10 days, a treatment that achieved normalization of hydroxyproline at an early stage, with a then still unchanged alkaline phosphatase. The remission rates were almost identical 2 years later, with complete remissions achieved in 90% of patients.[8,23] It is, therefore, to the benefit of the patient and the treating physician to achieve an early result with vigorous treatment. This prevents long, drawn-out periods of monitoring in the outpatient clinic.

The final biochemical criterion for complete remission is normalization of the serum alkaline phosphatase level. Since the effect of APD on serum alkaline phosphatase activity lags 3 months behind the effect on urinary hydroxyproline excretion, the former cannot normalize any earlier than 3 months after the start of treatment, even in those patients in whom normalization of urinary hydroxyproline excretion is immediate. Scrutiny of all the available treatment data indicates that normalization of the serum alkaline phosphatase level at 3 months is achieved with a total dose of 200 mg of APD intravenously in almost all patients in whom the initial serum alkaline phosphatase level did not exceed 3.5 times the upper limit of normal. In addition to the possibility that daily doses of APD as high as 30 mg intravenously may cause osteomalacia, an unduly high frequency of early fever and rigors has also been observed when the daily dose exceeds 45 mg.[24]

For monitoring long-term results, measurements of the serum alkaline phosphatase level are sufficient. A practical follow-up schedule is to assess the serum alkaline phosphatase level every 6 to 9 months, or earlier if the patient notes a recurrence of bone pain.

THE FUTURE

Our uniform experience with APD suggests that it is possible to suppress Paget's disease completely in a predictable fashion in the great majority of patients. The treatment period is short, the results are predictable and long-lasting, and the patient does not require maintenance therapy. Only infrequent follow-up is required. These results are of such a nature that progression of severe, widespread Paget's disease is probably entirely preventable if treatment is given early. Secondary prevention of severe Paget's disease is achievable, and the aim of treatment should no longer be restricted to immediate pain relief but should include an attempt to arrest future disease progression.

Unfortunately, only partial beneficial results occur in a minority of patients, and complete resistance, although rare, has been observed. The yet more potent third-generation bisphosphonates now becoming available have in our hands already been shown to be beneficial in patients in whom APD has not induced a remission. Their main advantage, however, may be that they will allow one to achieve early and complete suppression with a mere oral course and so even eliminate the impracticalities associated with the prolonged bisphosphonate infusions.

REFERENCES

1. Fleisch H: Bisphosphonates: Mechanism of action and clinical application. In: WA Peck (ed.) *Bone and Mineral Research.* Annual 1. Amsterdam, Excerpta Medica, 1983, pp. 319–357.
2. Boonekamp PM, Löwik CWGM, van der Wee-Pals LJA, et al: Enhancement of the inhibitory action of APD on the transformation of osteoclast precursors into resorbing cells after dimethylation of the amino group. *Bone Mineral* 1987;2:29–42.
3. Boonekamp PM, van der Wee–Pals LJA, van Wijk-van Lennep M, et al: Two modes of action of bisphosphonates on osteoclastic resorption of mineralized matrix. *Bone Mineral* 1986;1:27–40.
4. Löwik CWGM, van der Pluym G, van der Wee-Pals LJA, et al: Migration and phenotypic transformation of osteoclast precursors into mature osteoclasts: The effects of a bisphosphonate. *J Bone Mineral Res* 1988;2:185–192.
5. Shinoda H, Adamek G, Felix R, et al: Structure-activity relationships of various bisphosphonates. *Calif Tiss Int* 1983;35:87–99.
6. Reitsma PH, Bijvoet OLM, Verlinden-Ooms H, van der Wee-Pals L: Kinetic studies of bone and mineral metabolism during treatment with (3-amino-1-hydroxypropylidene) -1,1-bisphosphonate (APD) in rats. *Calcif Tissue Int* 1980;32:145–157.
7. Reitsma PH, Bijvoet OLM, Potokar M, et al: Apposition and resorption of bone during oral treatment with (3-amino-1-hydroxypropylidene)-1,1-bisphosphonate (APD). *Calcif Tissue Int* 1983;35:357–361.
8. Harinck HIJ, Bijvoet OLM, Blanksma HJ, Dahlinghaus-Nienhuis PJ: Efficaceous management with aminobisphosphonate (APD) in Paget's disease of bone. *Clin Orthop* 1987;217:79–98.
9. Douglas DL, Duckworth T, Kanis JA, et al: Biochemical and clinical responses to dichloromethylene diphosphonate (Cl_2MDP) in Paget's disease of bone. *Arthritis Rheum* 1980;23:1185–1192.
10. McCloskey EV, Yates AJP, Beneton MNC, et al: Comparative effects of intravenous diphosphonates on calcium and skeletal metabolism in man. Bone 1987;8:[Suppl 1] pp 35–41.
11. Attardo-Parrinello G, Merlini G, Pavesi F, et al: Effects of a new aminodiphosphonate (aminohydroxybutylidene-diphosphonate) in patients with osteolytic lesions from metastases and myelomatosis. *Arch Int Med* 1987;147:1629–1633.
12. Bijvoet OLM, Frijlink WB, Jie K, et al: APD in Paget's disease of bone: Role of the mononuclear phagocyte system? *Arthr Rheum* 1980;23:1193–1204.

13. Harinck HIJ, Papapoulos SE, Blanksma HJ, et al: Paget's disease of bone: Early and late responses to three different modes of treatment with aminohydroxypropylidene bisphosphonate (APD). *Brit Med J* 1987;295:1301–1305.
14. Bijvoet OLM, Vellenga CJLR, Harinck HIJ. Paget's disease of bones: Assessment, therapy, and secondary prevention. In Kleerekoper M, Krane SM (eds.): *Clinical Disorders of Bone and Mineral Metabolism.* New York, Mary Ann Liebert, Publishers, 1989, pp 525–542.
15. Frijlink WB, TeVelde J, Bijvoet OLM, Heynen G: Treatment of Paget's disease of bone with (3-amino-1-hydroxy-propylidene)-1,1-bisphosphonate (APD). *Lancet* 1979;i: 799–803.
16. Dodd GW, Ibbertson HK, Fraser TR, et al: Radiological assessment of Paget's disease of bone after treatment with the bisphosphonates EHDP and APD. *Br J Radiol* 1987; 60:849–860.
17. Maldague B, Malghem J: Dynamic radiologic patterns of Paget's disease of bone. *Clin Orthop Rel Res* 1987;217:126–151.
18. Vellenga CJLR, Bijvoet OLM, Pauwels EKJ: Bone scintigraphy and radiology in Paget's disease of bone. *Amer J Physiol Imaging* 1988;3:154–168.
19. Adami S, Frijlink WB, Bijvoet OLM, et al: Regulation of calcium absorption by 1,25 dihydroxyvitamin D3. Studies of the effect of bisphosphonate treatment. *Calc Tiss Int* 1983;35:357–361.
20. Papapoulos SE, Harinck HIJ, Bijvoet OLM, et al: Effects of decreasing serum calcium on circulating parathyroid hormone and vitamin D metabolites in normocalcaemic and hypercalcaemic patients treated with APD. *Bone Mineral* 1986;1:59–78.
21. Vellenga CLJR, Pauwels EKJ, Bijvoet OLM, et al: Quantitative bone scintigraphy in Paget's disease treated with APD. *Brit J Radiol* 1985;58:1165–1172.
22. Dinarello CA: Interleukin-1 and the pathogenesis of the acute phase response. *N Engl J Med* 1984;311:1413–1418.
23. Heynen G, Delwaide P, Bijvoet OLM, Franchimont P: Clinical and biological effects of low dose of (3-amino-1-hydroxypropylidene)-1,1-bisphosphonate (APD) in Paget's disease of bone. *Europ J Clin Invest* 1982;12:29–35.
24. Gallacher SJ, Ralston SH, Pastel U, Boyle IT: Side effects of pamidronate. *Lancet* 1988;ii:42–43.

CHAPTER **10**

Treatment of Paget's Disease with the New Bisphosphonates

John A. Kanis, Eugene V. McCloskey, Declan O'Doherty, Neveen A. T. Hamdy, Derek Bickerstaff, Monique Beneton, and Maniccam Thavarajah

INTRODUCTION

The increased availability of the bisphosphonates over the past 15 years has revolutionized the medical treatment of Paget's disease and also stimulated renewed interest in its surgical management. Etidronate is the most widely available bisphosphonate, and it is against a wide experience of this agent that new bisphosphonates are being evaluated.

The development of etidronate and its use in Paget's disease represented a major advance in drug treatment for several reasons. Unlike the calcitonins and mithramycin, the drug could be given by mouth. The escape phenomenon and the development of drug resistance were seldom observed, and not only was the activity of Paget's disease markedly suppressed, but this suppression could be maintained for many months and sometimes years after the end of treatment.

There are, however, some problems with its use. High doses of etidronate (for example, 20 mg/kg/d) have more certain effects in terms of disease suppression,[1-3] but such doses also impair the mineralization of bone. For this reason, lower doses than are optimal for disease suppression in all patients are usually recommended (for example, 5 mg/kg/d). Because of the variable experience with the use of recommended doses, there has been a great deal of interest in developing new treatment regimens with etidronate[3-6] and in developing new bisphosphonates that inhibit bone resorption but have less marked effects than etidronate on the mineralization of bone. This paper reviews the activity of some of these new bisphosphonates, with the exception of pamidronate, which is reviewed by Drs. Bijvoet and Burckhardt (Chapters 9 and 12).

THE NEW BISPHOSPHONATES

Three bisphosphonates have been used extensively in Paget's disease. These are etidronate, clodronate, and pamidronate (Figure 10.1). Four further bisphosphonates, aminohexane bisphosphonate, aminobutane bisphosphonate, residronate, and tiludronate are undergoing clinical investigation, and many more have been synthesized and are likely to become available over the next 10 years. They all share the same backbone structure of the geminal bisphosphonates, namely a P-C-P bond, and are thus analogues of pyrophosphate.[4]

The structure of the bisphosphonates is clearly important in determining their activity. Indeed, in experimental systems there is a greater than 1,000-fold range in the ability of various bisphosphonates to inhibit bone resorption,[7,8] but as far as is known their effects on bone remodeling in humans are similar. This contrasts with their effects in vitro, where quite varied metabolic effects have been shown for different bisphosphonates, for example, in biochemical effects in bone cell culture systems.[7–9] This is one of the reasons why we do not yet have clear ideas on the precise

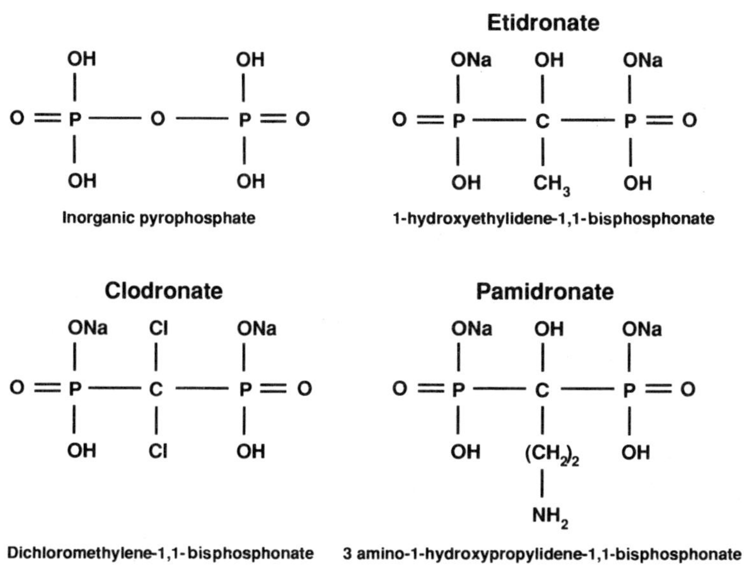

FIGURE 10.1. Structural formula of pyrophosphate and the geminal bisphosphonates used in Paget's disease.

mechanisms of action of the various bisphosphonates, even though the final common pathway is their ability to inhibit osteoclast-mediated bone resorption. Despite marked differences in their potency, the pharmacokinetics and effects of the various bisphosphonates in Paget's disease of bone share more similarities than differences in terms of their influence on bone remodeling, and for this reason these aspects are reviewed together. Characteristics of the individual agents are considered subsequently.

Pharmacokinetics

The intestinal absorption of all bisphosphonates tested in humans is low. Their bioavailability ranges from 1% to 10%, but in individuals it also varies markedly.[10,11] This is one of the reasons why responses to treatment may vary widely from center to center when doses of bisphosphonate close to their minimum effective dose are utilized, for example, in the case of etidronate. Gastrointestinal absorption is low for clodronate and for tiludronate but has not been directly studied for the other bisphosphonates. Indirect evidence, from their comparative activity when administered orally and intravenously, suggests that they too are poorly absorbed[12] (Kanis JA, O'Doherty D, unpublished observations). The development of formulations that would enhance intestinal absorption would be a significant advance, and recently, formulations of tiludronate that increase its bioavailability from the gastrointestinal tract have been developed.

Since the bisphosphonates have a strong affinity for calcium and for bone, their disappearance from the circulation is extremely rapid.[10] They are thought not to be metabolized, and in healthy individuals approximately 75% is excreted by the kidney unchanged and the remainder taken up by the skeleton.[13] There are small differences in skeletal uptake between the different bisphosphonates, but this is unlikely to be of importance for Paget's disease. On the other hand, the skeletal uptake of bisphosphonates in Paget's disease is remarkably heterogeneous, and indeed bisphosphonate retention is one of the techniques exploited in bone scintigraphy. Uptake appears to be dependent in part on blood flow but is particularly related to the degree of bone formation and mineralization. In Paget's disease scintigraphy provides a very sensitive method for examining the extent of pagetic bone lesions.

The preferential uptake of bisphosphonates at pagetic sites may have some therapeutic relevance in that the drug is targeted selectively to sites of disease activity. This poses some problems in the choice of dose, since with a fixed dose more bisphosphonate is targeted to skeletal sites in patients with the less extensive disease activity.

Activity of Bisphosphonates on Bone

In Paget's disease, all the bisphosphonates tested to date induce a dose-dependent suppression of bone resorption that can be measured by histologic studies, by tracer kinetics, and by indirect biochemical indexes of bone resorption. A decrease in hydroxyproline excretion, an indirect index of bone resorption, is seen within days of administration, particularly when the bisphosphonates are given intravenously. The decrease in hydroxyproline excretion is exponential, with a half-time of several days, but is dose dependent with any one bisphosphonate regimen (Figure 10.2).

In Paget's disease, rates of bone formation and mineralization are accelerated in addition to the focal increases in the rate of bone resorption. This is an amplification of the normal remodeling mechanism whereby areas of fatigue damage in bone are removed by resorption and new bone is laid down predominantly at sites of previous resorption (coupling). In the case of Paget's disease this coupling mechanism is intact, even though the rates of resorption and formation are much greater. Anarchic bone resorption is followed by anarchic formation at sites of previous resorption. As in

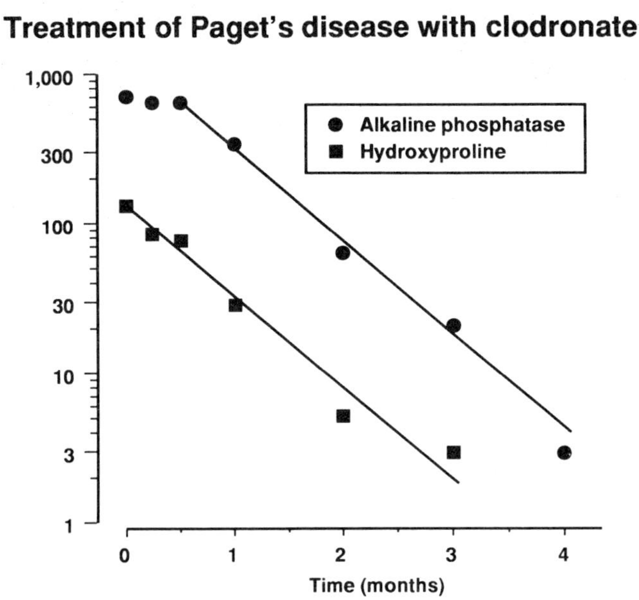

FIGURE 10.2. Responses of alkaline phosphatase (IU/L) and urine hydroxyproline (mmol/mol creatinine) to treatment with clodronate 800 mg daily by mouth. Values shown are observed values minus asymptotic values and plotted on a logarithmic scale. Both hydroxyproline and alkaline phosphatase values fell monoexponentially and had similar half-lifes, but the response of alkaline phosphatase lagged behind that of hydroxyproline.

the case of normal bone remodeling, these are surface-based events occurring on trabecular bone surfaces, within haversian canals, and on endosteal and periosteal surfaces of the cortex.

When bisphosphonates are given to patients with Paget's disease, the earliest effect noted is a decrease in bone resorption. The rate of onset of this effect is dose dependent but is relatively slow compared to that of the calcitonins. With calcitonin a decrease in hydroxyproline excretion occurs within hours of its administration, whereas the effects of the bisphosphonates take several days to complete (Figure 10.3). This suggests that a major effect of the bisphosphonates is to inhibit the recruitment of osteoclasts to bone surfaces but does not exclude a direct but slow action on osteoclasts within resorption cavities.

Irrespective of the precise mechanism of action, the end result is that the surfaces of bone that are undergoing resorption progressively diminish.

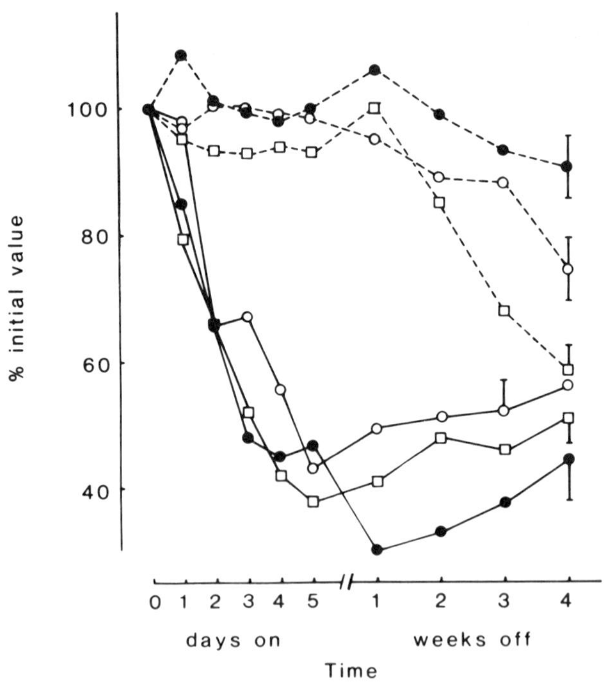

FIGURE 10.3. Effect of three bisphosphonates in Paget's disease. The bisphosphonates clodronate (squares), etidronate (closed circles), and aminohexane bisphosphonate (open circles) were given intravenously for 5 consecutive days. Note the early fall in hydroxyproline (solid lines). Serum alkaline phosphatase values began to fall 3–4 weeks after treatment (dotted lines).

Since osteoblasts or bone-forming cells are attracted primarily to sites of previous resorption by the coupling mechanism, a decrease in the resorption surface inevitably leads to a decrease in bone formation. For this reason the decrease in bone resorption induced by bisphosphonates is followed by a later decrease in bone formation, which can be documented either directly by histologic measurements or indirectly by biochemical markers of bone formation, such as serum activity of alkaline phosphatase (Figure 10.3).

This pattern of response is characteristic of all the bisphosphonates thus far tested.[12,14–16] The decrease in bone turnover is associated with a decrease in bone blood flow and a decrease in marrow fibrosis, both features of active Paget's disease. Of particular therapeutic relevance is that the new bone formed is characteristically lamellar in structure once turnover is diminished, whereas in active untreated Paget's disease, areas of woven bone formation occur. Woven bone formation is in part responsible for the anarchic appearance and together with increased vascularity gives rise to many of the clinical complications of Paget's disease. As might be expected, suppression of disease activity is associated with scintigraphic and in some cases radiographic indications of improvement, largely due to the decrease in bone turnover. Other changes include reduction in skin temperature over affected sites.

During the early phase of bisphosphonate treatment it would be expected that the inhibition of bone resorption with continued bone formation would decrease the net efflux of calcium from the skeleton to the extracellular pool. For this reason an early effect of treatment is a decrease in serum calcium. This in turn stimulates the secretion of parathyroid hormone (PTH), and such secondary effects have been well documented for clodronate, aminobutane, and aminohexane bisphosphonate[15–17] (Figure 10.4). The increase in PTH serves to minimize the hypocalcemic challenge by increasing the synthesis of calcitriol and thereby stimulating intestinal absorption of calcium. In addition, increased secretion of PTH decreases renal tubular reabsorption of phosphate and thereby decreases serum phosphate. This sequence of events has been well characterized for most of the new bisphosphonates and represents normal homeostatic responses to intervention rather than side effects. These changes disappear during the later phase of response when bone formation more closely matches bone resorption, albeit at a lower level than before treatment.

The pharmacodynamic effects of bisphosphonates described appear to be shared by all bisphosphonates that do not concurrently inhibit the mineralization of bone.[6] Specific characteristics of individual bisphosphonates are detailed in the following discussion.

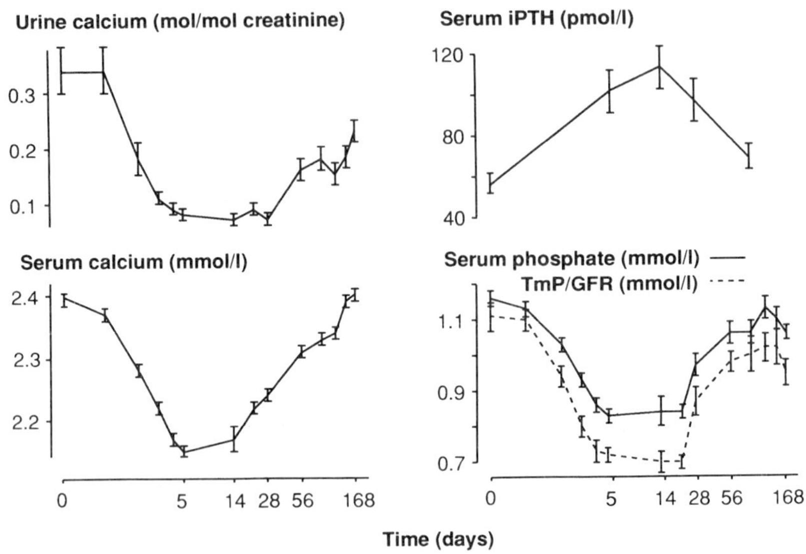

FIGURE 10.4. Effect of the aminobutane bisphosphonate on calcium and phosphate homeostasis. Intravenous treatment for 5 days resulted in a decrease in net efflux of calcium from bone and hence a decrease in mean (± SEM) serum calcium and fasting calcium excretion. Note the all in serum phosphate and TmP/GFR attributable to the secondary hyperparathyroidism. These effects persisted when treatment was stopped but reversed when bone formation and resorption became matched 6 months after the onset of treatment. TmP/GFR is the national renal tubular reabsorption of phosphate.

CLODRONATE

Dichloromethylene bisphosphonate (clodronate) inhibits bone resorption with much less marked effects than etidronate on the mineralization of bone. In humans its potency is similar to that of etidronate. Doses used in Paget's disease have varied from 400 mg to 3.2 g daily by mouth. A very effective regimen is 1,600 mg daily by mouth for 3 to 6 months (Figure 10.5). As is the case with all bisphosphonates, it is important to administer the drug with no calcium-containing foods or liquids since they impair drug absorption. A large number of studies have reported the effects of oral clodronate in Paget's disease. These studies indicate a rapid decrease in urinary excretion of hydroxyproline and a later fall in the activity of alkaline phosphatase. Histologic improvements in bone turnover are also observed (Table 10.1).[17-20] Suppression of disease activity is associated with the resumption of lamellar bone formation, which is normally mineralized.[19,20] There appears to be little difference in the degree of suppression of disease activity with doses between 800 and 1,600 mg daily given for 3 to 6 months.[19] However, the duration of remission appears to be longer with

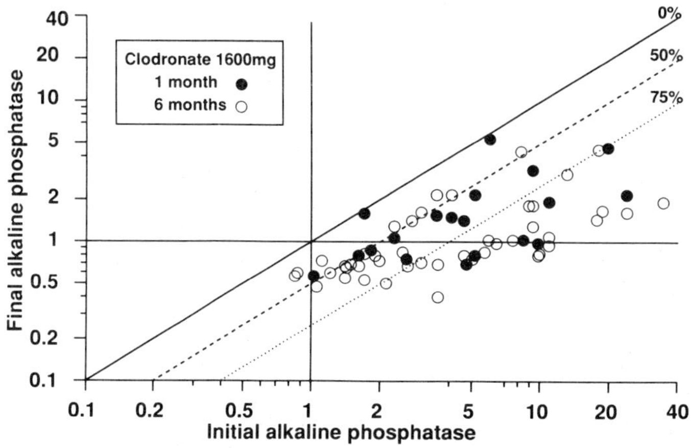

FIGURE 10.5. Serum activity of alkaline phosphatase (expressed as a ratio of the upper limit of normal) before and after treatment with clodronate using 1,600 mg daily by mouth for 6 months (○) or 1,600 mg daily for 1 month (●). Values after treatment are nadir values. Diagonal solid line, line of identity. Dotted line, values expected with 50% or 75% suppression of disease activity.

the higher doses.[1] Suppression of disease activity is associated with improvement in the bone scan[17,21] (Figure 10.6) and with clinical benefit.

As has been shown with other bisphosphonates, it is now evident that treatment for a 1-month period is capable of suppressing disease activity to a similar extent to that observed with 3- or 6-month treatment[1,22] (Figure 10.5). Similarly, the drug may be given intravenously (for example, 300 mg daily for 5 days).[14,23] The drug is infused in saline over 2 to 3 hours or longer. There is no marked difference in the degree of disease suppression when comparing the short treatments to the longer regimens, but the duration of response appears to be shorter (Table 10.2). Acquired resist-

TABLE 10.1 Effects of Clodronate on Histomorphometric Measurements in Iliac Trabecular Bone*

	Before treatment	After treatment	*P*<
Bone volume (% tissue volume)	37.4 ± 6.2	46.5 ± 8.5	0.01
Osteoid volume (% bone volume)	6.0 ± 1.3	2.4 ± 0.3	0.05
Osteoid thickness (μm)	11 ± 1	10 ± 1	NS†
Maximum number of lamellae	3.2 ± 0.3	3 ± 0.6	NS
Osteoblast density (/mm bone surface)	2.4 ± 1.2	0.7 ± 0.4	0.05
Osteoclast density (/mm bone surface)	1.14 ± 0.44	0.36 ± 0.18	0.05

*Ten patients were given 0.8 to 3.2 g clodronate for 3–6 months and had biopsy examinations 0–6 months after the end of treatment.

†NS, not significant.

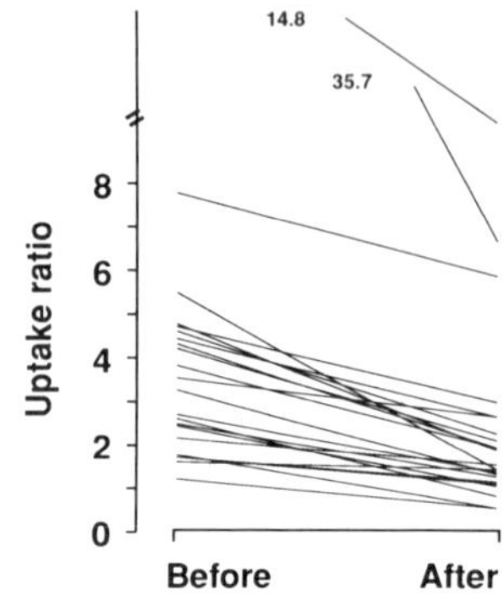

FIGURE 10.6. The effect of clodronate on scintigraphic uptake. Uptake was assessed from bone scans as the ratio of uptake at an affected site to that of a corresponding unaffected contralateral site using the same area of interest. Treatment (800–1,600 mg daily) was associated with a significant decrease in uptake ratio (5.32 ± SEM 1.5 to 2.39 ± 0.45; $P < 0.05$) 2–4 months after the beginning of treatment.

ance to clodronate has not been described, and the response to retreatment is similar.

There are few reported side effects. These include mild intestinal intolerance with treatment by mouth and transient proteinuria during intravenous infusion. Gastrointestinal intolerance is dose dependent and is nearly always resolved by dividing the daily dose.[24]

A potential concern with the bisphosphonates is their effects on the mineralization of bone. As mentioned previously, a problem with the use of etidronate has been the narrow range between the effective dose (to inhibit bone resorption) and the dose that inhibits mineralization. Decreased rates of mineralization induce osteomalacia and, if prolonged, increase the risk of fracture. Long-term studies with clodronate have shown no adverse effect of the drug on the mineralization of bone (Table 10.1). Bone formation rates decrease in pagetic bone but decrease to normal rather than to low values. Even when high doses of clodronate are given by intravenous infusion mineralization is not impaired, in sharp contrast to high doses of etidronate or to IV infusion of etidronate[6,14,23] (Figure 10.7). Clodronate thus fulfills a major requirement for a new generation of bisphosphonates.

There have been concerns that the use of clodronate may induce leukemia, and the occurrence of three cases (excluding a diagnostic error) led to the suspension of clinical studies in the United States in 1981. Since the suspension of these studies, no new cases of leukemia have been reported and many additional hundreds of patients have received clodronate without adverse effects in the rest of the world. These observations, together with predisposing factors identified in two of the three patients reported, indicated that the association was coincidental. In addition, studies of the long-term effects of clodronate on chromosomal damage have shown no increased incidence of chromosome or chromatid breaks.[25]

TABLE 10.2 Comparison of Five Treatment Regimens with Two Bisphosphonates*

Agent	Daily dose	Duration, months	Patients, Number	Responding, %	Normalizing, %†	Relapse-free, %†	
						1 year	2 years
Etidronate	5–10 mg/kg	6	24	71‡	65	61	15
	20 mg/kg	1	19	95	57	62	29
	20 mg/kg	6	41	95	59	51	20
Clodronate	800 mg	6	18	89	69	66	37
	1,600 mg	6	45	100	60	90‡	60‡
	1,600 mg	1	20	90	44	64	27

*There were no significant differences in disease activity between patients before treatment. Note that fewer patients responded given etidronate 5-10mg/kg/day for 6 months than with other regimens as judged by a 25% or greater decrease in disease activity. However, in patients in whom a response was evoked a similar proportion attained normal values of alkaline phosphatase (1).

†Proportion of patients who responded to treatment (i.e., excludes nonresponders).

‡Denotes significantly different results from other treatments.

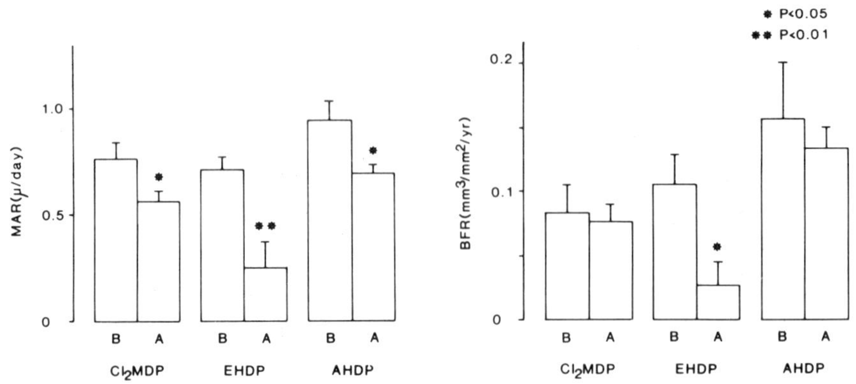

FIGURE 10.7. Effects of three bisphosphonates, clodronate, etidronate, and aminohexane bisphosphonate, on mean mineral apposition rate and bone formation rate. Rates were calculated before treatment and after intravenous treatment. Note the inhibitory effect of intravenous etidronate on mineralization. Neither AHDP nor Cl_2MDP decreased values below normal. Cl_2MDP, clodronate; EHDP, etidronate; AHDP, aminohexane bisphosphonate; MAR, mean mineral apposition rate; BFR, bone formation rate; B, before treatment; A, after intravenous treatment.

OTHER NEW BISPHOSPHONATES

Recently, four new bisphosphonates have been used experimentally in Paget's disease: tiludronic acid (4-chlorophenyl)-thiomethylene bisphosphonate alendronate, dimethylaminopropylidene bisphosphonate (dimethyl APD), aminohexane bisphosphonate (AHDP), and aminobutane bisphosphonate (ABDP)[15,16,26,27] (Figure 10.8).

Preliminary results with tiludronate using oral doses of 200 to 400 mg daily have suggested less complete suppression of Paget's disease than is commonly observed with clodronate.[26,28] The degree of response is similar to the effects of calcitonin (Figure 10.9). More recent but as yet unpublished data suggest that higher doses induce more complete effects.

The new amino derivatives appear to be highly potent agents. Daily intravenous infusions of ABDP for 5 days induce a dose-dependent suppression of disease activity over the range of 2.5 to 10 mg daily (Figure 10.10). Bone turnover decreases as expected of a bisphosphonate, with an early decrease in hydroxyproline and a later decrease in bone formation. Histologic studies have shown that the newly formed bone is lamellar in structure and that the rate of mineralization is not impaired.[16] The drug may also be given by mouth, and an oral formulation is currently being tested. With the exception of fever, no adverse effects have been observed.

A febrile reaction is observed in a minority of patients together with the other changes expected of an acute-phase response in much the same

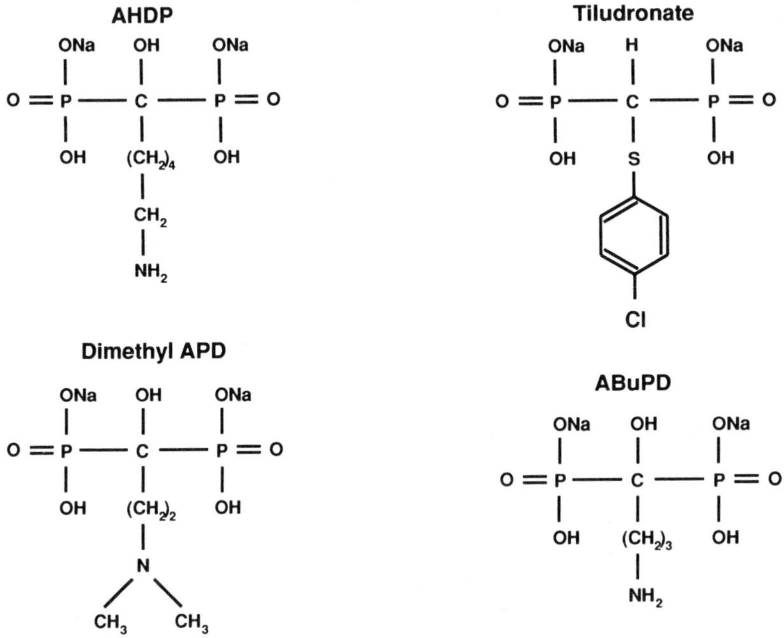

FIGURE 10.8. Structural formula of new bisphosphonates being tested for the treatment of Paget's disease.

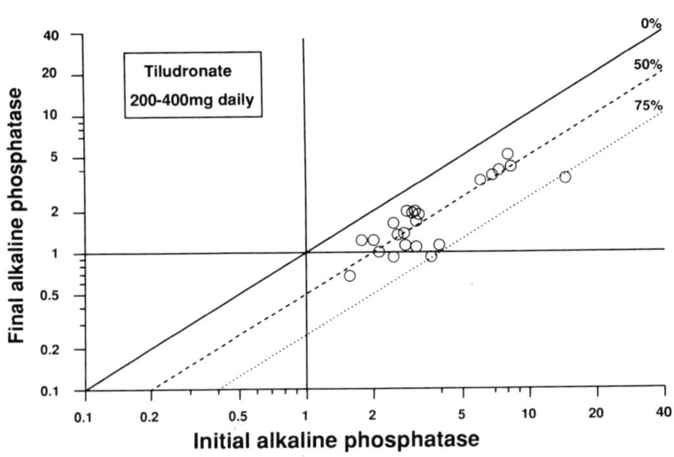

FIGURE 10.9. Serum activity of alkaline phosphatase (expressed as multiples of the normal range) before and after treatment with tiludronate 200–400 mg daily by mouth for 6 months. Compare Figure 10.5.[28]

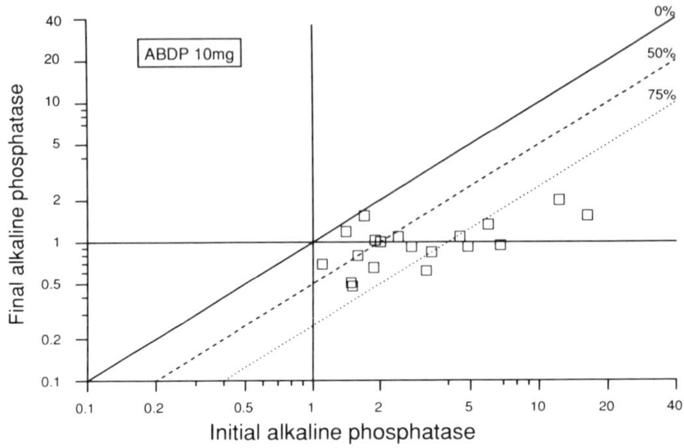

FIGURE 10.10. Serum activity of alkaline phosphatase before and after intravenous aminobutane bisphosphonate given daily for 5 days at a daily dose of 10 mg. See legend to Figure 10.5 for further explanation.

way as is observed with pamidronate. These include transient leukopenia, which is evident within 24 hours, particularly in the lymphocyte fraction, and is followed by a fall in neutrophils. The effect appears to be transient. It is of interest that even large doses do not consistently induce fever, though changes in white cell count are consistently observed.

It has been suggested that reexposure of patients to fever-inducing bisphosphonates does not induce a second reaction. A fever after a single infusion does not recur when further infusions are given, for example, weekly. Such desensitization does not appear to be permanent, however, and reexposure some months or years later may result in a further reaction. The mechanisms responsible for fever and leukopenia are unknown, but it is thought that this represents an acute-phase reaction and is associated with the expected changes in acute-phase proteins. The clinical significance of these effects is not known, but, in terms of the patient, it induces a mild flulike reaction that may persist for 1 or 2 days.

AHDP is ten time less potent than ABDP. A daily dose of 400 mg by mouth for 1 to 3 months induces marked biochemical suppression and healing of osteolysis and does not impair the mineralization of bone (Figure 10.7). Similar effects are reported with five daily intravenous infusions of 25 to 50 mg.[15] These regimens do not induce fever or lymphopenia, but higher intravenous doses (such as 75 mg intravenously) have been reported to induce fever in some patients.

Many other bisphosphonates are likely to become available shortly for testing in Paget's disease, but much more work is required to determine whether they offer advantages over the bisphosphonates currently being used or evaluated.

Comparative Aspects

Few studies have directly compared the efficacy of different treatments, and in many cases there is little information on dose response for any one treatment. In addition, there are problems reviewed elsewhere in the assessment of treatments between different centers.[1,29] In general, there is a remarkable similarity in response among bisphosphonates, as judged by changes in biochemical indexes of disease activity. As is the case for other therapeutic modalities, the proportion of patients in whom disease activity is restored to normal depends on the initial disease activity and dose. With extensive disease a higher proportion of patients attain normal values with bisphosphonates than with calcitonins. As the new bisphosphonates become available, the choice of bisphosphonate is likely to depend more on their side effects and ease of use than on differences in their efficacy as judged by the degree of disease suppression.

Despite the similarities of many treatment regimens in the degree of biochemical suppression of disease activity, there appear to be some differences, not only in the proportion of patients attaining a remission but in the duration of the response evoked. In general, short treatments appear to yield less prolonged remissions (Table 10.2). In addition, the length of remission appears to be related in part to the degree of suppression of Paget's disease induced over the first few months of treatment. Thus, in those patients who attain normal activity of alkaline phosphatase, remission is more prolonged irrespective of extent of disease activity.[1] This effect has some analogies with tumor chemotherapy in the sense that the greater the decrease in tumor burden the longer the remission expected. The more durable remissions obtained in Paget's disease in patients with the more complete biochemical responses may reflect the ablation of an abnormal osteoclast population. This suggests that treatment strategies for the future should include meticulous attention to maximal suppression of disease activity.

If the degree of disease suppression is a valid criterion of efficacy, then clodronate and the amino bisphosphonates seem to be the most effective. If the duration of remission is important, the most impressive long-term remissions have thus far been observed with clodronate. The extent to which biochemical control can be equated with clinical benefit is considered later.

CLINICAL EFFECTS OF TREATMENT

The aims of treatment are not to suppress abnormal biochemical or scintigraphic findings but to treat or prevent the complications that arise from Paget's disease (Table 10.3). The question arises whether or not the bio-

TABLE 10.3 Clinical Features and Complications of Paget's Disease

Common
Bone pain
Pagetic
Articular
Fracture
Long bones, vertebral bodies
Neurologic
Deafness
Deformity and enlargement of bones
Uncommon
Pain
Fissure fracture
Spinal neurologic syndrome
Hypercalcemia and calciuria of immobilization or fracture
Cardiovascular disease
Vascular bleeding from bone during surgery
Extraskeletal calcification
Urolithiasis
Rare
Gout
Epidural hematoma
Osteosarcoma and other bone tumors
Cranial nerve lesions (except VIII)
Brain stem and cerebellar syndromes
Hypercalcemia
Extramedullary hematopoiesis
Significance uncertain
Pseudogout
Angioid streaks
Hyperparathyroidism

chemical control of Paget's disease modifies the clinical consequences of the disorder. A great deal of evidence suggests that this is so.[29,30]

Pain

Pain is the most common complication of Paget's disease, but its cause is heterogeneous. Pain of bone origin may respond to simple analgesics or to one of the nonsteroidal antiinflammatory drugs. We prefer to give bisphosphonates for bone pain since a short treatment may induce prolonged pain relief. Pain relief has been noted in the vast majority of patients treated with the bisphosphonates reviewed. Most studies of Paget's disease report improvement in approximately 80% of patients, but there is a wide variation in response, almost certainly reflecting the different causes of pain. There have been no placebo-controlled trials with the new bisphosphonates in Paget's disease, but the persistence of pain relief suggests that in most instances it is not a placebo effect.[14,17,19] In addition, controlled studies of clodronate in other painful bone disorders have shown effects on bone pain significantly greater than any placebo response.[31-33] In Paget's disease pain relief with clodronate generally occurs later than with the calcitonins and may not be observed until several months after the start of treatment. In this respect it is interesting that the rate of decrease in bone blood flow induced by the bisphosphonates is also slower than that with calcitonin, suggesting a vascular basis for bone pain.

A common cause of pain in Paget's disease is osteoarthritis. Great difficulties may arise in distinguishing pain due to Paget's disease from pain due to osteoarthritis. We commonly give courses of specific treatment and reassess pain once disease activity has been adequately controlled. We have been surprised by the number of patients with pain thought to be due to osteoarthritis in whom a significant and sustained remission from pain was obtained by medical treatment.

In patients in whom osteoarthritis is of sufficient severity, surgical intervention is indicated. Pagetic bone is, however, highly vascular, and bleeding may be profuse.[33] For this reason it has been suggested that pretreatment of underlying Paget's disease would be advantageous to decrease bone blood flow before surgery.[34] In addition, it is possible that the outcome of surgery might be improved by prolonged preoperative and postoperative treatment maintaining a more normal bone quality, but this topic has not been specifically studied.

Bone Quality, Enlargement, and Deformity

The decrease in bone turnover induced by the bisphosphonates reviewed here is associated with a resumption of lamellar rather than woven bone formation. In addition, the new bone formed is normally mineralized. If lamellar bone formation were to continue with adequate long-term management and be subject to the normal factors that regulate bone modeling and remodeling, it might be supposed that long-term treatment would result in a gradual improvement of bony enlargement and deformity. Such improvement in skeletal architecture would, however, be a slow process.

Few centers have been involved in the systematic radiographic assessment of the response of Paget's disease to treatment.[35,36] These have mainly examined the effects of the calcitonins and pamidronate. Such studies have shown reductions in bone size, widening of the medullary cavity, improved corticomedullary differentiation, more uniform cortical density, and halt of the resorption front. Similar but anecdotal observations indicate a comparable effect of the new bisphosphonates. In particular, both clodronate and ABDP halt the resorption front and increase skeletal radiodensity.[13,29,37] When relapse occurs after bisphosphonate treatment, there may be a characteristic rim of radiotranslucency evident at the site of advance of the resorption front.

In our own studies we have been interested in whether deformity may regress. For this purpose we have undertaken sequential stereophotography of superficial bony sites of the skull and face.[29,38] These studies indicate that long-term suppression of disease activity by the bisphosphonates is associated with decrease in skull or facial volume and restoration of a more normal shape (Figure 10.11). Comparable changes are not observed at sites unaffected by Paget's disease. These observations have extremely important implications for the long-term medical management of Paget's dis-

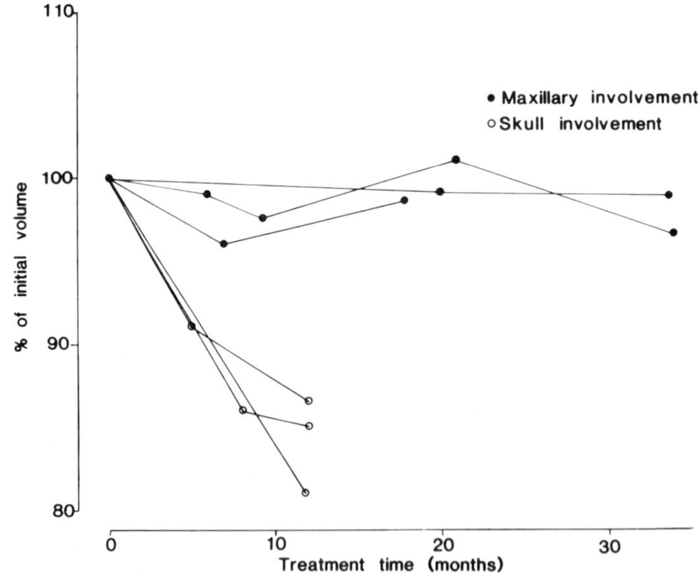

FIGURE 10.11. Effects of suppression of disease activity in six patients with Paget's disease treated with bisphosphonates. Three patients with Paget's disease affecting the anterior skull vault (open circle) showed a decrease in volume, whereas skull volume did not change in those patients with Paget's disease elsewhere (closed circle).[38]

ease. Not only may progressive deformity be arrested but adequate modeling of bone may also occur.

Fracture

There is no convincing evidence that medical treatment, either with the calcitonins, the bisphosphonates, or mithramycin, significantly alters the natural history of fissure fractures. The effects of medical treatment on the natural history of complete fractures is also uncertain and has not been well investigated, principally because of the large patient numbers that would be required to be studied. However, the risk of fracture appears to be increased in the presence of marked osteolytic disease, particularly of the lower limb, and the reversal of such abnormalities with the new bisphosphonates suggests that fracture frequency is likely to be decreased. Apparently normal rates of fracture healing have been observed in patients given clodronate immediately before their fracture or throughout their conservative management.[20]

Neurologic Syndromes

No long-term studies are yet available for the new bisphosphonates, with the exception of clodronate. Until recently most patients with progressive spinal syndromes underwent surgery, and this appears to have been beneficial in about 85% of patients. There is now considerable evidence to suggest that effective medical management with the bisphosphonates can improve spinal neurologic syndromes.[17,24,39] The response in these syndromes is comparable to that observed after laminectomy without the hazards of surgical intervention and without the mortality. After medical treatment the clinical improvement correlates remarkably with the degree of disease activity, as judged by biochemical estimates of bone turnover, and provides perhaps the most convincing evidence for the relationship between the clinical and biochemical indexes of disease activity.

The rate of neurologic improvement seen with bisphosphonates (and calcitonins) is surprisingly rapid (Figure 10.12), occurring within days or weeks of beginning of treatment. It is not, therefore, associated with changes in spinal canal diameter. The rapidity of response to medical treatment suggests that the response cannot have been due to the remodeling of bone, but rather to decrease in soft tissue swelling or to redistribution of blood flow. The latter mechanism is consistent with a known anatomic relationship between blood supply to the vertebrae and that to the spinal cord.

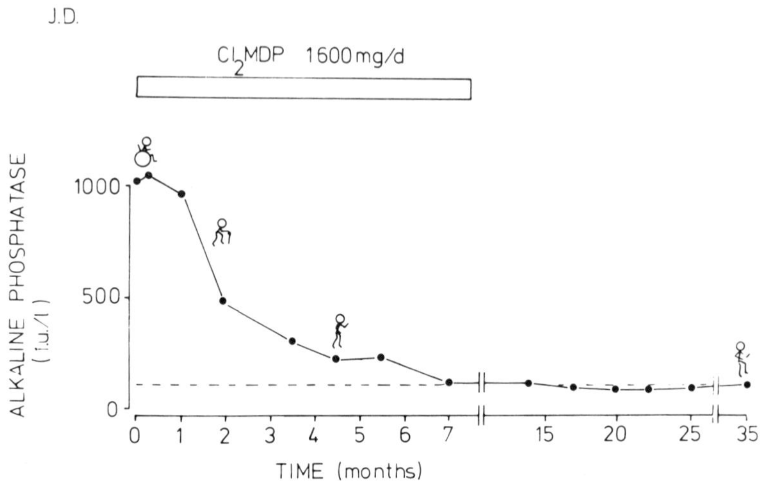

FIGURE 10.12. Sequential changes in alkaline phosphatase in a patient with slowly progressive paraparesis. Motor power improved within 1 month and was completely restored by 5 months. The patient has remained in remission now for 11 years.[24]

Sarcoma

There is no evidence that medical treatment alters the natural history of established sarcoma.

Other Complications

Immobilization bone loss and hypercalciuria and hypercalcemia have been effectively treated with clodronate. In the presence of coexisting hyperparathyroidism, the fall in serum calcium may be incomplete and may alert the physician to associated primary hyperparathyroidism.

Paget's disease significantly increases the cardiac output when the disorder is extensive. Since this is largely due to an increase in bone blood flow, a decrease in vascularity resulting from treatment decreases bone blood flow.

CONCLUSIONS

Despite the difficulties of assessing the effects of medical treatment on the complications of Paget's disease, it is now clear that the new bisphosphonates are capable of inducing marked suppression of disease activity and that this suppression can be maintained for many months or years after the

TABLE 10.4 Suggested Indications for Bisphosphonate Treatment of Paget's Disease

Indication	Evidence of Efficacy
Long-term suppression of disease activity	
Progressive neurologic syndromes	
Vascular steal	Yes, rapid improvement
Cord compression	Yes, slow improvement
Root compression	Yes, probable slow improvement
Nerve compression, deafness, and tinnitus	Rarely improves
Progressive deformity of skull or weight-bearing bones, especially in young	Likely
Healing of fissure fractures	Unproven but unlikely
Prophylaxis	
Juvenile hyperphosphatasia	Unproven but likely
Familial expansile osteolysis	Unproven but likely
Severe disease in young patients	Unproven but likely
Extensive osteolysis in weight-bearing long bones	Yes
In preparation for orthopedic surgery (more stable or normal skeletal environment)	Unproven but likely
High-output cardiac failure	Yes
Reduced risk of fracture	Unproven but likely
Short-term treatment	
Bone pain	Yes
Immobilization hypercalcemia and hypercalciuria and bone loss	Yes, not with etidronate
Before orthopedic surgery (to decrease bone vascularity)	Anecdotal but bone blood flow known to diminish
Improve fracture healing	No evidence
Sarcoma	No evidence

end of treatment. The new bisphosphonates thus far tested do not adversely affect mineralization of bone at the doses that effectively suppress bone turnover. In this respect they represent a significant advance over etidronate. Once relapse has occurred, retreatment induces a similar response. The suppression of disease activity is associated with histologic and radiographic improvements, and increasing evidence suggests that suppression of disease activity is associated with marked clinical benefit (Table 10.4). The most convincing and dramatic examples are the sustained remission from neurologic syndromes and the alteration in bone shape induced by clodronate. Nevertheless, a need clearly exists for well-designed long-term prospective studies to determine the optimal manner of using the new bisphosphonates and to determine whether or not the long-term suppression of disease activity now attainable decreases the incidence of other complications, particularly of fracture.

ACKNOWLEDGMENTS

Our studies in Paget's disease have been supported by the Medical Research Council, Norwich Eaton Pharmaceutical Industries, Merck Sharp and Dohme, Rorer Central Research, and Huhtamaki Oy Leiras.

REFERENCES

1. Gray RES, Yates AJP, Preston CJ, et al: Duration of effect of oral diphosphonate therapy in Paget's disease of bone. *Q J Med* 1987;64:755–767.
2. Russell RGG, Smith R, Preston C, et al: Diphosphonates in Paget's disease. *Lancet* 1974;1:894–898.
3. Canfield R, Rosner W, Skinner J, et al: Diphosphonate therapy of Paget's disease of bone. *J Clin Endocrinol Metab* 1977;44:96–106.
4. Siris ES, Canfield RE, Jacobs TE, et al: Long-term therapy of Paget's disease of bone with EHDP. *Arthritis Rheum* 1980;23:1177–1183.
5. Preston CJ, Yates AJP, Beneton MNC, et al: Effective short term treatment of Paget's disease with oral etidronate. *Br Med J* 1986;292:79–80.
6. Kanis JA, Urwin GH, Gray RES, et al: Effects of intravenous etidronate disodium on skeletal and calcium metabolism. *Am J Med* 1987;82(suppl 2A):55–70.
7. Fleisch H: Experimental basis for the use of bisphosphonates in Paget's disease of bone. *Clin Orthop* 1987;217:72–78.
8. Fleisch H: Bisphosphonates: Mechanisms of action and clinical applications, in Peck WA (ed): *Bone and Mineral Research Annual 1.* Amsterdam, Excerpta Medica, 1989; pp 319–357.
9. Shinoda H, Adamek G, Felix R, et al: Structure-activity relationship of various bisphosphonates. *Calcif Tissue Int* 1983;35:87–99.
10. Yakatan GL, Poynor WJ, Talbert RL, et al: Clodronate kinetics and bioavailability. *Clin Pharmacol Ther* 19892;31:402–410.
11. Fogelman I, Smith L, Mazess R, et al: Absorption of oral diphosphonate in normal subjects. *Clin Endocrinol* 1986;24:57–62.
12. Harinck HIJ, Bijvoet OLM, Blanksma HJ, Dahlinghaus-Nienhuys PJ: Efficacious management with aminobisphophonate (APD) in Paget's disease of bone. *Clin Orthop* 1987; 217:79–98.
13. Michael WR, King WR, Wakim JM: Metabolism of disodium ethane-1-hydroxy-1,1-diphosphonate (disodium etidronate) in the rat, rabbit, dog, and monkey. *Toxicol Appl Pharmacol* 1972;21:503–515.

14. Yates AJP, Percival RC, Gray RES, et al: Intravenous clodronate in the treatment and retreatment of Paget's disease of bone. *Lancet* 1985;1:474-477.
15. Atkins RM, Yates AJP, Gray RES, et al: Aminohexane disphosphonate in the treatment of Paget's disease of bone. *J Bone Mineral Res* 1987;2:273-279.
16. O'Docherty DP, Bickerstaff DR, McCloskey EV, et al: The treatment of Paget's disease with aminobutylidene diphosphonate. *J Bone Mineral Res* In Press.
17. Delmas PD, Chapuy MC, Vignon E, et al: Long-term effects of dichloromethylene diphosphonate in Paget's disease of bone. *J Clin Endocrinol Metab* 1982;54:837-844.
18. Meunier PJ, Salson C, Mathieu L, et al: Skeletal distribution of Paget's disease. *Clin Orthop* 1987;217:37-44.
19. Douglas DL, Duckworth T, Kanis JA, et al: Biochemical and clinical response to dichloromethylene diphosphonate (Cl2MDP) in Paget's disease of bone. *Arthritis Rheum* 1980;23:1185-1192.
20. Meunier PJ, Alexandre C, Edouard C, et al: Effects of disodium dichloromethylene diphosphonate on Paget's disease of bone. *Lancet* 1979;2:489-492.
21. Espinasse D, Mathieu L, Alexandre C, et al: The kinetics of 99mTc labelled EHDP in Paget's disease before and after dichloromethylene-diphosphonate treatment. *Metab Bone Dis* 1981;2:321-324.
22. Chapuy MC, Charon SA, Meunier PJ: Sustained biochemical effects of short treatment of Paget's disease of bone with dichloromethylene diphosphonate. *Metab Bone Dis* 1983;4:325-328.
23. McCloskey EV, Yates AJP, Beneton MNC, et al: Comparative effects of intravenous diphosphonates on calcium and skeletal metabolism in man. *Bone* 1987;8(suppl 1): 35-42.
24. Douglas DL, Duckworth T, Kanis JA, et al: Spinal cord dysfunction in Paget's disease of bone: Has medical treatment a vascular basis? *J Bone Joint Surg* 1981;63-B:495-503.
25. Borgstrom GH, Elomaa I, Blomqvist C, Porkka L: Cytogenetic investigations of patients on clodronate therapy for Paget's disease of bone. *Bone* 1987;8(suppl 1):85-86.
26. Reginster JY, Lecart MP, Deroisy R, et al: Treatment of Paget's disease of bone with high oral doses of oral tiludronate given during a five-day course therapy. *J Bone Mineral Res* 1990;5(suppl 2):170.
27. Papapoulos SE, Frolisch M, Hoekman K, Bijvoet OLM: Dimethyl-APD treatment modifies osteoblastic function in patients with Paget's disease. *Calcif Tissue Int* 1989; 44(suppl):s108.
28. Reginster JY, Jeugmans-Huynen AM, Albert A, et al: One year's treatment of Paget's disease of bone by synthetic salmon calcitonin as a nasal spray. *J Bone Mineral Res* 1988;3:249-252.
29. Kanis JA, Heynen G, Paterson A, et al: Endogenous secretion of calcitonin in physiological and pathological conditions, in Pecile A (ed): *Calcitonin.* Amsterdam, Elsevier, 1985, pp 81-88.
30. Kanis JA, Gray RES, McCloskey EV: Treating Paget's disease. *Br Med J* 1987; 294:1612-1613
31. Elomaa I, Blomqvist C, Grohn P, et al: Long-term controlled trial with diphosphonate in patients with osteolytic bone metastases. *Lancet* 1983;1:146-149.
32. Siris ES, Hyman GA, Canfield RE: Effects of dichloromethylene diphosphonate in women with breast carcinoma metastatic to the skeleton. *Am J Med* 1983;74:401.
33. Dove J: Complete fractures of the femur in Paget's disease of bone. *J Bone Joint Surg* 1980;62B:12-17.
34. Bowie HIC, Kanis JA: Calcitonin in the assessment and preparation of patients with Paget's disease for surgery, in Kanis JA (ed): *Bone Disease and Calcitonin.* Eastbourne, England, Armour Pharmaceutical, 1977, pp 61-69.

35. Doyle FH, Banks LM, Pennock JM: Radiologic observations on bone resorption in Paget's disease. *Arthritis Rheum* 1980;23:1205–1214.
36. Nagant de Deuxchaisnes C, Rombouts-Lindemans C, Huaux JP, et al: Treatment of Paget's disease with the diphosphonate APD: A biological and radiological study, in Donath A, Courvoisier B (eds): *Diphosphonates and Bone.* Geneva, Editions Medicine et Hygiene, 1982, pp 303–327.
37. Altman RD: Long-term follow up of therapy with intermittent etidronate disodium in Paget's disease of bone. *Am J Med* 1985;79:583–590.
38. Bickerstaff D, Douglas DL, Burke PH, et al: Improvement in facial deformity of Paget's disease treated with diphosphonates. *J Bone Joint Surg* 1990;728:132–136.
39. Douglas DL, Kanis JA, Duckworth T, et al: Paget's disease: Improvement of spinal cord dysfunction with diphosphonates and calcitonin. *Metab Bone Dis* 1981;3:327–336.

CHAPTER **11**

Alternative Modes of Administration of Salmon Calcitonin in Paget's Disease of Bone

Charles Nagant de Deuxchaisnes and Jean-Pierre Devogelaer

Calcitonin (CT) has an antiosteolytic action[1] with a clear therapeutic role in the treatment of Paget's disease as well as the prevention and treatment of osteoporosis.[2–4] The parenteral mode of administration of CT is a deterrent to its use in both Paget's disease and osteoporosis and is even less unacceptable in the prevention of osteoporosis. The advent of a nasal spray of salmon CT (SCT), which was studied in human volunteers for the first time in our unit in May 1983 and shown to have bioactivity,[5,6] has opened a new frontier in the therapeutic application of this peptide. Although the main purposes of intranasal insufflation of SCT (INSCT) are prevention and treatment of osteoporosis, Paget's disease of bone remains the model by which it is possible to judge its effectiveness, by monitoring parameters of bone turnover. This is an exceedingly reliable method to test the efficacy of INSCT and allows comparison of different doses as well as different forms of INSCT (with or without absorption promoters).

There are also other ways of administering SCT, such as intrarectal administration (IRSCT) by suppository. We also tested this mode of administration in our unit on both volunteers and patients with Paget's disease, and the preliminary results have been published.[6] We have used various suppositories with various excipients, and although these studies are still in progress, the findings for the first two formulations of the suppository will also be reported.

NASAL SPRAY

The nostril has at least two physiologic functions: respiration (80%) and olfaction (20%). However, the nasal mucosa is being used increasingly for drug administration, especially of small peptides, despite poor mucosal permeability and rapid clearance of peptide drugs from the mucosal surface. This trend began with antidiuretic hormone (synthetic lysine vasopressin) and has continued with luteinizing hormone-releasing hormone (LH-RH), insulin, glucagon, growth hormone-releasing hormone (GH-RH), corticotropin-releasing hormone (CRH), propanolol, gentamicin, and oxytocin, among others. Since the absorption of a peptide by the nasal mucosa is inversely related to its molecular weight, effective nasal absorption of CT bearing 32 residues cannot be taken for granted. Even short peptides (10 amino acids or fewer), which should be ideal candidates for effective nasal absorption, may have low bioavilability, for example, 1% for LH-RH and 6% for desmapressin, an analogue of vasopressin. Larger polypeptides such as GH-RH (44 residues) and CRH (41 residues) are even less well absorbed (0.2% to 0.6% and 0.1% to 1.0%, respectively). This subject has been reviewed recently by Pontiroli et al.[7]

The first attempts to administer CT intranasally in Paget's disease were made more than a decade ago by Ziegler et al,[8] using human CT (HCT), but with poor results at the dosage employed (0.5 mg/d), which was similar to the dosage commonly used parenterally. Later, SCT, which is more potent[9] by a factor of 20 to 40 and has a longer biologic half-life,[10] higher affinity for the CT receptors on the osteoclasts,[11] and lower susceptibility to oxidation than HCT, was prepared as an aerolized water solution and administered as a nasal spray. It is this spray that we initially tested.[5,6]

To increase the absorption of CT by the nasal mucosa, absorption enhancers, such as bile salts or their derivatives, can be added. Better absorption by the nasal mucosa is then achieved at the expense of local tolerance. There is a subtle balance to be achieved between enhanced absorption and local irritation. Sodium glycocholate has been used as a surfactant in conjunction with HCT,[12] giving rise to a surprisingly similar plasma peak concentration for intranasal versus intravenous administration. Besides using a plain spray, we have tested a spray with 1% sodium taurocholate as a surfactant.

Use of SCT Nasal Spray with 1% Sodium Taurocholate as an Absorption Promoter

Eighteen patients with Paget's disease were given the nasal spray during a 3-month period. They had not received specific antipagetic therapy for at least 6 months before treatment. Six patients received 100 IU/d, six 200 IU/d (100 IU in each nostril), and six 400 IU/d (100 IU in each nostril twice daily); these patients were referred to as the IN groups. Another five patients, referred to as the SC group, were treated by subcutaneous injections of 100 IU daily. Subjects were randomly assigned to the various treatment groups. The baseline level of alkaline phosphatase (AP) was determined on two occasions 2 weeks apart before the trial was begun. The coefficient of variation between these two measurements was 6.5 ± 1.1%. Initial AP levels (upper limit of normal 60 IU/L) were 265 ± 100 (range: 115 to 735), 174 ± 32 (range: 112 to 313), 249 ± 51 (range: 132 to 388), and 208 ± 46 IU/L (range: 122 to 355) in the four groups. These initial levels were not statistically different as determined by Mann-Whitney U-test.

Figure 11.1 shows the striking effect of the nasal spray on the AP level, irrespective of the dosage given and the mode of administration. In all groups, significance was achieved after 4 weeks for therapy (Wilcoxon

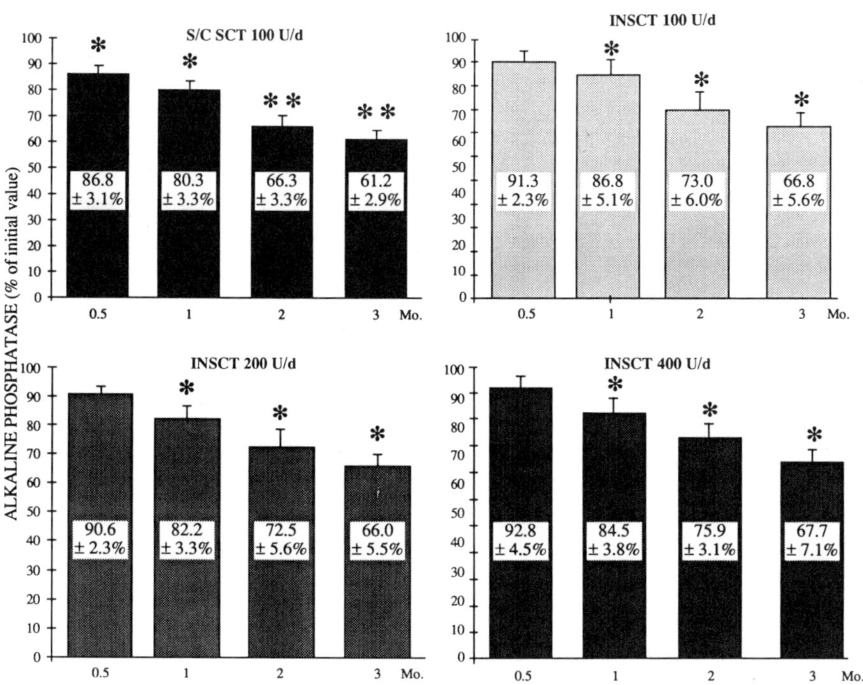

FIGURE 11.1. The effect of nasal spray of SCT (INSCT) with 1% taurocholate as surfactant (in three different dosages), as compared with a subcutaneous (SC) injections in patients with Paget's disease.*$P < 0.05$, **$P < 0.01$.

matched-pairs signed-rank test for the data for the IN groups and Student's paired *t* test for the SC group). The downward trend continued without evidence that a nadir had been reached. Figure 11.2 shows the individual responses after 3 months of therapy. If a 30% or greater decrease in AP is taken as an acceptable response, according to Russell et al,[13] a decrease in AP of 15% or less is essentially no response, and a decrease of 15% to 30% is an intermediate response, then for the entire group there were only two nonresponders (one receiving 200 IU and one receiving 400 IU daily intranasally). Thus 11% of those using the nasal spray did not respond. There were six other individuals with an intermediate response (three on 100 IU, one on 200 IU, and two on 400 IU daily), that is, 33% of all those on nasal spray. However, there was no indication that the continuing decrease in the AP level would not have put them among the acceptable responders had the therapy not been discontinued. In any event, 56% of those on the nasal spray were acceptable responders, as were all five on the daily subcutaneous injections.

Another way to look at the data is to divide the patients according to whether or not they have ever had therapy with SCT, as did Levy et al.[14] Among the 18 patients treated with INSCT, 10 had had parenteral SCT therapy before the study and 8 had not. The results obtained in these two

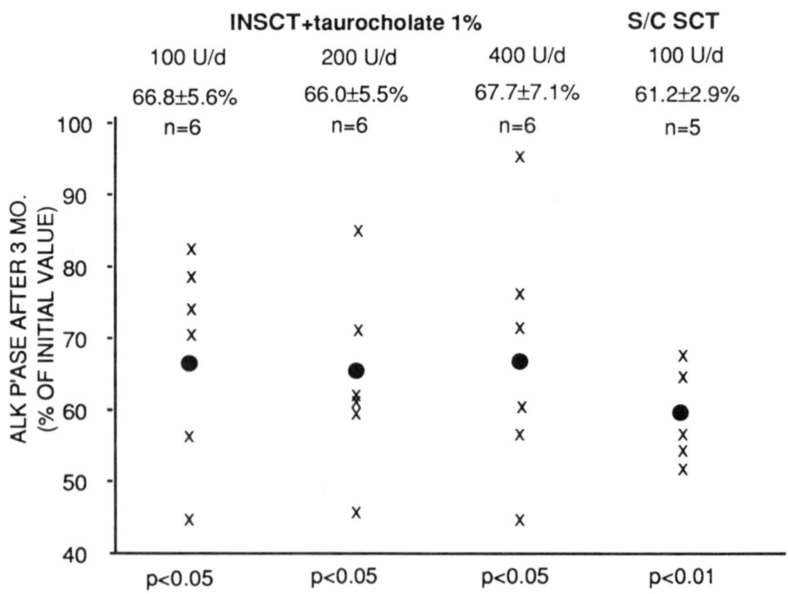

FIGURE 11.2. Individual and average results for the alkaline phosphatase after 3 months of therapy in the four groups defined in the caption for Figure 11.1.

groups were exactly the same: the AP level decreased to 66.0 ± 3.6% of initial value at 3 months for the pretreated group, versus 66.4 ± 5.7% for the group who had never been treated previously. Not only did previous therapy with SCT seem irrelevant, but previous therapy with EHDP (2 patients) did not seem to affect the efficacy of the spray since in these patients the AP levels at 3 months were 57% and 46% of the initial value, respectively. One course of EHDP had lasted 6 months and had been given 15 months earlier, and the other had lasted 4 months and had been given 4 years earlier. Treatment outcome was also unaffected in a patient who had a 6-month course of treatment with APD 4 years earlier. In this patient, the AP value was at 71% of the initial value at 3 months.

Stored patient sera were sent to Dr. F. R. Singer at the Bone Center of the Cedars-Sinai Medical Center, Los Angeles, California, for SCT antibody analysis. The presence or absence of SCT antibodies was determined in 8 patients at the onset of intranasal therapy, 1 of whom had positive findings. In 10 patients studied at the end of intranasal therapy, 6 had a positive result. One of these (on 400 IU) had a high antibody titer (>1 : 1,000). Six pairs of sera before and after 3 months of intranasal therapy were tested, 4 of which continued to yield negative results. One initially antibody-negative patient became antibody positive, and 1 increased his titer. If we compare the 4 patients without antibodies at 3 months with the 7 patients with antibodies (final AP; 66.9 ± 8.7% of initial value versus 71.9 ± 4.5%), there was no significant difference in response. Among the 5 patients in the SC group, three pairs of sera were available. Results of one remained negative for SCT antibodies, results of one became positive, and one pair showed increased positivity. Figure 11.3 shows the AP levels at 3 months for the patients whose SCT antibody status was determined.

In this short-term study, it did not appear to matter whether the patients had antibodies or not, nor whether they had been pretreated with parenteral SCT. It is possible that when SCT penetrates the nasal mucosa in high concentrations, it overcomes existing antibodies, which under these circumstances may not yet have neutralizing capacity. An alternative hypothesis is that the study was too short for the effect of the antibodies to manifest themselves. Whether their presence forebodes later resistance remains an unanswered question.

The classical systemic side effects of calcitonin were recorded in two patients on subcutaneous SCT (1 nausea, 1 flushing) but were transient and not severe. These side effects were also encountered in 4 patients on the nasal spray (2 on 100 IU, 1 on 200 IU, and 1 on 400 IU daily), that is, in 22%. The side effects were mild and transient. Two patients complained of both nausea and flushing, 1 of nausea only, and 1 of flushing only. Three

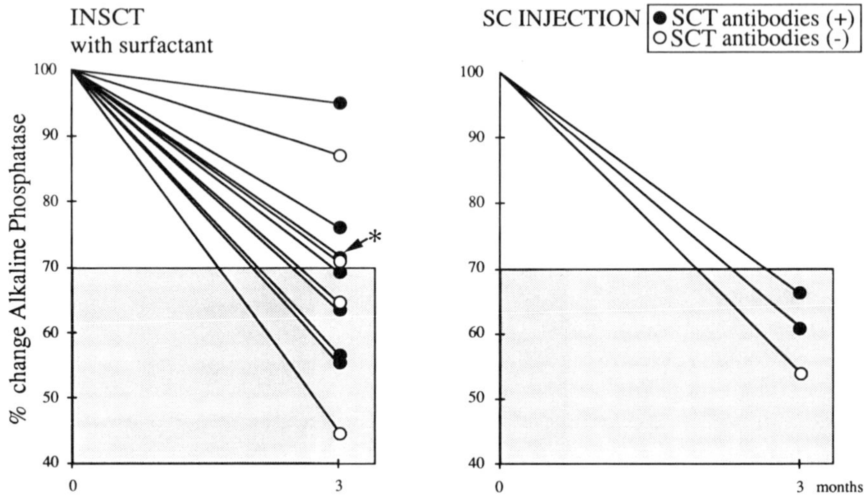

FIGURE 11.3. Individual changes of alkaline phosphatase after 3 months in those patients, in whom SCT antibodies could be determined at the end of the trial. x = high antibody titer (>1/1000). Shaded area is considered a satisfactory response (a decrease of at least 30% of initial value).

of these 4 patients were acceptable responders; the fourth had an intermediate response. As far as local irritation is concerned, only 4 patients (22%) had no adverse effects during the 3 months of intranasal administration. The other 14 complained of nose itching ($n = 7$), sneezing ($n = 12$), tears ($n = 2$), rhinorrhea ($n = 3$), or nasal obstruction ($n = 1$). These symptoms were often mild and transient, lasting a few seconds to a few minutes. Although no patient dropped out of the study, this high incidence of nasal side effects was considered unacceptable, and the nasal spray with 1% taurocholate was withdrawn from experimentation. The bile salts and their derivatives are excellent absorption promoters but are also ciliotoxic.[15] Taurocholate is less ciliotoxic than glycocholate,[15] the surfactant used by Pontiroli and colleagues[12] at a concentration of 15 mg in 0.5 ml of water, which enhances the bioavailability of HCT from approximately 3% to 27%.[7] This surfactant appears to be sufficiently potent that intranasal administration produces systemic side effects similar to those obtained with parenteral CT,[12] thus losing one of the advantages of the nasal route.[16] A lower concentration of taurocholate or another surfactant might achieve satisfactory nasal absorption without harming the nasal mucosa and with fewer systemic side effects. The long-term histopathologic effects of surfactants are not well known, and more chronic toxicity studies will be required before they gain general acceptance.

Other authors have also reported their experience with this nasal spray preparation. Gagel et al,[17] in a similar 3-month trial, had results similar to ours, insofar as efficacy is concerned. Seven patients were treated with INSCT, 2 with 100 IU, 3 with 300 IU, and 2 with 400 IU daily (average: 230 IU/d). The average decline in AP (initial value: 394 ± 52 IU/L) was 33% after 3 months versus 40% (initial value: 959 ± 388 IU/L in another group of 8 patients treated for 3 months with 100 IU subcutaneously. Systemic symptoms characteristic of SCT administration (which we encountered in 40% of our cases) were noted in 80% of their cases. Local nasal symptoms (transient tingling and mild stinging sensation often followed by a sneeze and sometimes by rhinorrhea) occurred in all their patients. Slight to moderate erythema of the nasal mucosa was seen in every case and mild edema in 20% of cases, but there was no tendency to progression despite continuation of therapy. No nasal ulceration was observed. D'Agostino et al[18] treated 8 patients (2 with 100 IU, 3 with 200 IU, and 3 with 400 IU daily); after 3 months an average decrease of AP of 20% was observed. There were only 3 acceptable responders (38%). In the group on 400 IU/d, none of the subjects responded; these subjects had all been treated previously with SCT parenterally and had developed a pronounced rise in SCT antibody titer. These results are difficult to interpret because the initial AP levels in the various groups were different (410 ± 65, 616 ± 101, 2,089 ± 881, respectively). In those patients in whom previous therapy with SCT had been given, INSCT acted as a booster for SCT antibody production. In the mildest of these cases, subsequent parenteral therapy with 100 IU SCT subcutaneously for 2 months resulted in only a 19.6% decrease in AP. Mild nasal discomfort was noted in all patients; in 78% this proved transient, whereas in 22% it persisted. One patient with persistent discomfort associated with sneezing decided to drop out.

Thus, INSCT with 1% taurocholate as an absorption promoter is very effective and often gives results of the same order of magnitude as subcutaneous administration. However, it may be tolerated only by patients with symptomatic disease, where the local discomfort is compensated for by a notable improvement of the bone pain for which the INSCT was prescribed. In osteoporosis this preparation is not warranted and particularly not in prevention of the disease.

Nasal Spray Without Absorption Promoter

A study of INSCT without an absorption promoter was also undertaken since this was expected to decrease local toxicity. Furthermore, it is the only spray available in many countries. We first studied its activity in normal volunteers.[5,6] Intramuscularly injected SCT 100 IU was significantly more active than the 200-IU spray for the first 4 hours post administration for all three urinary electrolytes tested (Na/Cr, Cl/Cr, Ca/Cr ratios). Nevertheless, the 200-IU spray was significantly more active than the placebo spray. In contrast, the 100-IU spray was more active than the placebo only for the Na/Cr ratio and only during the first postadministration hour.[5,6]

Since we had not tested the effect of nasal spray on hydroxyproline excretion in the original study, we did this in a separate study on ten volunteers, who were in the fasting state and remained so for the rest of the test, except for drinking water. As shown in Figure 11.4, 100 IU given as a nasal spray did not significantly affect the hydroxyproline/creatinine ratio, whereas half this dosage administered subcutaneously significantly decreased this ratio from the second postadministration hour onward. The trend of this ratio to increase before decreasing (Figure 11.4) has also been observed by O'Doherty et al.[19] These authors hypothesized that CT directly decreases tubular reabsorption of hydroxyproline, but they could not rule out a nonrenal effect.

We have also tested the acute hypocalcemic response of 50 IU subcutaneously versus 100 IU intranasally in two patients with Paget's disease, as well as 50 IU subcutaneously versus 800 IU intranasally in two other

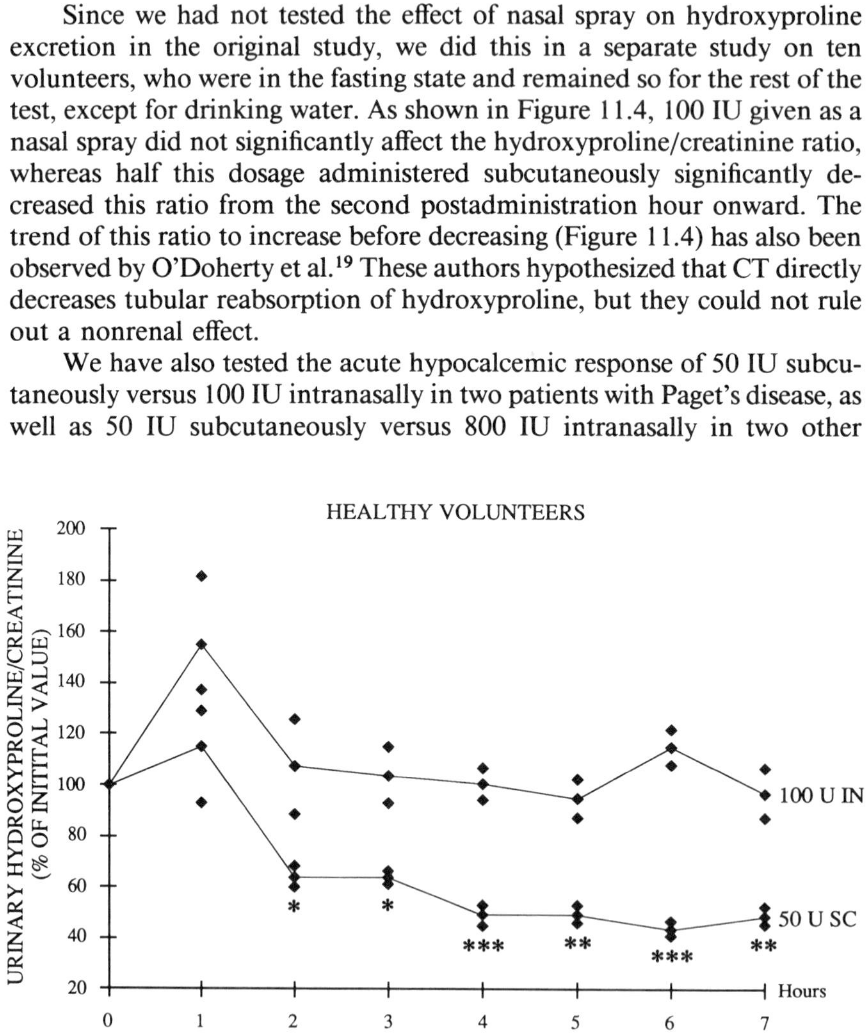

FIGURE 11.4. The effect of the plain nasal spray (IN) of 100 IU on the hydroxyproline/creatinine ratio in 10 healthy volunteers, as compared to the effect of a subcutaneous administration (SC) of 50 IU to the same volunteers ($n = 10$).$^*P < 0.5$; $^{**}P < 0.01$, $^{***}P < 0.001$. Test performed with subjects in the fasting state throughout.

patients (Figure 11.5). Since the action of the spray fell short of the action of SCT administered subcutaneously, this was not pursued further. It is well known that the absorption of the nasal spray correlates with the dosage used from 50 to 200 IU in one study[20] and from 150 to 700 IU in another study.[21] Therefore, no saturation of the nasal mucosa is expected at higher dosages. In these particular cases, therefore, the bioavailability of the nasal spray must have been lower than 6%. No general conclusion can be drawn from these two cases, except that the nasal mucosa may represent an effective barrier.

It was thus logical to test the activity of the nasal spray in Paget's disease at higher dosages. Two dosages have been tested: 200 IU/d in 13 patients and 400 IU/d in 9 patients, with the aim to treat for 12 months. The results have been reported in detail for both groups.[6,22] Figure 11.6 shows the results obtained at 3 months. Both dosages seem to be equally effective in achieving a significant lowering of the AP. Upon cessation of therapy, the increase in AP was more pronounced in the 400-IU/d group, as compared to the 200-IU/d group, an indication that the former dosage was more effective than the latter.[6] The proportion of responders, as

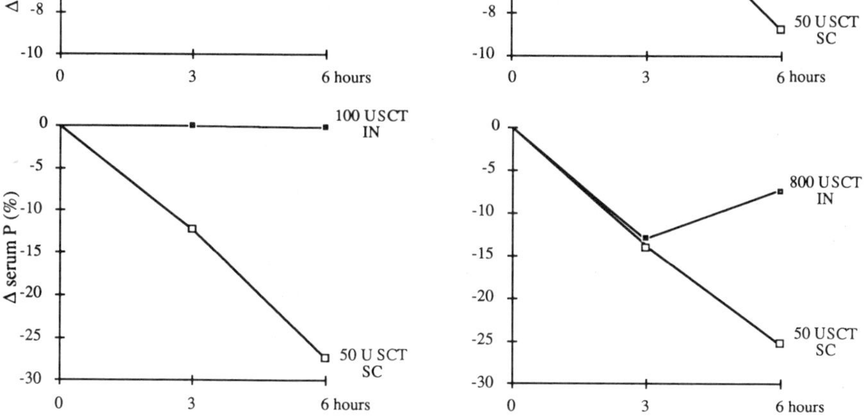

FIGURE 11.5. The effect of the plain spray (IN) of 100 IU and 800 IU on serum calcium and serum phosphorus levels in two patients with Paget's disease, as compared to the effect of a subcutaneous administration (SC) of 50 IU to the same patients.

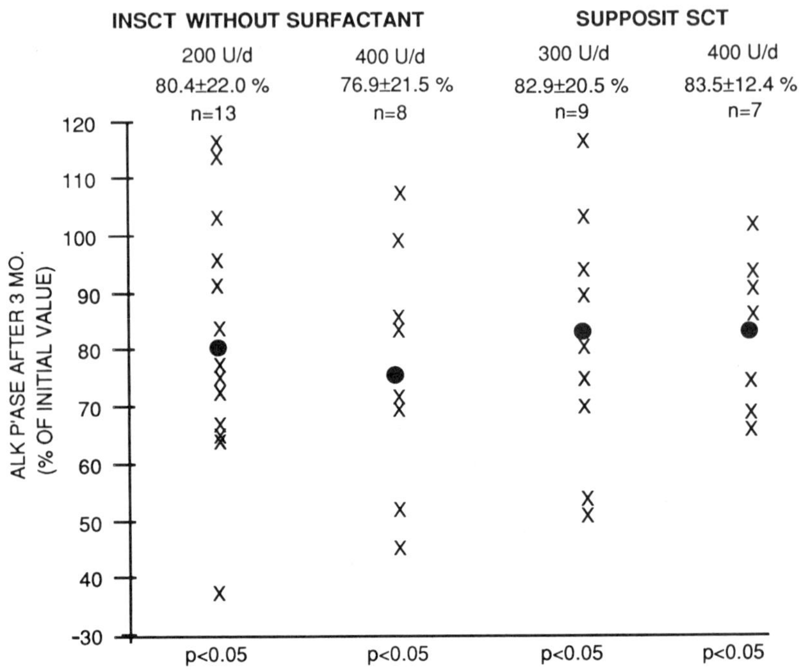

FIGURE 11.6. Individual and average results for the alkaline phosphatase after 3 months of therapy with the same plain spray (two dosages), and the suppository (two dosages).

defined previously, was 6/13 (40%) in the 200-IU group versus 5/9 (56%) in the 400-IU group, a difference that was not statistically significant.

When these results were published,[6] we had not analyzed separately the subjects who had been treated previously with SCT compared to those who had never had SCT, nor had we sent the few sera that had been saved to Dr. Singer in Los Angeles for SCT antibody analysis.

When the results of the two groups are pooled and analyzed according to whether the patients had ever been treated with SCT and considering only those patients who were present consistently without missing a visit until at least the eighth month, it was apparent that the 9 patients (5 on 200 IU and 4 on 400 IU/daily) who had never had SCT previously responded significantly better from the first month onward to the eighth month (Figure 11.7), with an AP value of 67 ± 4.5% of the initial level. In contrast, the 8 patients (5 on 200 IU, and 3 on 400 IU daily) who had received SCT previously did not respond significantly to the INSCT (Figure 11.7): the AP value at 8 months was 96 ± 7.1% of the initial value. The difference between the two groups at 8 months is statistically significant ($P < 0.05$), One potential confounding factor could be that the patients who had

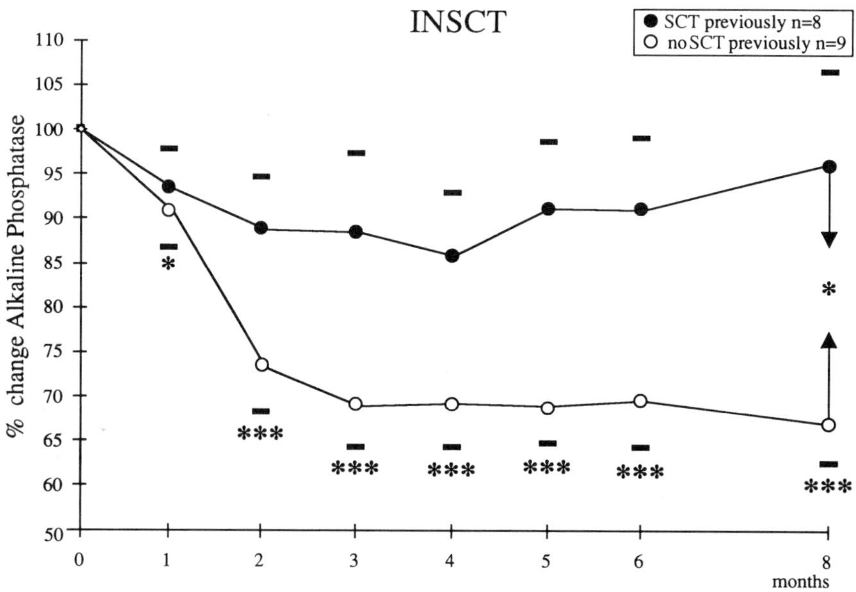

FIGURE 11.7. Effect of the administration of the plain spray (INSCT), with the two dosages pooled, on the alkaline phosphatase, according to whether or not the patients had SCT previously. Only the patients who consistently came to all visits have been considered. Asterisks are as in the caption of Figure 11.4.

received SCT previously had been so treated because their disease was more severe, as compared to the patients who had not been treated. There was indeed a trend for this to be so, but the difference was not statistically significant (AP at time 0: 234 ± 55 and 133 ± 15 IU/L, respectively, in the pretreated patients and in those who had never had SCT).

In the group who had never received SCT, two sera available from time 0, of course yielded negative results for SCT antibodies. Analysis of the two corresponding sera at the end showed one negative after 8 months (final AP: 68% of initial value), but the other had turned slightly positive (final AP: 82% of initial value). In the group that had been previously treated with SCT, of the two sera available from time 0, one had positive and one had negative results but yielded positive findings during therapy (final APS, respectively; 99% and 120% of initial value). A third serum was available at the end of therapy and yielded positive (final AP: 110% of initial value) results. Among the five patients who had an antibody determination at the end of the trial, the only acceptable response occurred in the single patient without antibodies. An intermediate response was noted in the subject with a low antibody titer (>1:5). The three cases with essentially no response had an antibody titer between 1:40 and 1:80. The individual data are depicted in Figure 11.8.

Pain was not evaluated systematically in the two groups of patients. However, whenever bone pain related to Paget's disease was present, it was partially alleviated, especially pain at night. Local tolerance to the nasal spray was excellent: only 1 patient in 22 withdrew (exacerbation of preexisting vasomotor rhinitis). No patient complained of systemic side effects such as flushing, nausea, abdominal cramps, diarrhea, or increased urinary frequency.

Thus both treatment regimens proved active in Paget's disease of bone, provided the patients has not been pretreated with SCT. The best proof of benefit is that one patient showed a positive focal bone balance at an osteolytic lesion of her distal tibia. This has been illustrated elsewhere[6] and is the ultimate proof of the beneficial action of any antiresorptive drug in Paget's disease.[23,24] In another more recent case with osteolytic lesions in the tibia, this could not be reproduced with the nasal spray to the same extent, despite the absence of antibodies. The radiologic changes that occurred in this case were in the right direction but remained short of what can be obtained with parenteral SCT in our experience.

Other authors have used this nasal spray without an absorption promoter in Paget's disease. Our results are similar but difficult to compare

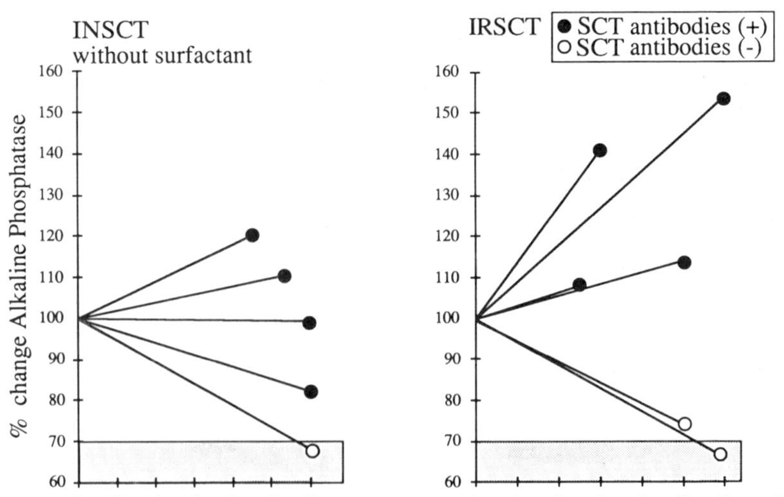

FIGURE 11.8. Individual changes in alkaline phosphatase in those patients where SCT antibodies could be determined at the end of the trial, with the plain spray and the suppository. Shaded area is considered a good response (a decrease of at least 30% of initial value).

with those of a similar study made by Reginster et al.,[25] who also used 200 IU/d in eight patients and 400 IU/d in nine patients. The latter dosage was reduced to 200 IU/d when the serum alkaline phosphatase fell to 50% of initial values. Another crucial difference, when compared to our study, was that no patient in the study had ever received SCT before entering the trial. Two patients were nonresponders and a third had a distinct relapse at 6 months of therapy. Overall, the parameters of bone turnover fell significantly to 63% of initial values after 12 months. These results compare well with what we have obtained in patients who had not been treated previously with SCT. The authors stressed the absence of systemic side effects for this mode of treatment.[26] Another study in nine patients was undertaken by Eisinger,[27] who employed another treatment schedule (200 IU three times weekly during the first 3 months, followed by 200 IU daily during 3 to 6 additional months). In this study, neither the level of AP nor the hydroxyproline excretion in the urine diminished significantly during the first 3 months or later. The latter parameter did change when we recalculated the date for hydroxyproline excretion by a Wilcoxon matched-pairs signed-rank test[6] but did not change for the alkaline phosphatase on recalculation. These findings are difficult to interpret since we do not know whether the subjects had been treated previously with SCT. Once more the good tolerance of the drug was stressed.[27]

Suppositories

We first studied the activity of a SCT suppository in human volunteers,[6] using the same method as for the nasal spray, that is, the stimulation of electrolyte excretion in the urine and inhibition of hydroxyproline excretion, studied in a double-blind fashion with two dosages (100 and 300 IU) versus placebo and compared with subcutaneous SCT (50 IU). The intrarectal route of administration (IRSCT) produced the expected dose-dependent result on electrolyte excretion. The subcutaneous 50-IU dose was superior to the 300 IU suppository, using the second postadministration hour as a test for this activity, in terms of Na, Cl, and Ca excretion. The potencies of the two modes of administration could not be distinguished by their effects on P and K excretion, nor on hydroxyproline excretion. The subcutaneous dosage, however, had much more prolonged action. Therefore, the bioequivalence of the suppository was less than 17%.

We then administered the 300-IU suppository daily to ten patients (six men, four women) with Paget's disease (age: 66.5 ± 6.5; range: 55 to 82), whose initial AP was 270 ± 32 IU/L, for a planned duration of 12 months. Figure 11.6 shows the results in this group after 3 months. The AP dropped to 89.5 ± 20.6 of initial values ($P < 0.05$). Three patients of ten (30%) were acceptable responders, as defined previously. Among the responders, two had osteolytic lesions, lending themselves to radiologic evaluation, and both responded. A resorption cleft in a humerus filled in after 6 months of therapy, as illustrated elsewhere.[6] A resorption cleft in the inferior ramus of the pubis disappeared after 1 year of therapy (Figure 11.9). One year after withdrawal, the resorption cleft, as expected, reappeared.[23,24] The suppositories were well tolerated; only one patient complained of local irritation and another of dyspepsia. The absence of systematic side effects has also been stressed by others.[28]

We then tried another suppository containing 200 IU twice daily (400 IU/d total), which allows a comparison with the results of the nasal spray at the same dosage. This was administered to 13 patients (six men, seven women; age: 68 ± 2.8; range: 56 to 78) with Paget's disease, whose initial AP was 228 ± 30 IU/L, for a planned duration of 12 months. Figure 11.6 shows the effect on the AP level at 3 months (83.9 ± 12.4%; $P < 0.05$). The use of two suppositories per day was poorly tolerated by seven patients who had local irritation; two had intestinal cramps, one had diarrhea, and one reported dizziness. The response could be judged only in seven patients, two of whom proved to be acceptable responders (29%). The twice-daily IRSCT scheme of administration was not superior (see Figure 11.6) to the

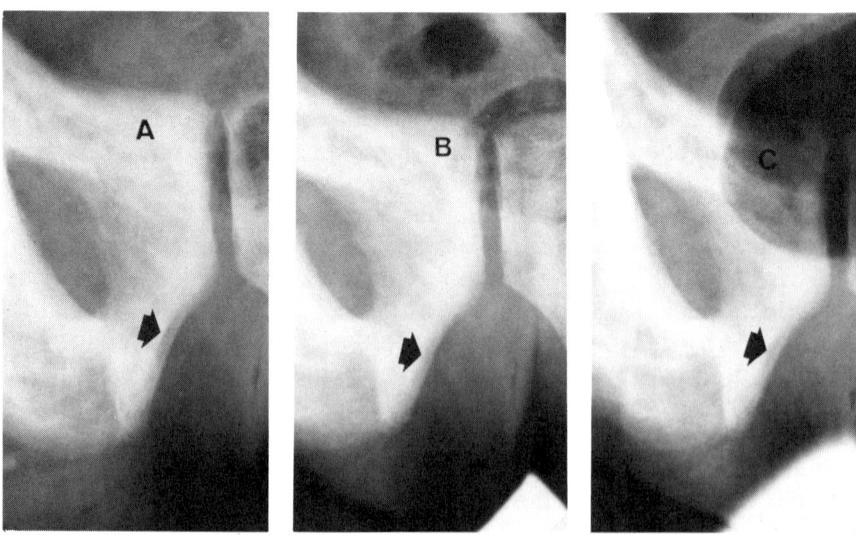

FIGURE 11.9. A resorption cleft at the inferior ramus of the pubis **(A)**. After 12 months of IRSCT (one daily suppository of 300 IU), the resorption cleft has been completely filled in **(B)**. After another year without therapy, the radiolucent area reappeared **(C)**.

previous trial, was less well tolerated, and was less acceptable to the patients.

Since there was no significant difference in the results between the two schemes of suppository administration and since there were many drop-outs in the second series, the results of the two groups were pooled, once more according to whether the subjects had been pretreated ($n = 8$) or not ($n = 9$) with SCT (Figure 11.10). As can be seen, the former group (pre-treated with SCT) had no significant drop in AP activity, whereas the latter showed a significant drop from the second month onward to the eighth month. The difference between the two groups was statistically significant ($P < 0.05$) at 8 months when 17 patients were still in the study. We also verified that the patients who had been treated previously with SCT were not afflicted with more severe disease than those who had never been treated. The initial AP levels in both groups were, respectively, 318 ± 40 and 269 ± 45 IU/L, a difference that was not statistically significant.

In the group that had never received SCT, six sera were available from time 0. All, of course, yielded negative SCT antibody findings. Sera of three of these cases were available at the end of the trial: findings for two

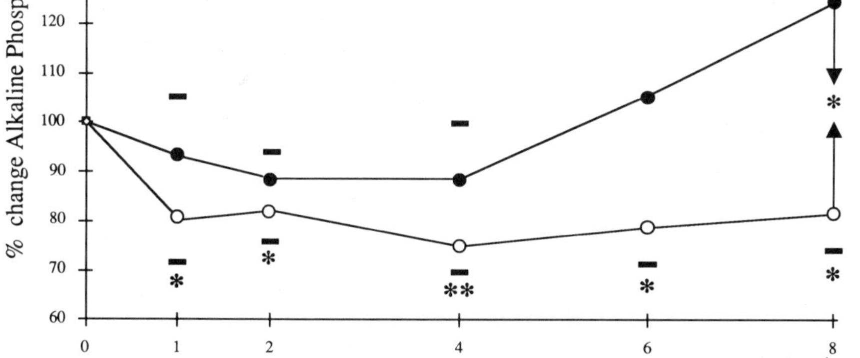

FIGURE 11.10. Effect of the administration of the suppository (IRSCT), with the two dosages pooled, on alkaline phosphatase, according to whether or not the patient had SCT previously. Only the patients who consistently came to all visits have been considered. Asterisks are as in the legend of Figure 11.4.

remained negative (final APs, respectively: 67% and 73% of initial levels), whereas those for one became positive (final AP: 141% of initial level). Among the patients who had been treated previously with SCT, there were three sera from time 0, one of which yielded negative results that became positive (final AP: 108% of initial value) and two, with initially positive results, that increased in positivity (final APs, respectively: 114% and 154%). None of the antibody titers was higher than 1:40. The individual data are shown in Figure 11.8.

If we pool the data in Figure 11.8 for the nasal spray and the suppository, we have three cases without SCT antibodies (final AP: 69 ± 2% of initial value) versus eight cases with SCT antibodies (final AP: 116 ± 8% of initial value). Although the numbers are too small to draw a definite conclusion, this difference is statistically significant ($P < 0.05$) in terms of the Mann-Whitney U-test.

The acute hypocalcemic responses to 50 IU of SCT and to 0.5 mg of HCT were compared in five patients who had been treated previously with SCT and whose response to either the nasal spray ($n = 4$) or the suppository ($n = 1$) was considered suboptimal. The tests were performed after cessation of therapy and were separated by 1 week. Figure 11.11 shows the results. The SCT injection induced moderate hypocalcemia, which was significant only after 6 hours, whereas HCT produced significant hypocalcemia at both the third and the sixth hour, at which time the serum calcium was significantly lower than that induced by SCT. Serum was significantly lower than that induced by SCT. Serum phosphate fell significantly at the sixth hour after HCT but did not fall significantly with SCT. Serum was saved in only two of these patients; both yielded positive results for SCT antibodies. The difference in response toward HCT is all the more

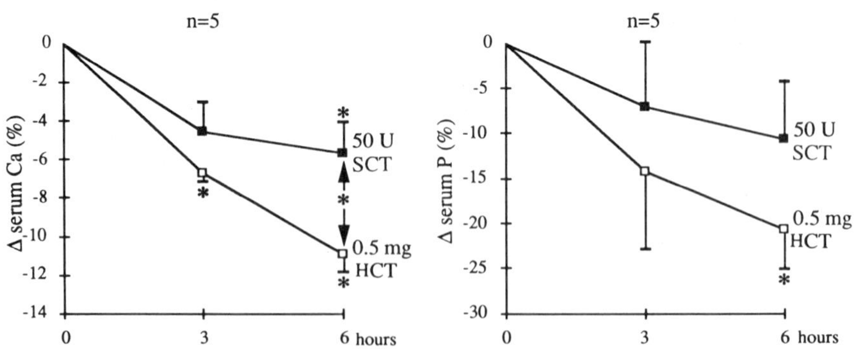

FIGURE 11.11. Acute hypocalcemic and hypophosphatemic responses in 5 subjects whose response to INSCT ($n = 4$) or IRSCT ($n = 1$) was considered unsatisfactory. Note the better response to HCT (0.5 mg) compared to SCT (50 IU), both given subcutaneously.

remarkable in that 0.5 mg of HCT is equivalent to 50 IU only in theory. According to Gennari et al,[29] 75 IU of HCT is required to produce calcium-lowering action equivalent to that of 50 IU of SCT. Thus, there was at least partial resistance to SCT.

In some cases, the SCT concentrations provided by the nasal or rectal route were not sufficient to cause a decrease in AP, as demonstrated by a subsequent reduction during parenteral therapy with SCT, as shown in Figure 11.12. In some cases, therefore, the apparent resistance can be overcome by resorting to the parenteral route. That this is not always the case is also apparent in Figure 11.12, since in some "resistant" cases HCT administered subcutaneously proved effective. In one of these cases, subsequent administration of SCT subcutaneously was unable to overcome the resistance. Clearly, in this instance SCT antibodies must have been operating.

When we consider all the treatments we have administered, dividing the patients into those who had or had not been treated previously with SCT and pooling all the dosages according to the mode of therapy, it is apparent that INSCT with surfactant, whether or not the patients had been pretreated with SCT, is significantly more active at 3 months than other forms of therapy (Figure 11.13). The nasal spray with surfactant is not significantly more effective than the plain spray or the suppository when given to patients who have never been treated by SCT. The plain spray, given to patients who have never been pretreated with SCT, also proved to

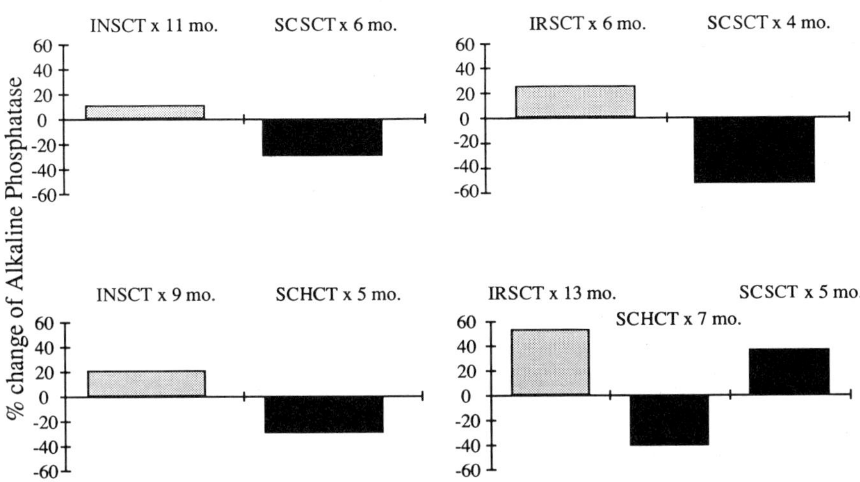

FIGURE 11.12. Cases resistant to INSCT or IRSCT that responded to SCT or HCT administered subcutaneously (SC). One case responded to HCT administered subcutaneously, but was resistant to SCT administered by the same route.

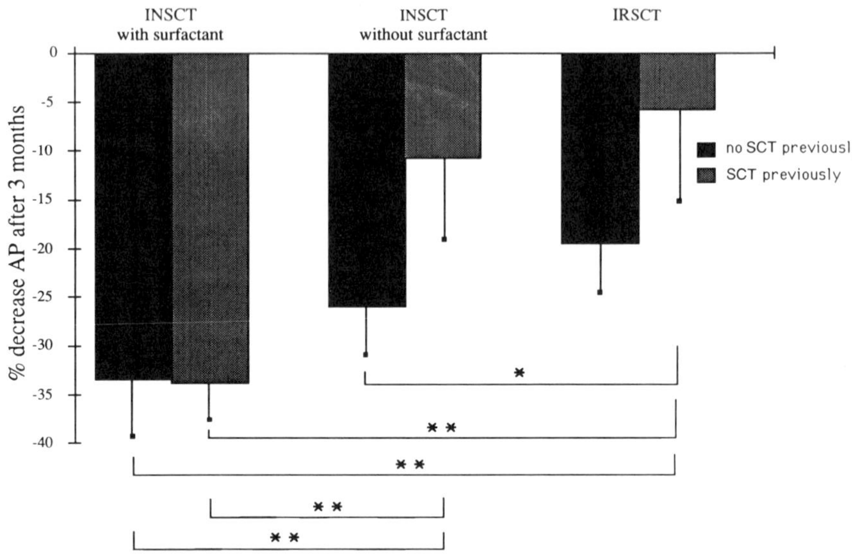

FIGURE 11.13. Activity of the various modes of therapy on the alkaline phosphatase after 3 months. The nasal spray with 1% sodium taurocholate as surfactant is effective whether or not the patient had SCT previously. This result was significantly greater than the plain spray and the suppository when these were given to patients who had SCT previously. No significant difference was seen in effectiveness if the patient had not had SCT before. The plain spray was significantly more active than the suppository in those patients who had SCT before, but this finding loses much of its significance if the baseline disease activity is taken into account.

be significantly more active at 3 months than the suppository in the patients who had been treated with SCT, but this finding loses much of its significance if the baseline disease activity, which is significantly higher ($P < 0.05$) in the latter group, is taken into account.

DISCUSSION

The need for alternative routes of administration of CT is obvious, especially in view of the demonstration that CT is able to prevent vertebral osteoporosis.[30] SCT administered as a nasal spray or as a suppository has biologic activity and is active in Paget's disease of bone.[5,6] Several problems nevertheless remain. First it is difficult to determine the bioavailability of the nasal spray since it depends on the model used in the evaluation. If we consider electrolyte excretion and compare 100 IU intranasally and 100 IU intramuscularly during the first postinjection hour, we estimate that the potency of the spray was of the order of 20%.[2] This is a generous estimation and does not take into account the more prolonged action of the parenteral mode of administration. On the other hand, electrolyte excretion is only one parameter by which to judge SCT activity, and it may not be the best, since what is actually sought is its action on bone. This is better reflected by the acute hypocalcemic response. Although most researchers have obtained significant hypocalcemia with parenteral CT, even in subjects with normal bone turnover,[29,31-33] with doses no higher than 100 IU of SCT and 0.5 mg of HCT, most authors have been unable to produce hypocalcemia with 200 IU INSCT,[20,34-36] with one exception.[37] Even at 400 IU INSCT, significant hypocalcemia was not observed,[34-36] except by those who determined the ionized calcium concentration.[34,36] That this depends on individual absorption characteristics of the nasal mucosa is suggested by the experience of Kurose et al,[35] who found that the subjects who had plasma SCT levels above 90 pg/mL did develop acute hypocalcemia, even when total plasma calcium concentrations were measured. Average SCT plasma levels after administration of 200, 300, and 400 IU INSCT reached 69 ± 18, 85 ± 34, and 97 ± 22 pg/mL, respectively, in these series.[35]

Hydroxyproline excretion is another parameter by the antiresorptive action of CT on bone is evaluated, even in subjects with normal bone turnover.[38] One study of patients with osteoporosis found that the 200 IU INSCT had no significant effect on hydroxyproline excretion, whereas the 400-IU spray significantly decreased this parameter by 10%, versus a significant 28% decrease for 100 IU by the intramuscular route.[36] No wonder we did not find an effect with 100 IU INSCT (Figure 11.4). In healthy volunteers, 400 IU INSCT was able to decrease the hourly hydroxyproline/creatinine ratio significantly with a compensatory increase during the night, so that the effect could not be seen in 24-hour urinary collections.[34]

Another parameter of CT action is the plasma cAMP concentration. Thamsborg et al[20] noted a significant increase in cyclic adenosine monophosphate (cAMP) concentration 15 minutes after the administration of 110 IU or 200 IU INSCT, whereas the 50-IU dosage and the placebo spray did not have this effect. The authors also stated that the 100- and 200-IU/d doses, but not the 50-IU/d dose, were able to increase lumbar bone mineral content significantly in their experience (Thamsborg G. et al, in preparation).

There are not many comparisons of the nasal and subcutaneous routes of administration in Paget's disease. Gonzales et al[39] saw essentially no effect of 200 IU INSCT on three patients with "severe" Paget's disease, as assessed by the hydroxyproline/creatinine ratio in the urine, compared to a significant diminution after intramuscular injection of 100 IU of SCT. In seven patients with "mild to moderately active" Paget's disease, there was a discernible effect on the hydroxyproline/creatinine ratio, which decreased by 8% with 200 IU INSCT versus 28% with 100 IU SCT intramuscularly.

The recent study by O'Doherty et al[19] is the most exhaustive investigation of this phenomenon in Paget's disease: 9 patients received 1, 10, and 100 IU SCT subcutaneously sequentially; 9 other patients received a placebo injection; 22 others received 400 IU INSCT. The groups were matched for disease activity. It was concluded that 400 IU of INSCT corresponded to approximately 30 IU of subcutaneous SCT, with considerable variation (from 0 to 111 IU), giving a mean bioequivalence of about 8%, using the acute "cumulative" hypocalcemic response as the measured parameter. The effect of 400 IU INSCT on the hydroxyproline/creatinine ratio was less than that of both 10 and 100 IU of subcutaneous SCT. On that basis, this effect indicates a bioequivalence of less than 2.5%, the same order of bioequivalence as that of the 3% estimated for HCT.[7] Interestingly, in the milder cases (hydroxyproline/creatinine ratio < 58 μmol/mmol, that is, 67 μg/mg) of Paget's disease, the nasal spray was more active and comparable to 100 IU given subcutaneously. The number of cases in this category that were studied is not stated but must not be large, since the group treated by INSCT had an average hydroxyproline/creatinine ratio of 71 μmol/mmol with 95% confidence estimates from 62 to 81. Only in the group receiving 100 IU subcutaneously was there a significant correlation between the acute hypocalcemic response and the decrease in hydroxyproline excretion. This corresponds to the experience of Eisinger[40] who, when administering 80 IU of SCT intravenously, found a significant correlation between acute hypocalcemia and both AP levels and hydroxyproline excretion. With 200 IU INSCT, there was no longer a significant correlation between acute hypocalcemia and both AP and hydroxyproline responses, and with 400 IU INSCT a correlation was present only for hydroxyproline excretion. In this series the acute hypocalcemic response was smaller with 400 IU INSCT, as compared to 80 IU intravenously, indicating bioavailability of less than 20%.

Most authors, like us, have usually administered the nasal spray in the morning in their physiologic studies. If it were true that an insufflation at midnight induces a 10-minute plasma level of SCT that is 70% greater than that achieved during daytime administration.[41] If this finding represents a general tendency of the nasal mucosa to absorb CT better late in the day, it would invalidate all the data obtained in these studies. However, the study making this claim was based on a single 10-minute plasma level. Full biochronological data, including C_{max}, T_{max}, and the area under the curve of plasma SCT, should be obtained before the notion of "nonabsorbant time" can be endorsed. Meanwhile, the clinician may as well favor "bedtime calcitonin" instead of "breakfast calcitonin" in daily practice.

Besides Paget's disease and normocalcemic states in which bone turnover is not elevated, as in normal volunteers or patients with osteoporosis, a third situation is represented by those conditions in which hypercalcemia prevails and CT is used for its calcium-lowering action. In cases of hypercalcemia of various origin, selected on the basis of an established calcium-lowering effect of 100 IU SCT given intramuscularly, three doses of INSCT were given to each patient in random order: 110, 200, and 400 IU. Only the latter dose had a calcium-lowering effect that was similar to that of an intramuscular injection of 100 IU SCT.[42] In primary hyperparathyroidism, using the area under the curve of the concentration of ionized calcium, 100 IU SCT given intramuscularly was more potent and more prolonged in its calcium-lowering action than the three doses of INSCT: 110, 200, and 400 IU.[43] Here, the bioavailability must also be less than 25%.

Whatever the reason, it is difficult to define precisely the bioavailability of the nasal spray without surfactant. The estimations vary from 8%[19] to 40%.[37] From the available data, our estimation[2] of 20% would seem to be a little high. Taking into account all the data in the literature as well as our own data, a revised estimate would be between 10% and 20%.

In subjects who have not been treated previously by SCT, the decline of AP activity to 67% of initial value (Figure 11.7), obtained by 200 to 400 IU INSCT, is successful treatment. How can one explain this despite the low bioavailability? With parenteral SCT, Wallach[44] reviewed 14 series in the literature totaling 328 patients with Paget's disease in whom the treatment had lasted an average 7.1 months with doses ranging from 10 to 160 IU/d, and calculated an average reduction in AP to 56% of the initial value. Hosking,[45] in his review of 10 series treated with SCT totaling 137 cases, obtained an average reduction of AP to 57% of initial value. A typical patient in these series might receive 50 to 100 IU/d, which is 25% of the dosage used in our studies with INSCT. Taking into account the fact that we eliminated subjects who had been previously treated with SCT, thus introducing a certain selection bias of milder cases, and also obtaining a slightly lesser reduction in the AP, the preceding data are compatible with a bioequivalence for the spray not higher than 20%. However, data during chronic therapy in Paget's disease are unavailable; the appropriate studies have not been made.

In any event, small doses of CT at times are effective in Paget's disease. One should bear in mind that the huge multinucleated osteoclasts that characterize Paget's disease can be extraordinarily sensitive to SCT to the extent that 1 IU given subcutaneously can induce mild but significant hypocalcemia.[19] In chronic administration, as little as 20 IU/d can produce impressive lowering of bone turnover.[46] Using 50 IU of SCT once a week in nine patients, Avramides et al[47] showed a maximal 49% and a final 33% decrease in AP values. In the experience of Wallach,[48] 25 IU three times weekly was unsatisfactory, whereas twice the dosage was effective. With

HCT the lowest effective dosage is 0.25 mg/d,[46] although at times, according to these authors, as little as 0.1 mg/d may be effective. One example of this was recorded by Evans,[49] who observed a biochemical response using 0.5 mg/wk "in what was supposed to be a control group." In the same cases, the osteoclast surface diminished in four of six patients.[50] These are the minimal doses needed to observe an effect, but the optimal doses are, of course, several times higher and of the order of 0.5 mg three times weekly to 1.0 mg/daily. This may explain why, despite low bioavailability, INSCT therapy may be active in Paget's disease, especially in mild cases. The implications of this for the primary or secondary prevention of spinal osteoporosis are clear. If all that is needed to prevent trabecular bone loss is 60 IU/wk of HCT[30] or 120 IU/wk of SCT,[51] then at 15% bioavailability 100 IU INSCT daily would provide the equivalent of 105 IU/wk parenterally.

Low bioequivalence might also explain a second problem with the plain spray and with the suppository: the apparent antibody-based resistance that occurs at low antibody titers in some cases and contrasts with the experience that prevails with parenteral SCT treatment, during which this event is exceptional and occurs at most in 22% of cases,[52] usually at much higher antibody titers. We have only indirect evidence that this is a problem. First, we did not encounter resistance to the spray with surfactant, whose effectiveness was indistinguishable from that of the parenteral route of administration. We have noted a high incidence of antibody formation (60%) in this group and also the highest titers ($<1:1{,}000$); however, these were not neutralizing. Of course, we do not know what would have happened if the study had lasted for more than 3 months. Nevertheless, this situation resembles that which we are accustomed to, using the parenteral route of administration: half the patients develop antibodies, but a minority of these exert a functionally effective neutralizing action. Also, it did not really matter whether the patients had had SCT previously. In contrast, with the plain spray (without surfactant), the presence or absence of antibodies seemed to yield different results, and, therefore, whether the patients had had SCT previously was of paramount importance, since reexposure to SCT is more likely to lead to renewed antibody formation than first exposure, as in the study of Levy et al.[14] It is apparent from Figure 11.13 that for patients treated previously with SCT, the nasal spray with surfactant is significantly more active at 3 months than either the nasal spray without surfactant or the suppository (also at 3 months), despite the lower average dosage of the nasal spray with surfactant (average: 240 ± 45 IU compared to an average of 280 ± 33 IU for the plain nasal spray, and an average 314 ± 15 IU for the suppository).

On the other hand, no clear-cut distinction among the groups can be made if we consider the results obtained in those patients who had never had SCT treatment. It would thus seem that the surfactant, by allowing maximal concentrations of SCT to enter the plasma, is able to overcome "low-titer antibody-based resistance." This, however, requires confirmation. An easy way to settle this problem, without using in vitro models, would be a systematic study in these patients, with repeated determinations of SCT antibody titers and in whom the administration of a plain SCT spray (200 IU/d) is followed by the parenteral administration of SCT (50 IU/d) in the resistant cases and in those showing resistance after initial success. This should, in turn, be followed by the administration of HCT (2 mg/d intranasally or 0.5 mg/d parenterally). In any event, Figure 11.12 shows that on occasion parenteral therapy with SCT is able to overcome resistance. Figures 11.11 and 11.12 show the superiority of parenteral HCT in this context. Whether this is due to low-titer antibodies, which low plasma concentrations of SCT are unable to overcome, is not definitely known.

There is one discordant point to this reasoning: the data collected by D'Agostino et al[18] in a smaller series than ours (8 versus 18 patients) in which antibody-based resistance seemed to exist, with the additional confounding factor that the resistant patients had disease activity many times higher than that of the others. It is well known that patients with severe disease activity do not respond to the nasal spray to the same extent as the milder cases.[19,39] On the other hand, there is no reason that an occasional patient may be resistant to a nasal spray with surfactant just as he or she may be resistant to parenteral SCT, on the basis of neutralizing antibodies, if the titer is high. Whether resistance in the patients studied by D'Agostino et al[18] occurred because the antibody titer and/or the disease activity was too high, or a combination of both, remains to be determined.

Our results with the plain spray are similar to those of Levy et al,[14] who treated nine patients with 200 IU/d INSCT, five of whom had received SCT parenterally previously. The previously untreated group had sustained inhibition of AP levels throughout the trial (12 months), whereas in the previously treated group an initial small and nonsignificant drop in AP, which soon returned to initial values, was observed. Three of the five patients previously treated had antibodies initially, and the other two developed high antibody titers during the trial. Three of four patients who had never been exposed to SCT also developed antibodies, albeit at a lower titer. Thus reexposure to SCT caused secondary antibody responses and clinical resistance in the patients who had been previously treated by SCT. In these patients, the administration if INHCT (2 mg/d) caused a significant lowering of AP to 66 $\pm$ 6% of initial value,[53] clearly demonstrating the neutralizing character of the SCT antibodies, as well as indicating that the nasal mucosa had remained permeable to CT. When these same sera were tested later, only low-titer SCT antibodies, which did not significantly affect the acute hypocalcemic response to SCT,[53] remained. Sera should not be tested for antibodies too early in the course of INSCT administration; ideally they should be tested after 6 months of therapy. After cessation of therapy, the antibody titers may fall and the hypocalcemic response may be restored.[53] This may explain why the authors who have tested for hypocalcemic responses after the trial was finished may have found it normal.[54] The findings reported in the latest paper of the group,[55] analyzing 16 sera after 3 months of therapy, are reminiscent of the data we obtained after 3 months with INSCT plus an absorption promoter. There may not have been enough time for the antibodies to exert or express their blocking action. Grauer et al,[55] during INSCT therapy with 400 IU/d in nine patients, saw antibodies develop in seven after an average 9.5 months; four had neutralizing activity with a subsequent rise in AP level. In the two patients with high-titer antibodies, the serum showed neutralizing activity, whereas in the five patients with low antibody titers, two also demonstrated neutralizing properties. Neutralizing activity, therefore, depends not only on the titer of the antibodies but also on affinity for the receptor, on the binding site, and on other factors. To demonstrate this, both the Zurich group[14,53] and the Heidelberg group[56] have used a cultured human breast cancer cell line, in which SCT normally stimulates cAMP production and which is inhibited when the antibodies have neutralizing ability. That neutralizing SCT antibodies can be bound to the hormone in such a manner as to interfere with the hormone-receptor interaction has long been known. The subject has been repeatedly reviewed.[45,52] In such cases, the administration of HCT, which is nonimmunogenic, invariably restores the responsiveness of the osteoclasts, as indicated by a number of studies.[52,57–60]

To overcome this problem and have higher CT concentrations in the plasma, one would wish to have a potent and harmless surfactant that increases the permeability of the nasal mucosa by acting on the mucous film or perhaps by decreasing the proteolytic enzyme activity of the nasal mucosa, thus allowing the peptide to remain intact in contact with the nasal mucosa. Other modes of administration should also be explored to obtain higher concentrations of CT in the circulation. The addition of sodium glycocholate to a nasal spray of HCT probably increases the bioavailability of HCT ninefold, from approximately 3% to 27%,[7] but the toxicity of this surfactant for the nasal mucosa probably precludes its systematic use in chronic conditions.

The future of CT therapy may reside in oral administration. Although the intestinal mucosa has very low passive permeability to large polypeptides such as CT, with its 32 amino acid residues, as well as high concentrations of luminal and intracellular peptidase enzymes, these problems can be resolved by selective enhancers of intestinal absorption. In the rat, a number of absorption promoters of HCT have been tested on the oral mucosa, that is, between the lower lip and gingiva.[61] The most successful were from the bile salt group, sodium deoxycholate and sodium tauroglycocholate; from the sodium straight-chain fatty acid group, sodium myristate; and from the saponin group, quillayasaponin, as well as surfactants from other groups, such as sucrose palmitate and sodium lauryl sulfate, the most potent of all surfactants tested. Another approach is to incorporate CT into bile salt–fatty acid mixed micelles and chylomicrons, thus exploiting the pathways of fatty acid and glyceride absorption. This approach has been used for oral insulin delivery,[62] with a formulation designed to mimic the cholesterol-glyceride-lecithin composition of the chylomicron. It is hoped that these compounds can deliver a SCT concentration in the blood stream that can overcome SCT "low antibody titer resistance" and be more cost-effective for the patient and society.

A third potential problem of the nasal spray is that it is not known whether the permeability of nasal mucosa is unaltered during chronic use, especially if a surfactant has been added. This problem was raised recently in a study of INSCT in Paget's disease in which five of nine patients on 200 to 400 IU/d had initial suppression of the parameters of bone turnover that later returned to pretreatment levels; a high antibody titer developed in only one.[63] An alternative hypothesis might be "low-titer antibody-based resistance." Whether the nasal mucosa retains its permeability can be resolved by studying the action of SCT on urinary electrolytes before the initiation of therapy and repeating this periodically (once a year) on therapy and off therapy. This could settle, in addition, the problem of down-regulation or modification of the receptors on the osteoclasts. There might be dissociation of the various responses to SCT after chronic exposure, as has been shown in the rat, in which after 6 months of therapy with 2 IU/kg SCT given intramuscularly (5 days out of 7), the 1-hour acute hypocalcemic response was maintained, whereas the 6-minute plasma cAMP peak was significantly blunted.[64]

In any event, and with all the reservations we have indicated, all of which require further investigation, the nasal spray, as it stands, represents a major advance in CT therapy. It is appropriate in the treatment of Paget's disease, especially the milder forms, and for individuals who have never been treated with SCT. It is especially useful in those elderly patients for whom parenteral therapy is unacceptable, impractical, or produces too many side effects. Occasionally, in pagetic osteolytic lesions the focal bone balance may turn positive, when appropriate radiographic techniques are employed. This mode of therapy is particularly well tolerated, and we had only 1 dropout among 22 cases because of a local problem (exacerbation of preexisting vasomotor rhinitis). Not a single patient complained of systemic side effects of CT, such as flushing, nausea, abdominal cramps, diarrhea, and/or increased urinary frequency. Local tolerance was studied in a 6-month trial with 200 and 400 IU/d given to patients with Paget's disease.[65] Nasal mucociliary clearance was unchanged; ciliary beat frequency increased slightly but significantly. Comparison to a control group at the end of a treatment period revealed no difference in ciliary beat frequency but a decrease in mucociliary clearance. ENT examination results remained normal. The authors concluded that the integrity of nasal mucosa was preserved.

Fewer data are available for the SCT suppository. Absorption of eel CT (ECT) in the rat's rectum was described as poor.[66] To obtain the same area under the curve in terms of plasma ECT concentration, the dose administered rectally had to be multiplied by a factor of 160 to simulate the concentrations provided by intramuscular administration. Fortunately, some surfactants were able to fill this gap, increasing the area under the curve by a factor of 180.[66] Surfactants are, of course, better tolerated by the rectal than the nasal mucosa.

Buclin et al[34] are the only authors who have studied the suppository and the nasal spray at the same doses in the same subjects. The SCT suppository delivers short-term high plasma levels, as compared to the low but long peaks produced by the nasal spray. Both forms of administration ultimately produce the same area under the curve for the plasma level of SCT. With the suppository, the sharp plasma peak is followed by a rapid decrease to less than 10% of the observed peak value within 1 hour. The peak after rectal administration occurred earlier than after intramuscular injection but was three to four times lower. The 200-IU suppository was unable to lower the total calcium concentration; it induced a significant fall in the plasma ionized calcium concentration, which the 200-IU nasal spray was unable to achieve, perhaps reflecting the early high peak by the rectal route. The suppository is more natriuretic and calciuretic than the nasal spray. The effect on hydroxyproline excretion was not evaluated in this study, but it is known from our study[6] that the 300-IU suppository significantly inhibits the hydroxyproline/creatinine ratio from the second to the sixth postadministration hour, and a 100-IU suppository exerts the same action from the second to the fourth postadministration hour. Whether the high peaks are clinically advantageous in our studies cannot be ascertained. When comparing Figure 11.7 to Figure 11.10, one may gain the impression that INSCT is more effective than IRSCT.This impression may be misleading since the initial value of AP in the INSCT group ($n = 9$) is significantly lower ($P < 0.001$) than the initial value in the IRSCT group ($n = 7$), when one considers those patients who had never had SCT. On occasion, the 300-IU suppository is very effective in filling in osteolytic areas in Paget's disease.[6] The 300-IU suppository is well tolerated when administered once a day, in contrast to the 200-IU suppository administered twice a day. Others have stressed the good systemic tolerance of the 300-IU suppository.[29] Other intrarectal formulations are being tested in the hope of finding one that will be more effective than the intranasal formulations. These studies are still in progress.

In mild cases of tumor-induced hypercalcemia, IRSCT proved able to reduce the serum calcium significantly from 2.96 ± 0.09 to 2.57 ± 0.09 mmol/L after 1 week.[67] This was followed by a rise after discontinuation to 2.86 ± 0.09 mmol/L 1 week later. The dosage used was 300 IU three times daily. During therapy, hydroxyproline excretion decreased slightly but significantly. The absence of significant side effects was stressed.

Thus, both INSCT and IRSCT are effective and useful modes of administration of CT. More research must be undertaken to optimize these routes of administration and to make other routes available to the clinician. We have now tested SCT delivery by oral inhalation (an aerosol without absorption promoter) and shown it to be effectively absorbed into the blood stream by this route.[68]

SUMMARY AND CONCLUSIONS

Alternative modes of administration of calcitonin have been used in the treatment of Paget's disease of bone; a nasal spray with surfactant (1% sodium taurocholate), a plain spray without surfactant, and two suppositories of different composition. All were very effective in patients with Paget's disease who had not been given SCT previously. The effectiveness of the nasal spray with surfactant was not conditioned in our experience either by previous SCT therapy or by SCT antibodies but entailed local toxicity to the nasal mucosa. Its potency was of the order of magnitude of SCT administered subcutaneously. However, treatment with this kind of spray was only pursued for 3 months. The plain spray without surfactant and the suppository seemed to have limited activity when patients had received SCT previously and when SCT antibodies, even at a low titer, were present. Perhaps this is linked to low bioavailability of the preparations. Nevertheless, in ordinary circumstances, the plain spray and/or the suppository can be extraordinarily useful and an ideal substitute for the parenteral mode of administration of SCT, even to the point of being able to affect focal bone balance of osteolytic lesions positively as indicated by radiograph in some patients. Furthermore, these modes of administration, especially the plain nasal spray, are well tolerated, both locally and systemically.

REFERENCES

1. Nagant de Deuxchaisnes C: Calcitonin in the treatment of Paget's disease. *Triangle* 1983;22:103–128.
2. Nagant de Deuxchaisnes C: Use of calcitonin in the treatment of postmenopausal osteoporosis, In DeLuca HF, Mazess R (eds.): *Osteoporosis. Physiological Basis, Assessment, and Treatment.* New York, Elsevier, 1990, pp 247–258.
3. Nagant de Deuxchaisnes C: Medical management of Paget's disease, In DeGroot LJ (ed.): *Endocrinology,* 2nd ed. Vol 2. Philadelphia, WB Saunders, 1989, pp 1211–1244.
4. Nagant de Deuxchaisnes C, Devogelaer JP: Surveillance et suivi à long terme de la maladie osseuse de Paget (except English summary), In Simon L, Sebert JL, Herisson C (eds.): *La Maladie Osseuse de Paget. Actualités.* Paris, Masson, 1989, pp 257–273.
5. Nagant de Deuxchaisnes C, Devogelaer JP, Huaux JP, et al: Effect of a nasal spray of salmon calcitonin in normal subjects and in patients with Paget's disease of bone, In Pecile A (ed.): Calcitonin 1984. Amsterdam, Elsevier Science Publishers BV, 1985, pp 329–343.
6. Nagant de Deuxchaisnes C, Devogelaer JP, Huaux JP, et al: New modes of administration of salmon calcitonin in Paget's disease. Nasal spray and suppository. *Clin Orthop* 1987;217:56–71.
7. Pontiroli AE, Calderara A, Pozza G: Intranasal drug delivery: Potential advantages and limitation from a clinical pharmacokinetic perspective. *Clin Pharmacokinet* 1989; 17:299–307.
8. Ziegler R, Holz G, Raue F, Streibl W: Nasal application of human calcitonin in Paget's disease of bone, In MacIntyre I, Szelke M (eds.): *Molecular Endocrinology.* Amsterdam, Elsevier/North Holland Biomedical Press, 1979, pp 293–300.
9. Guttman S: Chemistry and structure-activity relationship of natural and synthetic calcitonins, In Pecile A (ed.): Calcitonin 1980. Amsterdam, Excerpta Medica, 1981, pp 11–24.
10. Singer FR, Rude RK, Mills BG: Studies of the treatment and aetiology of Paget's disease of bone, In MacIntyre I (ed.): Human Calcitonin and Paget's disease. Bern, Hans Huber Publishers, 1977, pp 93–110.
11. Marx SJ, Woodard CJ, Aurbach GD: Calcitonin receptors of kidney and bone. *Science* 1972;178:999–1000.
12. Pontiroli AE, Alberetto M, Pozza G: Intranasal calcitonin and plasma calcium concentrations in normal subjects. *Br Med J* 1985;290:1390–91.
13. Russell RGG, Smith R, Preston C, et al: Diphosphonates in Paget's disease. *Lancet* 1974;1:894–898.
14. Levy F, Muff R, Dotti-Sigrist S, et al: Formation of neutralizing antibodies during intranasal synthetic salmon calcitonin treatment of Paget's disease. *J Clin Endocrinol Metab* 1988;67:541–45.
15. Duchateau GSMJE, Zuidema J, Merkus FWHM: Bile salts and intranasal drug absorption. *Int J Pharm* 1986;31:193–199.
16. Nagant de Deuxchaisnes C, Devogelaer JP, Huaux JP, et al: Intranasal calcitonin and plasma calcium concentrations. *Br Med J* 1985;291:544–545.
17. Gagel RF, Logan C, Mallette LE: Treatment of Paget's disease of bone with salmon calcitonin nasal spray. *J Am Geriatr Soc* 1988;36:1011–1014.
18. D'Agostino HR, Barnett CA, Zielinski XJ, Gordan GS: Intranasal salmon calcitonin treatment of Paget's disease of bone. *Clin Orthop* 1988;230:223–228.
19. O'Doherty DP, Bickerstaff DR, McCloskey EV, et al: A comparison of the acute effects of subcutaneous and intranasal calcitonin. *Clin Sci* 1990;78:215–219.

20. Thamsborg G, Storm TL, Brinch E, et al: The effect of different doses of nasal salmon calcitonin on plasma cyclic AMP and serum ionized calcium. *Calcif Tissue Int* 1990; 46:5–8.
21. Pun KK, Chan LWL, Lau P, et al: Absorption of intranasal salmon calcitonin in normal subjects and hypogonadic men. *Calcif Tissue Int* 1990;46:130–132.
22. Nagant de Deuxchaisnes C, Devogelaer JP: Alternative routes of administration of salmon calcitonin, In Mazzuoli GF (ed.): *Calcitonin '88*. Milan, Esi Stampa Medica SpA, 1989, pp 87–98.
23. Nagant de Deuxchaisnes C, Maldague B, Malghem J, et al: The action of the main therapeutic regimes on Paget's disease of bone, with a note on the effect of vitamin D deficiency. *Arthritis Rheum* 1980;23:1215–1234.
24. Maldague B, Malghem J: Dynamic radiologic patterns of Paget's disease of bone. *Clin Orthop* 1987;217:126–151.
25. Reginster JY, Jeugmans-Huynen AM, Albert A, et al: One year's treatment of Paget's disease of bone by synthetic salmon calcitonin as a nasal spray. *J Bone Min Res* 1988; 3:249–252.
26. Reginster JY, Franchimont P: Side effects of synthetic salmon calcitonin given by intranasal spray compared with intramuscular injection. *Clin Exp Rheumatol* 1985;3:155–157.
27. Eisinger J: Action de la calcitonine en spray nasal chez les pagétiques. *Lyon Mediter Med* 1985;221:9631–9634.
28. Eisinger J: Tolérance clinique de la calcitonine en fonction du mode d'administration: Intérêt des formes non injectables. *Rev Rhum Mal Osteoartic* 1987;54:65–67.
29. Gennari C, Chierichetti SM, Vibelli C, et al: Acute effects of salmon, human and porcine calcitonin on plasma calcium and cyclic AMP levels in man. *Curr Ther Res* 1981;30:1024–1032.
30. MacIntyre I, Stevenson JC, Whitehead MI, et al: Calcitonin for prevention of postmenopausal bone loss. *Lancet* 1988;1:900–901.
31. Langer B, Peytremann A, Rufener C, Jenny M: Effets comparés de l'administration d'une dose unique de calcitonine synthétique (de type humain et de type saumon), chez l'homme normal et les sujets atteints de maladie de Paget ou d'hypercalcémie. *Schweiz Med Wochenschr* 1971;101:69–80.
32. Blanc D, Chapuy MC, Meunier P: Evaluation de l'activité ostéaclastique par le test d'hypocalcémie provoquée par la calcitonine de saumon. *Nouv Presse Med* 1977;6:2489–2494.
33. Fournié A, Valverde C, Tap G, et al: Test d'hypocalcémie aiguë à la calcitonine de porc et de saumon. *Rev Rhum Mal Osteoartic* 1977;44:91–98.
34. Buclin T, Randin JP, Jacquet AF, et al: The effect of rectal and nasal administration of salmon calcitonin in normal subjects. *Calcif Tissue Int* 1987;41:252–258.
35. Kurose H, Seino Y, Shima M, et al: Intranasal absorption of salmon calcitonin. *Calcif Tissue Int* 1987;41:249–251.
36. Vega E, Gonzales D, Ghiringielli G, Mautalen C: Acute effect of the intranasal administration of salmon calcitonin in osteoporotic women. *Bone Miner* 1989;7:267–273.
37. Reginster JY, Denis D, Albert A, Franchimont P: Assessment of the biological effectiveness of nasal synthetic salmon calcitonin (SSCT) by comparison with intramuscular (I.M.) or placebo injection in normal subjects. *Bone Miner* 1987;2:133–140.
38. Krane SM, Harris ED Jr, Singer FR, Potts JT Jr: Acute effects of calcitonin on bone formation in man. *Metabolism* 1973;22:51–58.
39. Gonzales D, Vega E, Ghiringhelli G, Mautalen C: Comparison of the acute effect of the intranasal and intramuscular administration of salmon calcitonin in Paget's disease. *Calcif Tissue Int* 1987;41:313–315.

40. Eisinger J: Comparison de l'effet hypocalcémiant immédiat de la calcitonine de saumon par voie veineuse et par voie nasale. *Rev Rhum Mal Osteoartic* 1985;52:195.
41. Tarquini B, Cavallini V, Cariddi A, et al: Prominent circadian absorption of intranasal salmon calcitonin (SCT) in healthy subjects. *Chronobiologia* 1988;5:149–152.
42. Elomaa I, Azria M, Attinger M, Bleicher M: Pilot evaluation of the hypocalcemic effect of intranasal salmon calcitonin. *Calcif Tissue Int* 1985;37 (suppl):Abstract 383.
43. Sjöberg HE, Torring O: Effect of nasal calcitonin in mild primary hyperparathyroidism. *J Bone Min Res* 1986;1(suppl 1): abstract 369.
44. Wallach S: Comparative effects of salmon, human and eel calcitonins on skeletal turnover in human disease, in Gennari C, Segre G (eds.): *The Effects of Calcitonin in Man*. Milan, Masson Italia Editori, 1983, pp 141–151.
45. Hosking DJ: Practical implications of calcitonin antigenicity. In Gennari C, Segre G (eds.): *The Effects of Calcitonin in Man*. Milan, Masson Italia Editori, 1983, pp 67–74.
46. Singer FR, Rude RK, Mills BG: Studies of the treatment and aetiology of Paget's disease of bone. In MacIntyre I (ed.): *Human Calcitonin and Paget's Disease*. Bern, Hans Huber Publishers, 1977, pp 93–110.
47. Avramides A, Flores A, DeRose J, Wallach S: Treatment of Paget's disease of bone with once a week injections of salmon calcitonin. *Brit Med J* 1975;3:632.
48. Wallach S: Discussion after Singer et al.[52]
49. Evans IMA: Human calcitonin in the treatment of Paget's disease: Long-term trials, in MacIntyre I (ed.): *Human Calcitonin and Paget's Disease*. Bern, Hans Huber Publishers, 1977;111–123.
50. Bordier PJ, Woodhouse NJY, Maris PJ, et al: Treatment of Paget's disease with human calcitonin: Histological evidence of healing. *Eur J Clin Invest* 1972;2:275.
51. Palmieri GMA, Pitcock JA, Brown P, et al: Effect of calcitonin and vitamin D in osteoporosis. *Calcif Tissue Int* 1989;45:137–141.
52. Singer FR, Fredericks RS, Minkin C: Salmon calcitonin therapy for Paget's disease of bone: The problem of acquired clinical resistance. *Arthritis Rheum* 1980;23:1148–1153.
53. Muff R, Dambacher MA, Perrenoud A, et al: Efficacy of intranasal human calcitonin in patients with Paget's disease refractory to salmon calcitonin. *Am J Med* 1990; 89:181–184.
54. Reginster JY, Almer S, Gaspar S, et al: Hypocalcémie induite chez le sujet pagétique par la calcitonine salmine nasale: Effets des anticorps anticalcitonine salmine. *Rev Rhum Mal Osteoartic* 1989;56(7):563–567.
55. Reginster JY, Gennari C, Mautalen C, et al: Influence of specific anti-salmon calcitonin antibodies on biological effectiveness of nasal salmon calcitonin in Paget's disease of bone. *Scand J Rheumatol* 1990;19:83–86.
56. Grauer A, Raue F, Schneider HG, et al: In vitro detection of neutralizing antibodies after treatment of Paget's disease of bone with nasal salmon calcitonin. *J Bone Miner Res* 1990;5:387–391.
57. Rojanasathit D, Rosenberg E, Haddad JG Jr: Paget's bone disease: Response to human calcitonin in patients resistant to salmon calcitonin. *Lancet* 1974;2:1412–1415.
58. Hosking DJ: Calcitonin and diphosphonate in the treatment of Paget's disease of bone. *Metab Bone Dis Rel Res* 1981;3:317–326.
59. Haddad JG, Whyte MP, Murphy WA: Human calcitonin therapy: Efficacy in Paget's bone disease in patients with antibody resistance to heterologous calcitonins and in patients with lytic skeletal lesion. In Caniggia A (ed.): *Human Calcitonin*. Milan, Ciba-Geigy SpA, 1983, pp 87–93.
60. Scuro LA, Lo Cascio V, Adami S: Therapeutic use of human calcitonin in patients with Paget's disease resistant to heterologous calcitonins. In Caniggia A (ed.): *Human Calcitonin*. Milan, Ciba-Geigy SpA, 1983, pp 181–191.

61. Nakada Y, Awata N, Nakamichi C, Sugimoto I: The effect of additives on the oral mucosal absorption of human calcitonin in rats. *J Pharmacobiodyn* 1988;11:395–401.
62. Cho YW, Flynn M: Oral delivery of insulin. *Lancet* 1989;2:1518–1519.
63. Singer FR, Villanueva R, Ginger K: Acquired resistance to salmon and human calcitonin during treatment of Paget's disease of bone. *Calcif Tissue Int* 1989;44 (suppl):S-87 (N32).
64. Zanelli JM, Salmon M, Lane E, et al: Chronic treatment of rats with salmon calcitonin: A model for clinical resistance. *Calcif Tissue Int* 1984;34:480 (abstract).
65. Acezat-Mispelmer F, Boucherat M, Souchet T, et al: Evaluation of nasal tolerability of synthetic salmon calcitonin solution administered by nasal route. *J Bone Min Res* 1989; 4:S192 (abstract 300).
66. Miyake M, Nishihata T, Nagano A, et al: Rectal absorption of [ASU]-EEL calcitonin in rats. *Chem Pharm Bull* 1985;33:740–745.
67. Thiébaud D, Burckhardt P, Jaeger P, Azria M: Effectiveness of salmon calcitonin administered as suppositories in tumor-induced hypercalcemia. *Am J Med* 1987;82:745–750.
68. Nagant de Deuxchaisnes C: Development of alternative modes of administration of calcitonin, in Christiansen C, Overgaard K (eds.): Osteoporosis 1990. Copenhagen, Osteopress ApS, 1990, pp 1958–1962.

CHAPTER 12

Treatment of Paget's Disease with Short Courses of Bisphosphonates

Peter Burckhardt and D. Thiébaud

INTRODUCTION

Since calcitonin has become available, the treatment of Paget's disease has required continuous administration of the drug until a maximal effect is obtained. Interruption of the treatment is usually followed by eventual relapse. When bisphosphonates were introduced, the regimen was not changed; the drugs were given over prolonged periods of at least several months. However, it appeared that the bisphosphonates, especially those of the second generation, were more efficient than calcitonin in that they had a greater ability to lower the biochemical parameters of Paget's disease into the normal range.[1] When the drugs were given until normalization was obtained, the effect was sustained for a relatively long period, with complete remission in some cases. Since it was not possible to relate sustained inhibition of abnormal pagetic bone remodeling to the total amount of bisphosphonates given, it was theorized that shorter periods of treatment might still have a prolonged effect, so long as the total dose administered was sufficiently high. Given the low and rather erratic intestinal absorption of bisphosphonates, such short courses had to be administered by the parenteral route.

SHORT COURSES OF BISPHOSPHONATES

The first therapeutical trials were published in 1985 involving short courses of 5 days only.[2] Treated patients showed an immediate drop in urinary hydroxyproline excretion and a slower but constant decrease of alkaline phosphatase that continued over several months after the administration of clodronate (Cl2MBP), accompanied by sustained clinical improvement. This effect was also demonstrated with very short courses of other bisphosphonates, such as AHBP,[3] APD,[4] EHDP,[5] and AHBuBP,[6] given over 4 to 7 days (Table 12.1). Therefore it became possible to achieve treatment of Paget's disease with a small series of infusions and to obtain positive effects that were sustained for at least several months.

However, these short courses of bisphosphonates, were not necessarily sufficient for healing severe cases of Paget's disease. In addition, they were not practicable on an outpatient basis, and for this reason they would have been economically unacceptable to many countries. Therefore, it was important to demonstrate that the efficacy of short courses of treatment was not due to the parenteral administration of the drug but to the fact that the total dose of bisphosphonates was sufficient. Assuming that the absorption rate of APD is between 2% and 3%, 1,200 mg/d given orally would correspond to 30 mg/d given intravenously and a short course of 5 days with this oral dose should yield results comparable to those of intravenous treatment with 30 mg for 5 days. The results of such treatment indeed corresponded to that which would be expected with intravenous treatment: a decrease in hydroxyproline excretion within 7 days and of alkaline phosphatase within 3 months, with a sustained effect for 6 months or

TABLE 12.1 Short Intravenous Treatments with Bisphosphonates

Ref.	Author	Drug*	Daily Dose	Duration of Treatment, days	Total Dose	No.	Infusion h/day
2	Yates	Cl_2MBP	300 mg	5	1500 mg	31	3
4	Vera	APD	25 mg	7	175 mg	9	2
8	Delmas	APD	10 mg	7	70 mg	9	3
			25 mg	7	175 mg	17	7
3	Atkins	AHBP	25 mg	5	125 mg	17	3
4	Cantrill	HEBP	300 mg	5	1500 mg	7	3
5	Ibbertson	APD	15 mg	5	75 mg	11	1
14	Cantrill	APD	±26 mg	5	±130 mg	(61)	2
6	Adami	AHBuBP	2.5–25 mg	4	10–100 mg	14	2
8	Delmas	APD	60 mg	3	180 mg	9	24
11	Thiébaud	APD	60 mg	1	60 mg	11	24

*Cl_2MBP = dichloromethylene biphosphonate (clodronate); APD = aminohydroxy-propylidene biphosphonate (pamidronate, AHPrBP); AHBP = aminohexame-bisphosphonate; HEBP = hydroxy-ethylidene biphosphonate (etidronate); AHBuBP = aminohydroxy-butylidene biphosphonate.

longer[7] (Figure 12.1). Scintigraphic skeletal studies showed a significant effect after 6 months. It was concluded that with a sufficiently high dose, orally or intravenously, the accelerated bone turnover could be normalized for a period of several months or more.

Sustained efficacy after a short oral treatment course was seen in mild cases but more severe cases of Paget's disease probably require higher bisphosphonate doses to achieve remission. These higher doses could hardly be administered within a few days. Because of the uncertain pharmacodynamics and toxicity of these agents during prolonged oral administration of high doses, most specialists still depend on 5-day intravenous courses, administering a total of 75 to 250 mg of APD, 125 to 250 mg of AHBP, 1,500 mg of HEBP, or 1,500 mg of Cl_2MBP (Table 12.1).

LONG-TERM EFFECTS

In many cases, the biochemical data, specifically hydroxyproline excretion and serum alkaline phosphatase activity, showed prolonged normalization for up to 1 year or more.[7] More importantly, there was also a prolonged

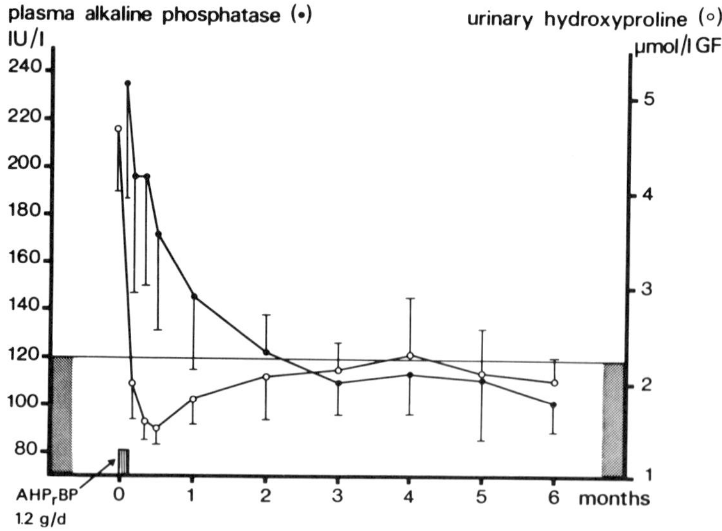

FIGURE 12.1. Sustained normalization of biochemical parameters after a short course with APD (AHPrBP), 1.2 g/d per os for 5 days. Six patients with Paget's disease were studied. *Reproduced from Thiébaud et al,[7] with permission.*

normalization of the pagetic bone structure, histomorphometrically and radiologically. When APD was given for only 3 days at a rate of 60 mg/d intravenously, normalization of bone structure could be observed radiologically 6 months after the treatment (P. J. Meunier, personal communication), in agreement with significant histologic improvement of pagetic bone in bone biopsy findings 3 months after treatment with APD for only 5 days.[8]

Clinical effects that are obvious at the beginning of the treatment and are usually parallel to biologic effects, are more difficult to quantify on a long-term basis. Since biochemical relapse is usually accompanied by clinical and radiologic relapse, a sustained biochemical effect usually means real remission. Clinical relapse can precede a recrudescence of the biochemical parameters, but this is exceptional.

SINGLE-DAY TREATMENT

In the treatment of malignant hypercalcemia, which is a model for bone disease with increased bone resorption, a single infusion of APD is as effective in normalizing plasma calcium as more prolonged APD treatment,[9] although patients with severe hypercalcemia needed a relatively higher doses for full effectiveness. After a low dose, plasma calcium did not completely normalize or hypercalcemia returned soon afterward.[10] This dose dependency in malignant hypercalcemia suggests that a single low-dose infusion might represent a suboptimal dose, whereas prolonged treatment might result in supraoptimal doses. By analogy, it was assumed that a single infusion of a bisphosphonate might be sufficient for mild cases of Paget's disease. Indeed, when 60 mg of APD was given in a single infusion to patients with mild Paget's disease, an immediate normalization of hydroxyproline and subsequent normalization of alkaline phosphatase were followed by a prolonged period of remission of up to 1 year[11] (Figure 12.2). Although small acute decreases in plasma and urinary calcium and phosphorus within the normal range were rapidly reversed within a few days, it was several months until they had returned to initial levels (Figure 12.3). Osteocalcin (bone Gla protein) increased at first and then showed a constant decrease over the next 4 months until it stabilized at a lower level (Figure 12.4). These subtle biochemical changes over several months illustrate the prolonged effect on bone metabolism exerted by a single administration of APD. Although no radiologic and histomorphometric data are available to demonstrate a long-term effect after a single infusion, it can be assumed that the effects are not necessarily different from those demonstrated several months after a treatment of 3 days' length.

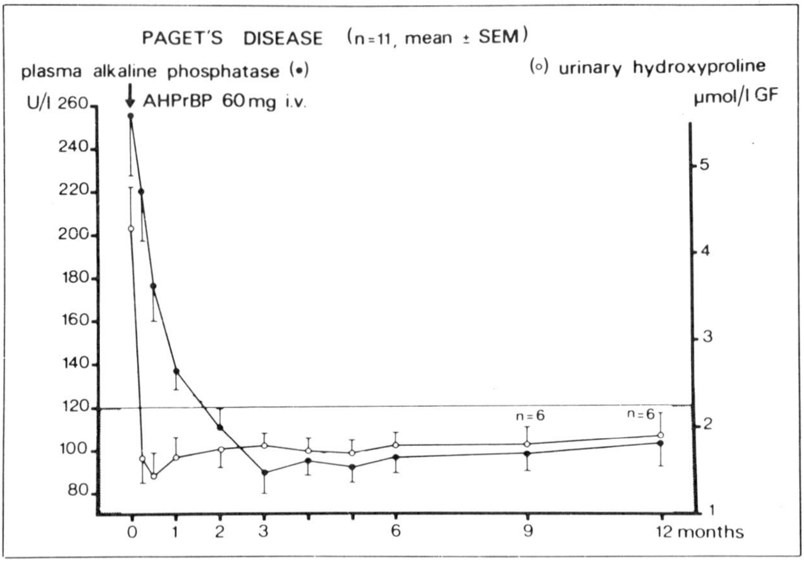

FIGURE 12.2. Sustained normalization of biochemical parameters after a single infusion of 60 mg APD (AHPrBP) intravenously in 11 patients with Paget's disease. *Reproduced from Thiébaud et al,[12] with permission.*

TREATMENT OF RELAPSES

The advantages offered by a treatment with a single infusion are obvious: no hospitalization and no problems with compliance. The disadvantages are in the risk of an insufficient dose with insufficient effectiveness and a higher relapse rate. This is especially likely to occur in severe cases of Paget's disease. Indeed, in some patients, a single infusion was capable of normalizing some of the features of pagetic bone, but the advancing zone of bone lysis persisted and expanded again after a couple of months. In the treatment of malignant hypercalcemia, it has been shown that relapses of hypercalcemia can be treated by further infusions of APD, although efficacy is slightly less satisfactory.[12] When biochemical parameters of Paget's disease relapse to above the normal range, a second course with bisphosphonates has been shown to be very effective.[2,6,11] In this regard, a single infusion may also be effective (Figure 12.5).

STRATEGIES BASED ON SHORT TREATMENTS

Since short treatments (including single infusions) can easily be repeated, it is acceptable that the first course not completely normalize hydroxyproline

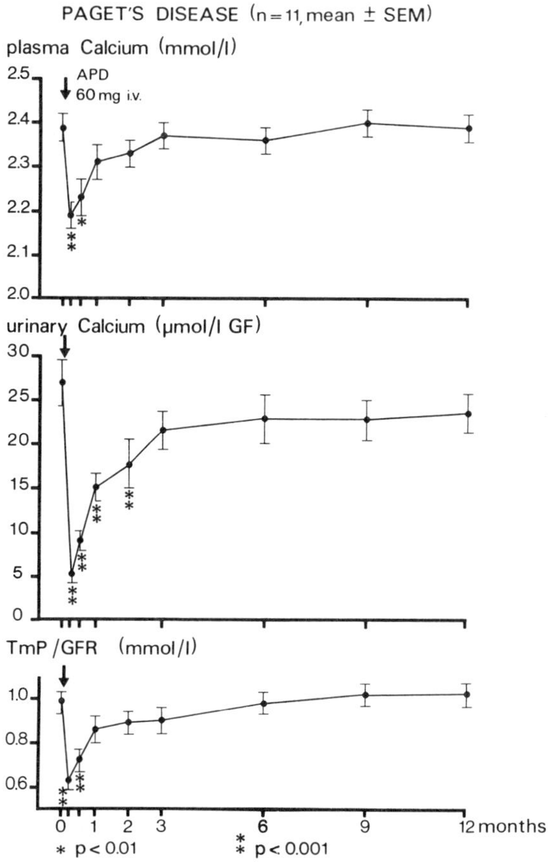

FIGURE 12.3. Plasma and urinary calcium before and after a single infusion of 60 mg APD (AHPrBP) intravenously in 11 patients with Paget's disease. *Reproduced from Thiébaud et al,*[12] *with permission.*

excretion, although such normalization is the ultimate goal of the treatment. It is therefore reasonable that severe cases be treated with two or three infusions of bisphosphonates whereas mild cases need only a single infusion (Figure 12.6). Monthly or at least 3-month reassessments will reveal whether normalization has occurred. It must be remembered that the normalization of alkaline phosphatase may take 3 months longer than hydroxyproline excretion. In the case of partial responses a second infusion or series of infusions can be undertaken. How often this procedure can be repeated successfully is still open. Since total doses absorbed during continuous oral treatments usually exceed the doses given by repetitive short intravenous courses and show no side effects or resistance it can be pre-

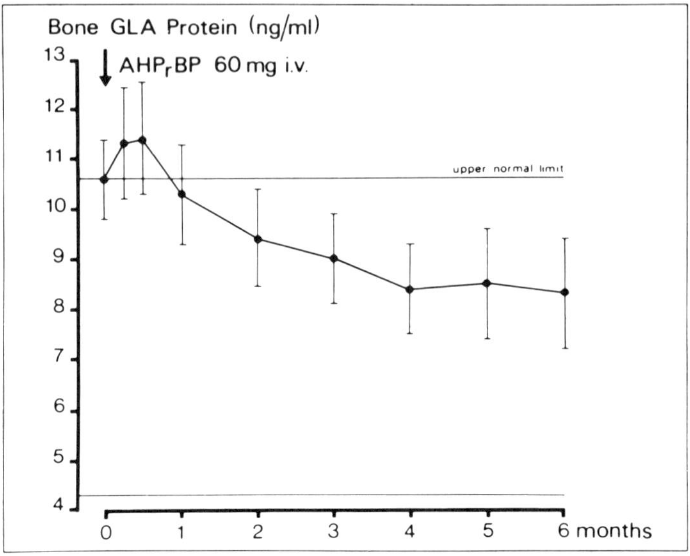

FIGURE 12.4. Sustained normalization of plasma osteocalcin (bone Gla protein) after a single infusion of 60 mg APD (AHPrBP) intravenously in 7 patients with Paget's disease. *Reproduced from Thiébaud et al,[12] with permission.*

sumed that short intravenous courses can be repeated several times. One research group[13,14,15] gave five consecutive infusions of 15 mg APD each, probably an insufficient dose for all cases. This was followed by a protocol of weekly infusions of 15 mg for 12 weeks, then 30 mg for 6 or 12 weeks; finally a protocol evolved of biweekly infusions of 60 mg, three to six times according to the severity of the case, on the basis of values greater or less than 500 units/L of alkaline phosphatase. They observed a complete remission after one course in 63% of patients, and 80% when the protocol was repeated three or four times. Although it is somewhat demanding on an outpatient to return every second week for an infusion, this sequential approach offers the advantage of observing the effectiveness of each dose and adding progressively more bisphosphonate until total remission. Alternatively, higher doses per infusion or grouping of two or three infusion into a single course would permit the patient to return for reassessment less often, every 3 months.

CONCLUSION

Short intravenous courses of bisphosphonate have a sustained effect on Paget's disease. The immediate and sustained effect of a single infusion of

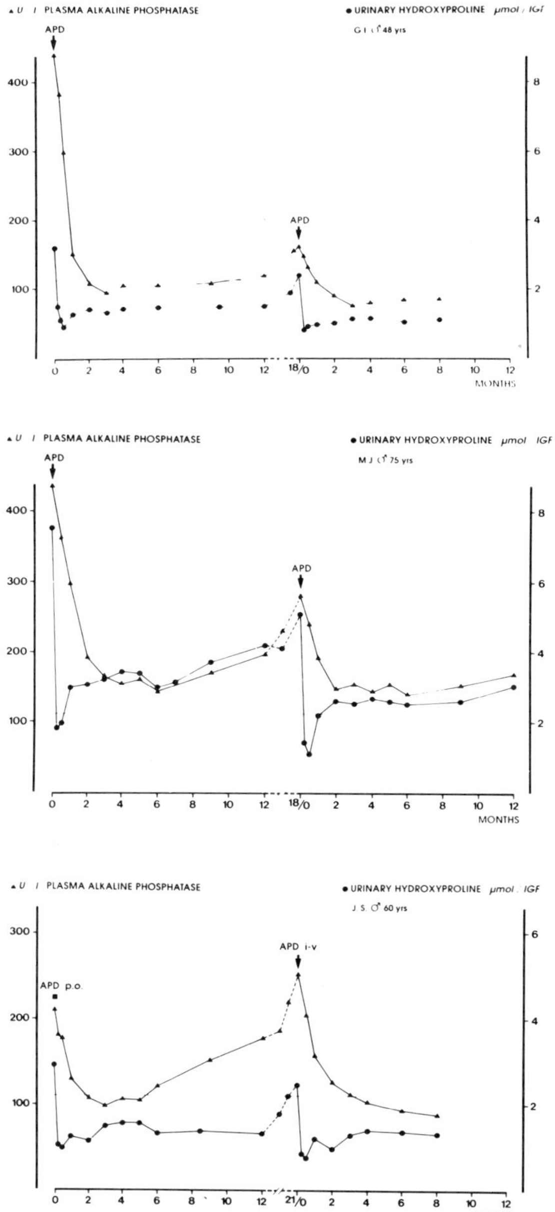

FIGURE 12.5. Efficacy of retreatment of recurrent Paget's disease with single infusions of APD (AHPrBP). The upper normal range of plasma alkaline phosphatase is 120 U/L, and the upper normal range of urinary hydroxyproline is 2.2 μmol/GF.

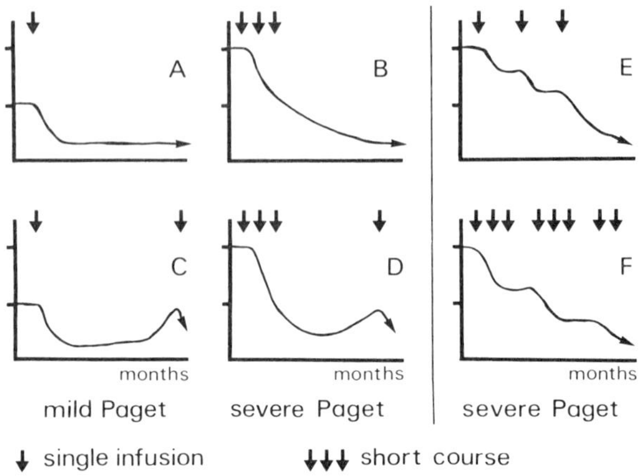

FIGURE 12.6. Therapeutic strategies using short treatments of bisphosphonates: single infusion or single course of several infusions with remission in mild (A) and in severe (B) disease, with recurrence in mild (C) and in severe (D) disease; repeated infusions (E) or courses (F) in severe disease.

bisphosphonates in malignant hypercalcemia motivated therapeutic trials of a single infusion of APD in Paget's disease. In mild cases, this was sufficient for immediate and sustained normalization of biochemical parameters. Severe cases need several infusions or repeated single infusions. Therapeutic strategies based on single or repeated infusions can be used in outpatient clinics and prevent difficulties with compliance and uncertain intestinal absorption. This approach permits adapting the total dose to the severity of the disease and its evolution.

REFERENCES

1. Frijlink P, Velde JTE, Bijvoet OLM, Heynen G: Treatment of Paget's disease with (3-amino-1-hydroxypropylidene)-1, 1-bisphosphonate (APD). *Lancet* 1979;1:799–803.
2. Yates AJP, Percival RC, Gray RES, et al: Intravenous clodronate in the treatment and retreatment of Paget's disease of bone. *Lancet* 1985;1:1474–1477.
3. Atkins RM, Yates AJP, Gray RES, et al: Aminohexane diphosphonate in the treatment of Paget's disease of bone. *J Bone Mineral Res* 1987;2(4):273–279.
4. Vera E, Gonzalez D, Ghiringhelli G, Mautalen C: Intravenous aminopropylidene bisphosphonate (APD) in the treatment of Paget's bone disease. *J Bone Mineral Res* 1987;2(4):267–271.
5. Lawson-Matthew PW, Guilland-Cumming DF, Yates AJP, et al: Contrasting effects of intravenous and oral etidronate on vitamin D metabolism in man. *Clin Sci* 1988;74:101–106.
6. Adami S, Salvagno G, Guarrera G, et al: Treatment of Paget's disease of bone with

intravenous 4-amino-1-hydroxybutylidene-1,1-bisphosphonate. *Calcif Tissue Int* 1986; 39:226–229.

7. Thiébaud D, Jaeger P, Burckhardt P: Paget's disease of bone treated in five days with AHPrBP (APD) per os. *J Bone Mineral Res* 1987;2(1):45–52.
8. Delmas PD, Casez JP, Arlot MA, et al: Long term effects of intravenous (IV) aminopropylidene diphosphonate (APD) in patients with refractory Paget's disease of bone. *Calcif Tissue Int* 1989;44(suppl):5104.
9. Thiébaud D, Jaeger P, Jacquet AF, Burckhardt P: A single-day treatment of tumor-induced hypercalcemia by intravenous amino-hydroxypropylidene bisphosphonate. *J Bone Mineral Res* 1986;1(6):555–562.
10. Thiébaud D, Jaeger P, Jacquet AF, Burckhardt P: Dose-response in the treatment of hypercalcemia of malignancy by a single infusion of the bisphosphonate AHPrPB. *J Clin Oncol* 1988;6(5):762–768.
11. Thiébaud D, Jaeger P, Gobelet C, et al: A single infusion of the bisphosphonate AHPrBP (APD) as treatment of Paget's disease of bone. *Am J Med* 1988;85:207–212.
12. Thiébaud D, Jaeger P, Burckhardt P: Response to retreatment of malignant hypercalcemia with the bisphosphonate AHPrBP (APD): Respective role of kidney and bone. *J Bone Mineral Res* 1990;5(3):221–226.
13. Richardson PC, Cantrill JA, Anderson DC: Experience of treating 218 patients with Paget's disease of bone using intravenous 3-aminohydroxy-propylidene 1-1 bisphosphonate (pamidronate, APD). *J Bone Mineral Res* 1989;4(suppl 1):S198.
14. Cantrill JA, Buckler HM, Anderson DC: Primary treatment of 133 patients with Paget's disease of bone with intravenous 3-amino-hydroxy-propylidene-1-1-,bisphosphonate (APD). *Calcif Tissue Int* 1988;42(suppl):52.
15. Ibbertson K, Dodd G, Holdaway I, et al: Paget's disease of bone: Reversal of bone lysis with pamidronate. *J Bone Mineral Res* 1989;4(suppl 1):S359.

CHAPTER 13

Two Decades of Experience in the Treatment of Paget's Disease of Bone with Plicamycin (Mithramycin)

Will G. Ryan

INTRODUCTION

Although Sir James Paget described the bone disease bearing his name in 1876, almost a century elapsed before effective therapies were developed. Now there are several and effective treatment of most if not all patients with the disorder will likely be possible within the next several years. Thus within the past 20 years, rapid strides have been made in our understanding of and ability to manage this disease.

Our introduction of mithramycin (now known as plicamycin to avoid confusion with mitomycin) in the late 1960s[1] was almost simultaneous with the introduction of the calcitonins and was followed shortly thereafter by the introduction of the bisphosphonates. The development of these later therapies has generally relegated plicamycin's use, because of its toxicity,[2,3] to a secondary role in treatment of Paget's disease resistant to the other agents and it remains a useful agent in that regard.

Plicamycin was widely used in the 1960s for treatment of a variety of cancers[4] and was most successful in the treatment of embryonal[5] and testicular cancer[6,7] at that time. Our selection of a cancer chemotherapeutic agent for therapy of Paget's disease was based on the premise that it resembled, in many respects, a low-grade neoplastic process. The osteoclasts in the areas of the skeleton involved in Paget's disease appear to have escaped from the factors that normally regulate their activity, similar to that seen in cancer. Thus it seemed that a cancer chemotherapeutic agent might be effective for treatment. What causes this loss of regulatory processes is at present unclear although there is evidence that it may be induced by a virus.[8,9] In considering a chemotherapeutic agent that might be active against the osteoclast we initially chose actinomycin D because it had been shown to block the effects of vitamin D- and parathyroid hormone-induced hypercalcemia in rats.[10,11] We cautiously administered this agent (in approximately one third the dose used in chemotherapy of cancer) to two subjects with advanced Paget's disease and saw a modest effect on serum alkaline phosphatase (SAP) and urinary hydroxyproline (OHP). The effect was not impressive enough for us to consider further use although it was subsequently used by another group.[12] At about that time[13] it was reported that hypocalcemia was occurring in some subjects in whom plicamycin was being used for cancer chemotherapy. This observation made us think that it would be useful to try it in Paget's disease in that the observed hypocalcemia was possibly caused by osteoclast toxicity. Subsequent experience has borne this out, and plicamycin is very useful in treatment of hypercalcemia of various causes.[14]

We cautiously administered plicamycin to several patients with advanced Paget's disease and observed dramatic effects on SAP and OHP

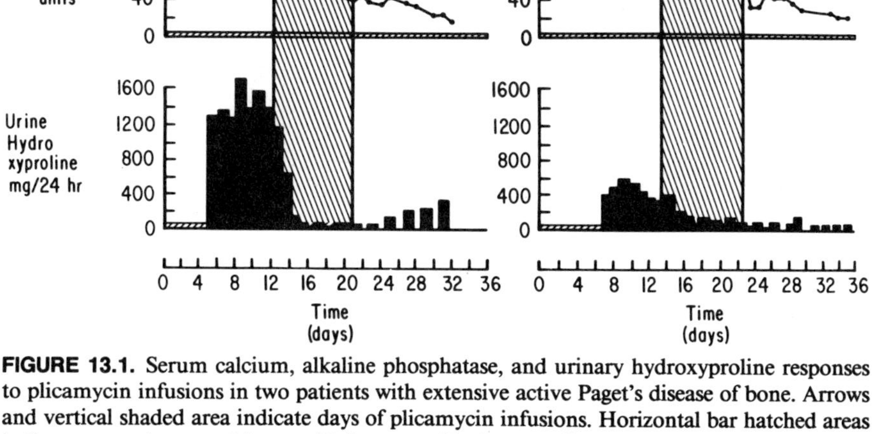

FIGURE 13.1. Serum calcium, alkaline phosphatase, and urinary hydroxyproline responses to plicamycin infusions in two patients with extensive active Paget's disease of bone. Arrows and vertical shaded area indicate days of plicamycin infusions. Horizontal bar hatched areas indicate normal ranges. Note rapid decrease of hydroxyproline accompanied by lowering of serum calcium and slower reduction in serum alkaline phosphatase. *Reproduced from Ryan et al,[15] with permission from the American Medical Association.*

with symptomatic relief as well.[1,15] Figure 13.1 is representative of the effects seen at a dose of 25 μg/kg/d for 10 days. Note the rapid decrease in OHP and serum calcium indicating the effect on osteoclastic activity, followed by the slower decline in SAP reflecting the compensatory decline in osteoblast activity.

Encouraged by these initial results we expanded its use over the next several years to approximately 200 patients.[16] On average, there was a two-thirds reduction in the level of SAP (Figure 13.2) and OHP (Figure 13.3) by the end of the treatment period with a variable further decline in SAP for 1 to 2 months thereafter (Figure 13.4). We have not used OHP extensively for evaluation of the therapeutic effect because of its expense and inconvenience to the patient, as well as our impression that SAP

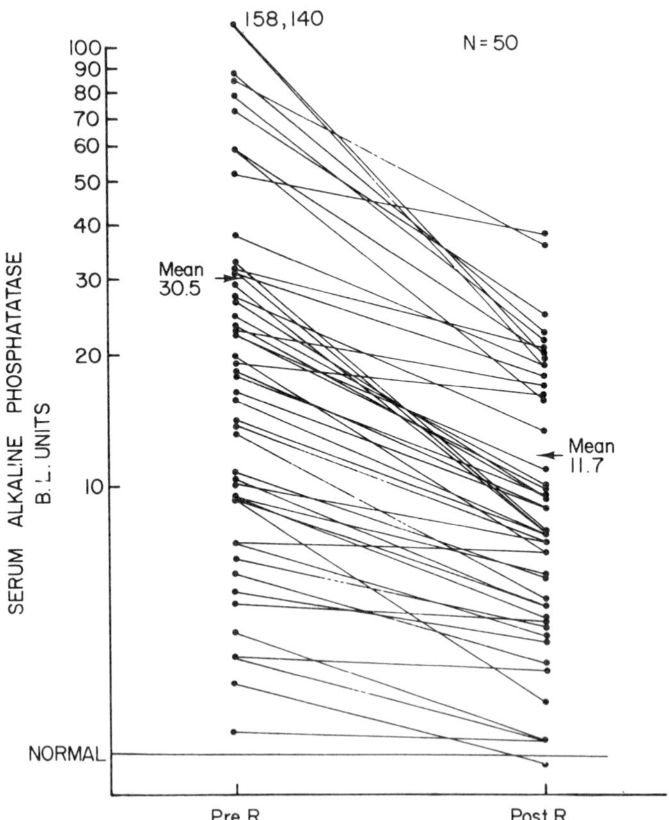

FIGURE 13.2. Individual pretreatment and immediate posttreatment serum alkaline phosphatase values in the first 50 subjects treated with plicamycin (25 μg/kg/d for 10 days). Note the log scale. *Reproduced from Ryan et al,[16] with permission.*

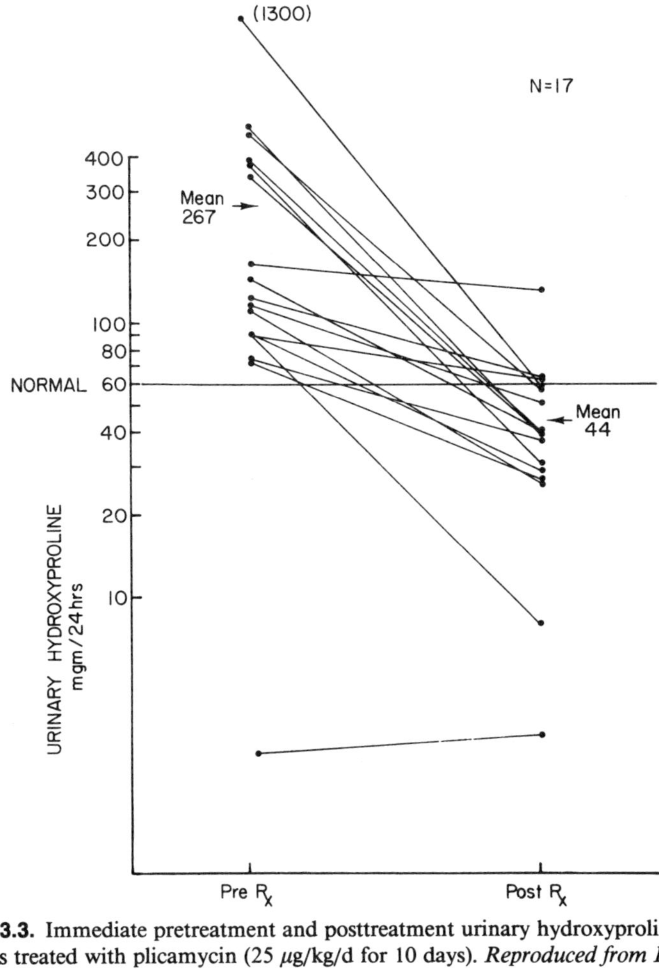

FIGURE 13.3. Immediate pretreatment and posttreatment urinary hydroxyproline values in 17 subjects treated with plicamycin (25 μg/kg/d for 10 days). *Reproduced from Ryan et al,[16] with permission.*

generally gives a more sensitive reflection of disease activity, except for evaluation of early stages of therapy. The overall effects were generally salutary (subjectively in relief of pain as well as objectively by SAP and bone scans) but generally lasted only 1 to 2 years. Roentgenographic evidence of bone remodeling was seen[17] but was unusual, as might be expected in the adult (Figure 13.5). Similar experiences have been reported by others, generally with lower doses and/or less frequent administration[18-21] with less toxicity, good symptomatic effects, but generally a less dramatic effect on the objective parameters of disease activity (SAP, OHP, and bone scan results). Russell et al[22] reported the effects of a 10-day

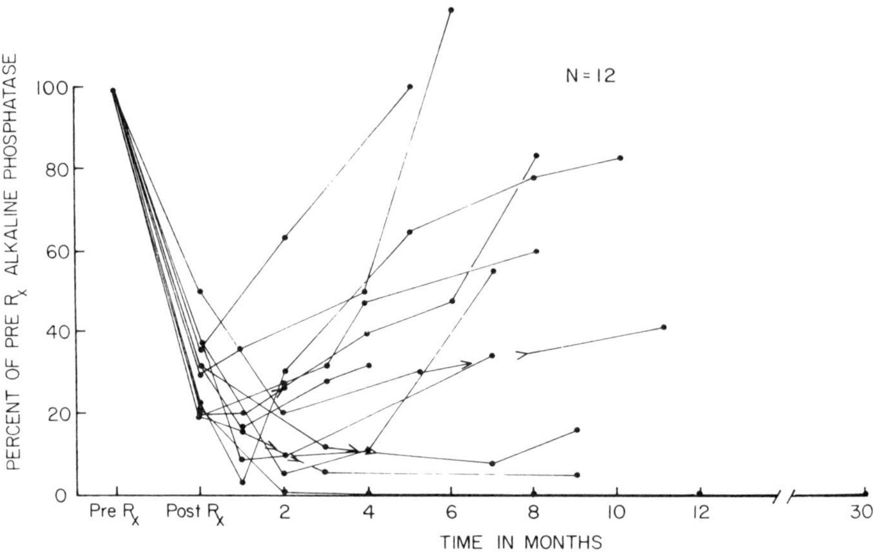

FIGURE 13.4. Pretreatment and posttreatment serum alkaline phosphatase values in 12 subjects, with subsequent values off treatment over the following months. *Reproduced from Ryan et al[16] with permission.*

course of plicamycin at 15 μg/kg/d in nine patients showing good symptomatic relief, lowering of SAP and OHP and improvement in results of bone scan performed with technetium-99m stannous phosphonate. Subsequently he reported[23] the long-term effectiveness of low-dose therapy (15 μg/kg/d for 3 days, reducing to 10 μg/kg/d "for a further week"). Symptomatic effectiveness was maintained, but "objective measures of disease activity were less favorable" and there was no evidence of long-term toxicity. He continues to use this regimen as the treatment of choice in patients with severe or significant Paget's disease and remains impressed by the dramatic results found. Russell believes that it is also a useful diagnostic test in patients with concomitant hip osteoarthritis to determine which is the more significant problem, the Paget's disease or the osteoarthritis (personal communication).

Heath[24] reported effective and rapid relief of bone pain in 18 patients who had received 27 courses of plicamycin therapy at a dose of 10 μg/kg/d for 10 days. He concluded, however, that long-term relief is unusual unless calcitonin or sodium etidronate is added. Condon et al[18] discussed treatment of Paget's disease with plicamycin and later he and his colleagues[25] reported on treatment in 12 patients using glucagon, calcitonin, and plicamycin. They concluded that calcitonin and glucagon have additive proper-

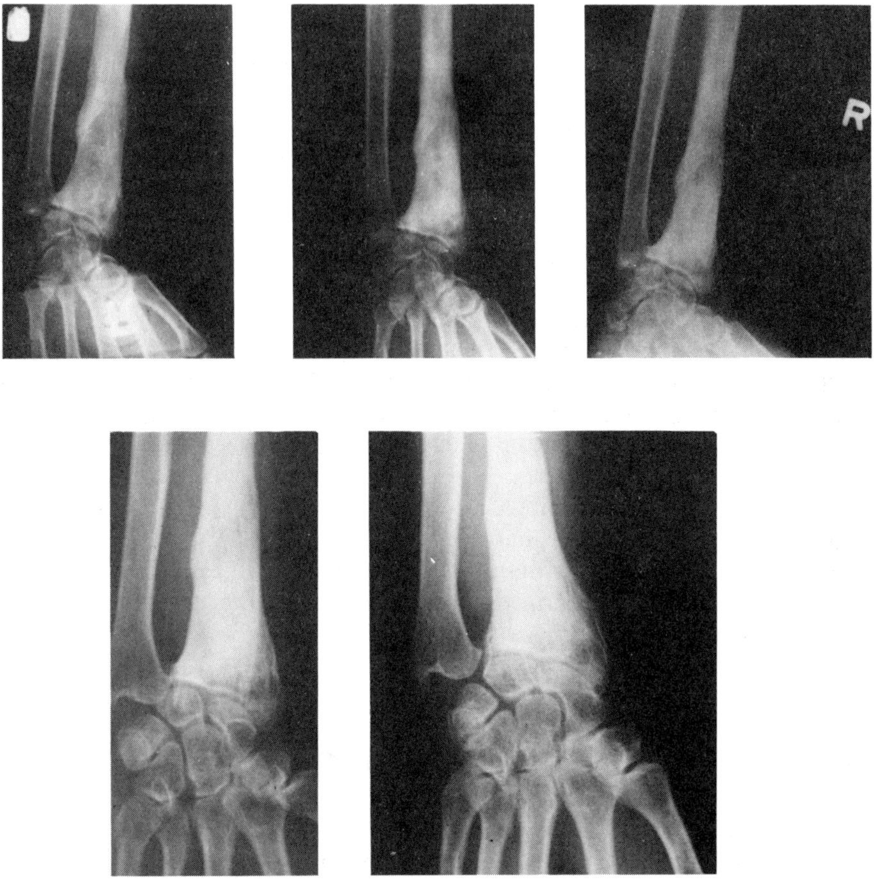

FIGURE 13.5. Serial radiographs of the distal forearm before and at approximately 6-month intervals during 2 years following plicamycin treatment. The patient's Paget's disease remained in remission during that interval. Radiographs taken during relapse several years later showed reversion toward the pretreatment appearance. *Reproduced from Ryan,[17] with permission.*

ties in Paget's disease and that the use of the three drugs in combination may reduce the incidence of side effects and development of "drug resistance."

Hadjipavlou et al.[26] reported on similar combinations and concluded that calcitonin combined with plicamycin was the most effective therapy. They also found plicamycin the most effective drug for achieving rapid control of pain. In view of the excellent results obtained in their patients with spinal stenosis caused by Paget's disease they advocated a trial of plicamycin therapy before any surgical decompression was begun.

Pembrook et al.[27] reported a favorable response of congestive heart failure to successive courses of therapy with plicamycin and calcitonin similar to that observed in our initial patient treated with plicamycin alone.[1] Ajlouni and Theil[28,29] reported detailed studies of calcium, phosphorus, parathyroid hormone, SAP, and OHP responses in several similarly treated patients. Their data essentially confirmed our previous observations.

Several patients have shown a continuation of the favorable effects over several years. One patient treated with plicamycin alone in 1972 and without subsequent antipagetic therapy[30] is still in complete remission as judged by serial bone scan results (Figure 13.6) and normal SAP and represents the longest remission and, possibly, the first documented cure of the disease.

Subsequently we embarked on trials of less intensive outpatient regimens and could show reasonable effects (Figure 13.7)[31] but subsequently abandoned these trials, primarily because of the nauseagenic side effect. Several patients even developed anticipatory nausea, as has been seen with various chemotherapies for cancer.

ADMINISTRATION OF PLICAMYCIN

The optimal dose and duration of administration of plicamycin are not firmly established. When originally used for cancer chemotherapy, doses of 25.5 to 50.0 μg/kg/d or every other day were commonly employed.[2] These doses, however, were associated with considerable toxicity, and hemorrhagic diatheses, sometimes resulting in death, were commonly encountered. Plicamycin use at lower doses is commonly associated with some degree of hepatic, renal, and platelet toxicity. We have the impression that 24-hour infusions are associated with the least toxicity and the greatest therapeutic effect. However, shorter infusion periods may be used, and we have commonly used intravenous injections under outpatient circumstances. Toxicity and therapeutic effect are closely related to frequency and amount of dosing. There does not appear to be significant delayed or cumulative toxicity. Nausea (and even anticipatory nausea as seen in other forms of chemotherapy) is a limiting factor with prolonged outpatient use of lower-dose therapy, even though other measures of toxicity are uncommon. Prolonged infusion periods are more commonly associated with extravasation into tissue surrounding the site of intravenous administra-

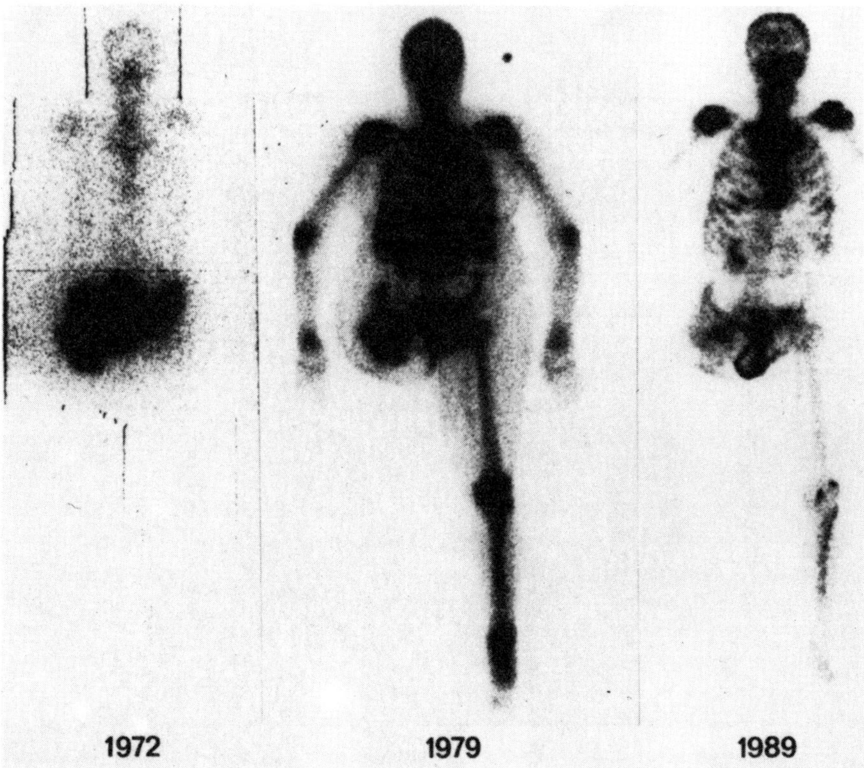

FIGURE 13.6. Bone scans made in 1972 (before treatment with plicamycin) and in 1979 and 1989 (7 and 17 years after treatment) in a patient who has had a prolonged remission of disease activity. Subsequent serial serum alkaline phosphatase values have remained normal, as have results of bone scans repeated in 1983 and 1989. Deformity in right pelvis is secondary to prior osteomyelitis complicating Paget's disease. Amputation was done several years before 1972. *Reproduced from Ryan and Schwartz[32] with permission.*

tion and are accompanied by a moderately severe and prolonged (several weeks to months) tissue reaction. We have never observed sloughing.

In lower doses (15 to 25 μg/kg of ideal body weight/d), reversible hepatotoxicity is almost invariably seen and is of little consequence as long as carefully monitored by daily determination of serum enzymes. The serum glutamic-pyruvic transaminase (SGPT) and isocitric dehydrogenase (ICD) increase over baseline to a greater extent and possibly occur about a day earlier than the increases of serum glutamic-oxaloacetic transaminase (SGOT) or lactate dehydrogenase (LDH). Thus, one or the other of the former should be included in the chemistry panels used to monitor toxicity. We commonly allow the SGPT to increase to approximately ten times

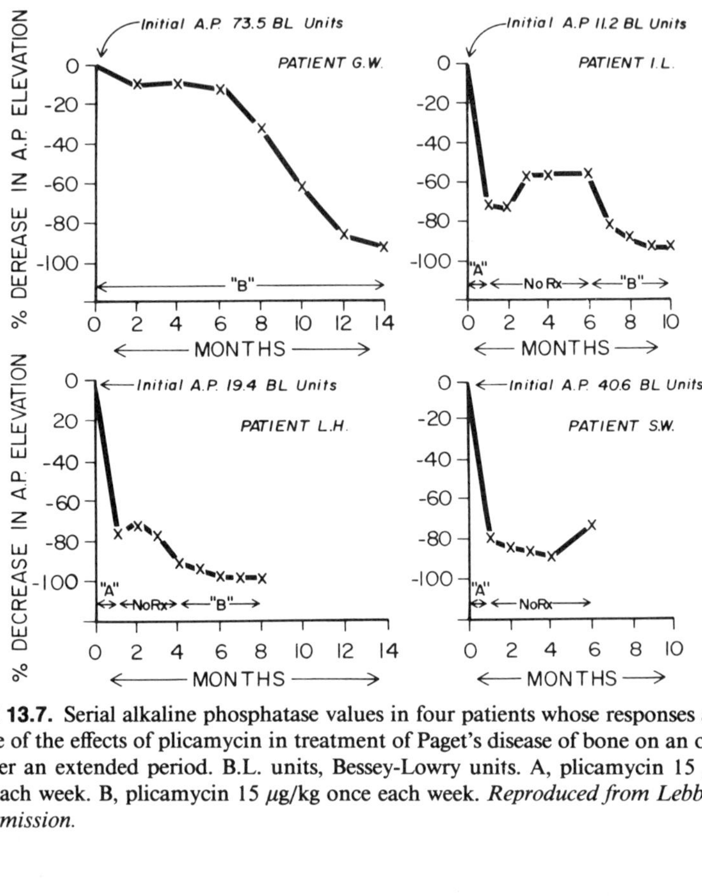

FIGURE 13.7. Serial alkaline phosphatase values in four patients whose responses are representative of the effects of plicamycin in treatment of Paget's disease of bone on an outpatient basis over an extended period. B.L. units, Bessey-Lowry units. A, plicamycin 15 μg/kg for 5 days each week. B, plicamycin 15 μg/kg once each week. *Reproduced from Lebbin et al,*[31] *with permission.*

the upper limit of normal before interrupting plicamycin administration. Also, we usually increase the dose of plicamycin until we see a significant increase in serum levels of hepatic enzymes and thus to some extent titrate the dose used, depending on the degree of enzyme increase seen. In this manner we believe we give the patient maximum therapeutic effect without encountering undue toxicity. Usually by the second day after withholding plicamycin because of toxicity, the enzyme levels are returning toward baseline values and therapy may be resumed. We have never seen evidence of residual hepatic damage.

Nephrotoxicity is less commonly seen at these doses (approximately 5%) but tends to be of longer duration (1 to 2 weeks), and we have seen a few patients with mild residual renal damage as indicated by a persistent increase in serum creatinine of 0.2 to 0.5 mg/dL. We monitor for renal toxicity during therapy by daily determinations of serum creatinine and interrupt therapy if an increase of 0.3 mg/dL or greater is seen. It is important not to use blood urea nitrogen (BUN) as an indicator of nephrotoxicity since it frequently decreases as a result of diminished food intake because of nausea during therapy. Thus an increase in BUN may not be seen until relatively late in nephrotoxicity. We believe it important to maintain hydration of the patient (with intravenous fluids if necessary) to minimize nephrotoxicity.

We have seen evidence of platelet toxicity (thrombocytopenia) on only two occasions. In one instance the patient received 50 μg/kg/d by error for 5 days. The platelet count decreased to a nadir of 75,000/mm^3 but recovered uneventfully and the patient suffered no untoward effect. There did not appear to be any increased therapeutic benefit produced by this increase over the usual dose. On the other occasion in which we saw significant thrombocytopenia, there was a therapy-associated disaster. An elderly man (age 78) whose severe back pain had been unresponsive to all other available therapeutic measures developed severe hepatic, renal, and platelet toxicity late in the course of therapy and died of ensuing complications. This has been our only very bad experience during 20 years of plicamycin therapy for Paget's disease, but it does emphasize the potential hazards of this mode of therapy. Although we have never used plicamycin casually, this experience has made us even more conservative and cautious in its use.

In Table 13.1 are the guidelines we use during intensive daily therapy

TABLE 13.1 Precautions and Observations During Hospital Treatment with Plicamycin

1. Complete blood count, platelet count, SGOT, SGPT, LDH, calcium, creatinine, and alkaline phosphatase daily.
2. Baseline coagulation profile. Repeat if platelet count decreases to < 150,000/mm^3.
3. Observe daily for signs of bleeding, plethora, fever, anorexia, nausea, or vomiting (indicative of possible excessive toxicity).
4. Withhold treatment if liver enzymes increase to more than ten times the upper limit of normal, if platelets decrease rapidly or < 150,000/mm^3, if serum creatinine rises by more than 0.3 mg/dL, or if fever, severe nausea, or vomiting develops or the patient appears unduly toxic.
5. Treat only symptomatic hypocalcemia with oral or intravenous calcium if necessary.
6. Use antinausea drugs liberally; orally, rectally, or intravenously as indicated.
7. Keep the patient well hydrated with oral or intravenous fluids.
8. Withdraw other medications (particularly nephrotoxic or antiplatelet agents) if possible during treatment.
9. DO NOT GIVE A DOSE OF PLICAMYCIN WITHOUT KNOWING THE MORNING'S LABORATORY VALUES FOR LIVER ENZYMES, CREATININE, AND PLATELET COUNT.

in hospitalized patients. Faced with the prospect of repeated courses of therapy with a toxic agent, we began to explore possible combinations of agents in hopes of seeing longer-lasting effects or possible cure. The only combinations showing promise to date have been with sodium etidronate[32] or with vinblastine.

Treatment of 12 patients (Figure 13.8) with sodium etidronate followed by a course of plicamycin in the late 1970s and early 1980s resulted in complete or near-complete remissions of disease activity for several years in at least six in whom adequate follow-up was obtained and for over 10 years in two patients.

Our recent trial in four patients of intravenous sodium etidronate 300 mg/d in combination with plicamycin 10 to 15 μg/kg/d (both given as concurrent 24-hour infusions for 7 days) was disappointing in that the effect on SAP and OHP did not appear to be greater than with plicamycin alone.

In the middle to late 1980s we explored the use of vinblastine administered concurrently with plicamycin in five patients with severe disease unresponsive to other available therapies. Our reasoning for combining vinblastine with plicamycin was that the former appeared to be particularly toxic to the macrophage.[33,34] Since the osteoclast is thought to be derived from macrophages,[35] we reasoned that it might be toxic to the pagetic osteoclast as well. In addition, the two agents have differing toxicities: vinblastine has neurocyte and leukocyte toxicity, which are not usually seen with plicamycin. Our experience with this combination has been gratifying. One young woman with severe disease of the tibia resulting in two fractures and requiring subsequent osteotomy for straightening is still in complete remission as judged by low normal SAP and OHP values 3½ years post treatment (Figure 13.9). Two other patients have had gratifying relief of neural compression syndromes. One patient was barely able to stand by supporting most of his weight with his arms and now can walk with a cane. However, all but one patient are now showing signs of relapse, as judged by a slowly increasing SAP, and neural compression has reappeared in one. Two of the patients treated with this regimen developed severe septicemia, and one developed thrombocytopenia and leukopenia resulting in septicemia. Fortunately, all recovered uneventfully, but we judge this therapy too toxic for continued use except in extreme circumstances.

As new, more potent bisphosphonates appear and exert sufficient disease control in most patients, it appears likely that plicamycin will have a lesser role in therapy of Paget's disease. However, its combination with these agents in selected patients with particularly resistant disease may result in more effective control and possible cure. The ultimate role of

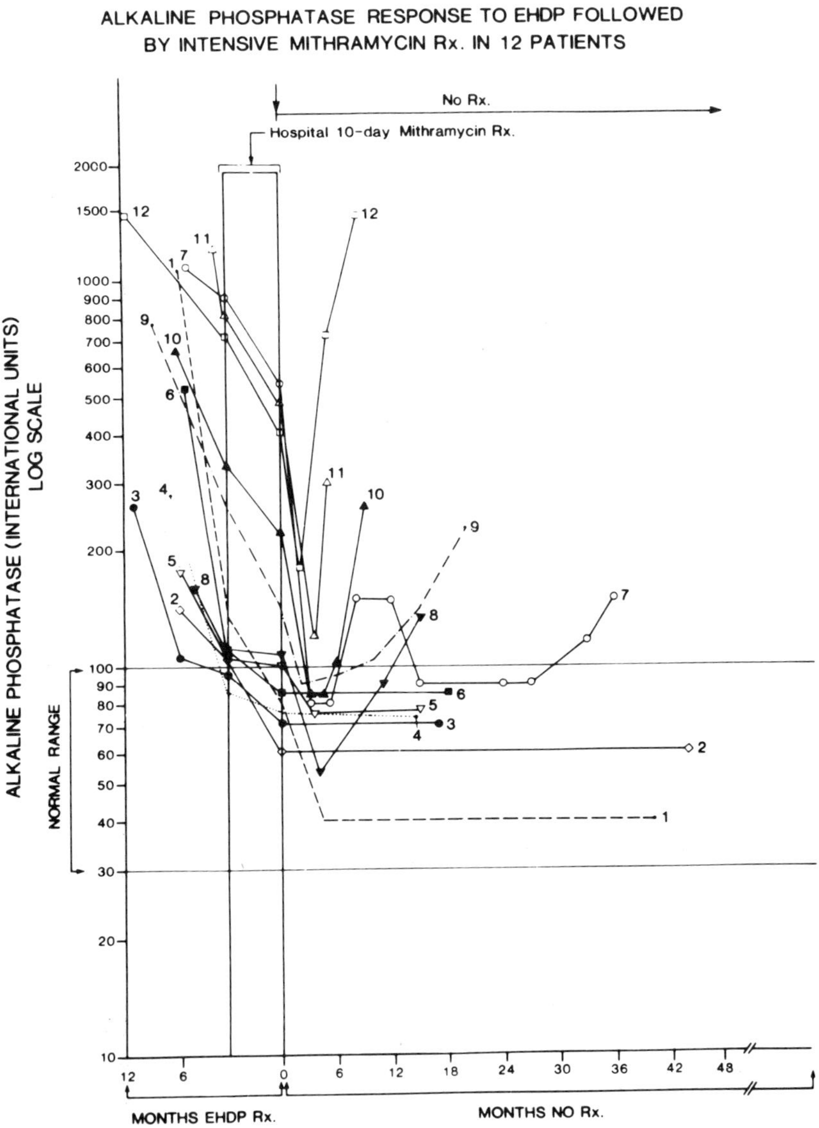

FIGURE 13.8. Serial alkaline phosphatase values following sodium etidronate plus plicamycin therapy in 12 patients. The 6 patients with normalization of alkaline phosphatase response have remained in remission for several years as judged by subsequent alkaline phosphatase values and bone scans.

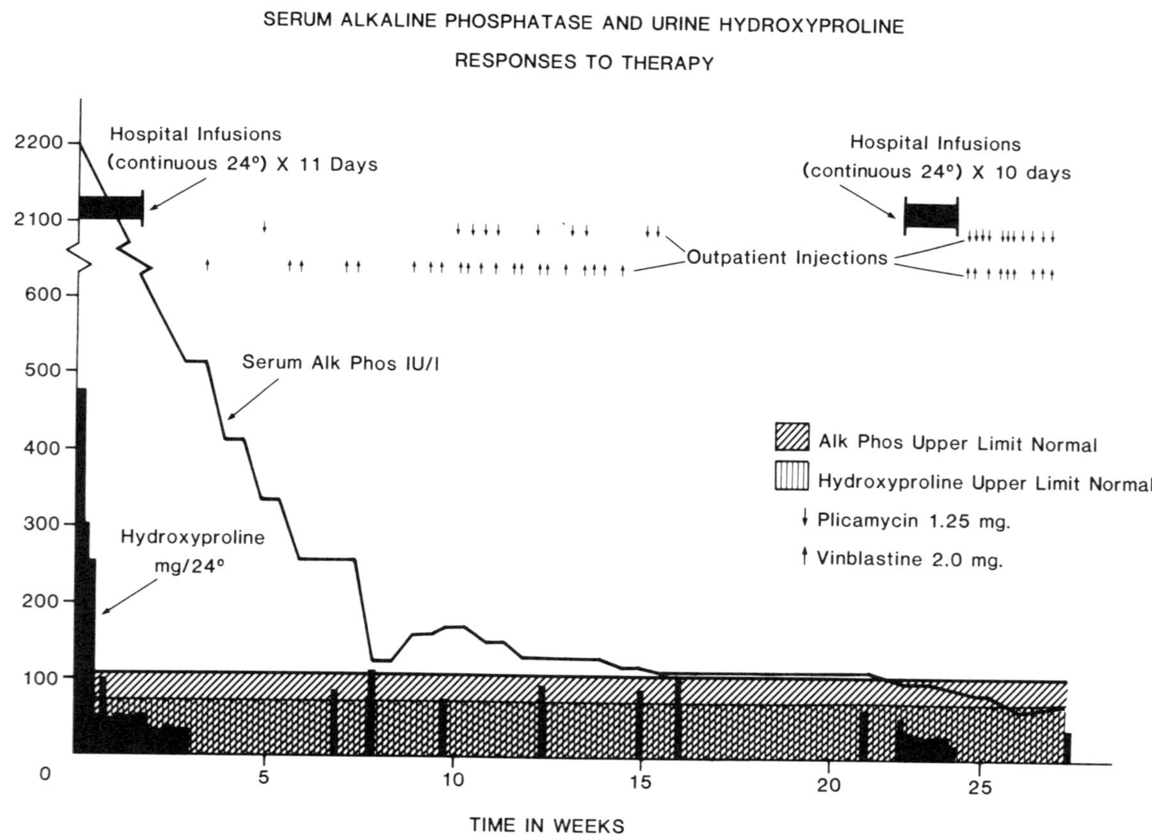

FIGURE 13.9. Serum alkaline phosphatase and urinary hydroxyproline responses to plicamycin combined with vinblastine therapy in one patient. The patient has continued to have normal serum alkaline phosphatase and urinary hydroxyproline values to the present without additional therapy since 1985.

plicamycin in the therapy of Paget's disease, like that of other agents, remains to be determined.

REFERENCES

1. Ryan WG, Schwartz TB, Perlia CP: Effects of mithramycin on Paget's disease of bone. *Ann Intern Med* 1969;70:549–557.
2. Kennedy BJ: Metabolic and toxic effects of mithramycin during tumor therapy. *Am J Med* 1970;49:494–503.
3. Monto RS, Talley RW, Caldwell MJ, et al: Observations on the mechanism of hemorrhagic toxicity in mithramycin therapy. *Cancer Res* 1969;29:697–704.
4. Kofman S, Eisenstein R: Mithramycin in the treatment of disseminated cancer. *Cancer Chemother* 1963;32:77.
5. Kofman S, Medrek TJ, Alexander RW: Mithramycin in treatment of embryonal cancer. *Cancer* 1964;17:938–948.
6. Brown JH, Kennedy BJ: Mithramycin in the treatment of disseminated testicular neoplasms. *N Engl J Med* 1965;272:111–118.
7. Ream NW, Perlia CP, Wolter J, Taylor SG III: Mithramycin therapy in disseminated germinal testicular cancer. *JAMA* 1968;204:1030–1036.
8. Rebel A, Malkani K, Basle M: Particularités ultrastructurales des osteoclasts de la maladie de Paget. *Rev Rhum Mal Osteo-Articulaires* 1974;41:767–771.
9. Mills BG, Singer FR: Nuclear inclusions in Paget's disease of bone. *Science* 1976;194:201–202.
10. Eisenstein R, Passavoy M: Actinomycin D inhibits parathyroid hormone and vitamin D activity. *Proc Soc Exp Biol Med* 1964;117:77–79.
11. Rasmussen H, Arnaud C, Hawker C: Actinomycin D and response to parathyroid hormone. *Science* 1964;154:1019–1021.
12. Fennelly JJ: Clinical and biochemical studies of Paget's disease of bone with emphasis on the effects of RNA inhibitors actinomycin D and mithramycin. *Ir J Med Sci* 1971;140:431–448.
13. Parsons V, Baum M, Self M: Effects of mithramycin on calcium and hydroxyproline metabolism in patients with malignant disease. *Br Med J* 1967;1:474–477.
14. Perlia CP, Gubisch NJ, Wolter J, et al: Mithramycin treatment of hypercalcemia. *Cancer* 1970;25:389–394.
15. Ryan WG, Schwartz TB, Northrop G: Experiences in the treatment of Paget's disease of bone with mithramycin. *JAMA* 1970;213:1153–1157.
16. Ryan WG, Schwartz TB, Northrop G: Treatment of Paget's disease with mithramycin: Further experiences. *Semin Drug Treat* 1972;2:57–64.
17. Ryan WG: Treatment of Paget's disease of bone with mithramycin. *Clin Orthop* 1977;127:106–110.
18. Condon JR, Reith SBM, Nassim JR, et al: Treatment of Paget's disease of bone with mithramycin. *Br Med J* 1971;1:421–423.
19. Elias EG, Evans JT: Mithramycin in the treatment of Paget's disease of bone. *J Bone Joint Surg* 1972;54:1730–1736.
20. Aitken JM, Lindsey R: Mithramycin in Paget's disease. *Lancet* 1973;1:1177.
21. Eisinger JB, Recordier AM: Traitment de la maladie de Paget par la mithramycine. *Lyon Med* 1975;11:627–629.
22. Russell AS, Lentle BC: Mithramycin therapy in Paget's disease. *Can Med Assoc J* 1974;110:397–400.

23. Russell AS, Chalmers IM, Percy JS, Lentle BC: Long term effectiveness of low dose mithramycin for Paget's disease of bone. *Arthritis Rheum* 1979;22:215–218.
24. Heath DA: The role of mithramycin in the management of Paget's disease. *Metab Bone Dis* 1981;4,5:343–345.
25. Condon JR, Surtees J, Robinson V: Control of osteitis deformans using glucagon, calcitonin and mithramycin. *Postgrad Med J* 1981;57:84–88.
26. Hadjipavlou AG, Tsoukas GM, Siller TN, et al: Combination drug therapy in treatment of Paget's disease of bone. *J Bone Joint Surg* 1977;59(A):1045–1051.
27. Pembrook RC, Chung CH, Carvallo AP: Effects of mithramycin and calcitonin in cardiovascular complications of Paget's disease of bone. *Conn Med* 1975;39:209–214.
28. Theil GB, Ajlouni K: Mithramycin effects on calcium phosphorus and parathyroid hormone in osseous Paget's disease. *Am J Med Sci* 1975;269:13–18.
29. Ajlouni K, Theil GB: Effect of mithramycin on hydroxyproline metabolism in Paget's disease. *J Lab Clin Med* 1977;90:803–808.
30. Ryan WG, Schwartz TB, Fordham EW: Mithramycin and long remission of Paget's disease of bone. *Ann Intern Med* 1980;92:129.
31. Lebbin D, Ryan WG, Schwartz TB: Outpatient treatment of Paget's disease of bone with mithramycin. *Ann Intern Med* 1974;81:635–637.
32. Ryan WG, Schwartz TB: Mithramycin treatment of Paget's disease of bone: Exploration of combined mithramycin-EHDP therapy. *Arthritis Rheum* 1980;23:1155–1161.
33. Ahn YS, Harrington WJ: Clinical uses of macrophage inhibitors. *Adv Intern Med* 1980;25:453–473.
34. Ahn YS, Harrington WJ, Mylvaganam R, et al: Slow infusion of vinca alkaloids in the treatment of idiopathic thrombocytopenic purpura. *Ann Intern Med* 1984;100:192–196.
35. Owen M: The origin of bone cells in the postnatal organism. *Arthritis Rheum* 1980;23:1073–1077.

CHAPTER 14

Arthritis and Paget's Disease of Bone

Stephen M. Krane and Susan F. Kroop

Although Paget's disease may be asymptomatic and recognized by physicians in the course of radiologic examinations for unrelated clinical problems or the finding of elevated serum alkaline phosphatase activity on routine chemical screening, symptomatic musculoskeletal manifestations are common. These clinical problems result from neural compression, pain over pagetic lesions near joints or referred to joints, joint disease secondary to pagetic involvement of subchondral bone or more distal bone deformities, or occurrence of other rheumatologic disorders on the background of Paget's disease. It is the purpose of this review to consider these rheumatologic manifestations and illustrate some of the clinical problems with examples from our own experience.

GOUT

A 70-year-old white man (J. G.) had known Paget's disease that involved the right humerus for 25 years (Figure 14.1). The disease resulted in a painful deformity of the right arm associated with decreased range of motion of the shoulder and elbow. The serum alkaline phosphatase value was approximately three times normal. J. G. was treated with calcitonin and later disodium etidronate, which resulted in both clinical and biochemical improvement. J. G. also complained of a 25-year history of intermittent episodes of right great toe pain, redness, and swelling. Physical examination revealed a swollen, red, and warm first metatarsal phalangeal joint with a yellow-white area consistent with tophus (Figure 14.2). Aspiration revealed chalky mate-

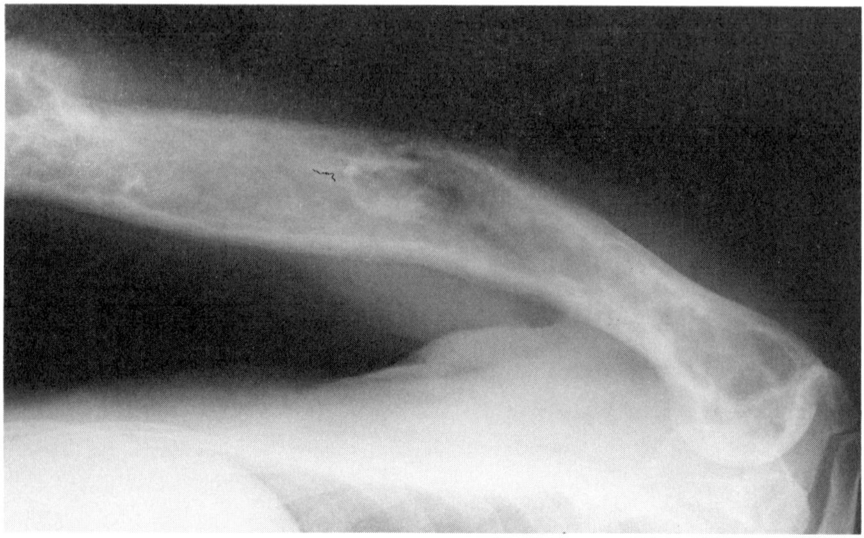

FIGURE 14.1. Radiographs of the right humerus (J. G.) with extensive lytic and blastic Paget's disease and a bowing deformity.

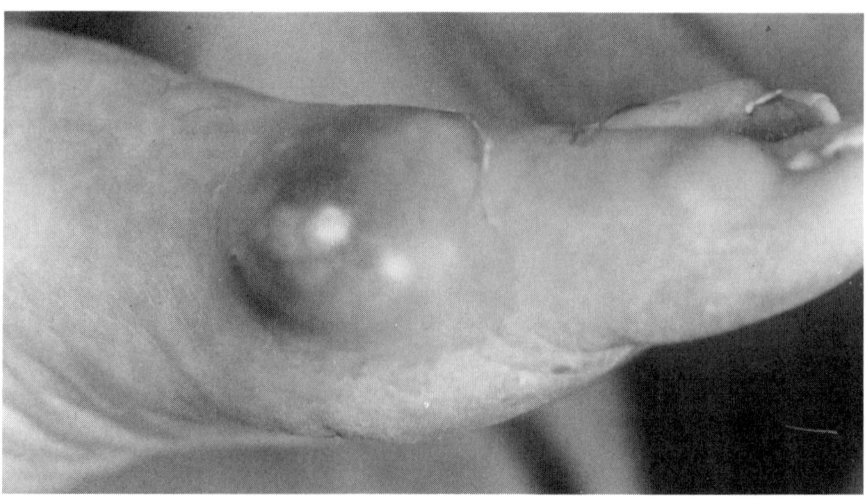

FIGURE 14.2. First metatarsal phalangeal joint (J. G.) with acute inflammation associated with a tophus consistent with gout.

rial that consisted of sodium urate crystals typical of gout. Serum uric acid was only mildly elevated on several determinations. J. G. was initially treated with phenylbutazone or colchicine during the acute episodes. Because of increased frequency of episodes, prophylaxis with daily colchicine and later allopurinol was begun. After 3 years of allopurinol administration, he was asymptomatic and the tophus had resolved.

The association of Paget's disease and gout was noted in some of the early descriptions of Paget's disease. Although there has been disagreement about whether there is more than chance association of these two disorders, more recent data support the concept of an interrelation. Franck et al.[1] in a review of 47 patients with Paget's disease found that 40% (19/47) were hyperuricemic. Seven of the 19 individuals with hyperuricemia (all men) also had clinical evidence of gouty arthritis. The serum uric acid concentration correlated with both the extent and the activity of bone disease, suggesting that the pagetic process contributes to the development of gout. In a later series the course of 149 patients with Paget's disease was reviewed.[2] Hyperuricemia was present in 20% of patients who were not being treated with allopurinol. Acute gouty arthritis was present in less than 10% (11/149) of the patients in this series. Winfield and Stamp[3] found hyperuricemia in 6 of 50 patients with Paget's disease. None of these had acute gouty arthritis. Most recently, Lluberas-Acosta et al[4] reviewed the incidence of Paget's disease as detected by abnormal bone scan with standard radiologic confirmation in patients with gout. Of their patients, 23% (6/26) had evidence of Paget's versus 2% (7/333) of a reference population who had undergone bone scans, supporting an increased incidence of gout in the pagetic population. There was no significant difference in the serum uric acid levels among the patients with gout alone, gout and Paget's disease, or Paget's disease alone. The populations studied in these four reports differed in the severity of their Paget's disease. This may explain the differences in incidence of gout if one postulates that greater skeletal turnover in more active, severe Paget's leads to increased degradation of nucleic acids and secondary hyperuricemia.

Certainly acute arthritis in the patient with Paget's disease should be evaluated by joint aspiration and microscopic examination of the synovial fluid for monosodium urate crystals. If such crystals are present, indomethacin or colchicine should be administered. In addition, when chronic joint pain is associated with hyperuricemia, erosive arthritis secondary to gout should be considered, evaluated radiographically, and treated by chronic suppression of serum uric acid levels with allopurinol and anti-inflammatory agents such as colchicine or indomethacin, if necessary.

CALCIFIC PERIARTHRITIS AND CHONDROCALCINOSIS

The incidence of calcific periarthritis in Paget's disease varies among the published studies. Franck et al.[1] reviewed radiographs of 55 patients with Paget's disease and identified periarticular calcifications in 36%. Altman and Collins[2] found only 8 patients of 290 patients reviewed with periarthritis. Two of these individuals had periarthritis of the shoulder with proximal humoral or scapular Paget's disease.

Chondrocalcinosis has also been reported in patients with Paget's disease. Franck et al[1] found only two incidences of chondrocalcinosis on examination of wrist and knee radiographs of 54 patients. Altman and Collins[2] reported chondrocalcinosis in only 4 of 290 patients. Winfield and Stamp[3] reported that only 2 individuals of 50 with Paget's disease studied developed acute pseudogout of the knee and had chondrocalcinosis revealed on plain radiographs. Although the available data do not support an increase in incidence of calcific periarthritis or chondrocalcinosis in patients with Paget's disease, it is clear that these conditions occur in patients with Paget's disease and must be considered in the differential diagnosis of an acute arthritis. Calcific periarthritis and chondrocalcinosis are treated with nonsteroidal antiinflammatory medications or intraarticular glucocorticoid injections.

SYSTEMIC INFLAMMATORY ARTHRITIS

The occurrence of several forms of inflammatory arthritis has been observed in patients with Paget's disease. Franck et al[1] reported that 2 of 55 patients had rheumatoid or psoriatic arthritis. Altman and Collins[2] described 3 patients with rheumatoid or psoriatic arthritis and 1 with Sjögren's syndrome and associated mild synovitis in the small joints. Case reports have also included patients with systemic lupus erythematosus[5] and dermatomyositis.[6] All patients described were treated for their inflammatory arthritis with chrysotherapy or glucocorticoids. Although the numbers of patients are few, there does not seem to have been an altered response to antiarthritic therapy in patients with inflammatory arthritis in the setting of Paget's disease.

Ankylosing spondylitis has been associated with Paget's disease in several studies. Franck et al[1] reported six patients with physical findings of limitation of chest expansion and spinal fusion that suggested ankylosing spondylitis. Syndesmophytes were not identified radiographically, but pagetic involvement of the pelvis was present in five of six and of the lumbosacral spine in four of six of these subjects. The HLA-B27 antigen was not present in the four subjects tested. Altman and Collins[2] described two individuals with symptoms of ankylosing spondylitis who had syndesmophyte formation coexisting with Paget's disease. Alarcon-Segovia and Martinez-Cordero[7] described one individual with Paget's disease, ankylosing spondylitis, and rheumatoid arthritis. The Paget's disease in this patient was asymptomatic. The rheumatoid arthritis responded to D-penicillamine and gold sodium thiomalate, and the ankylosing spondylitis responded to indomethacin. Both HLA-B27 and DR4 antigens were present in this individual.

DEGENERATIVE JOINT DISEASE

D. H. is a 56-year-old white man who had a 10-year history of intermittent lower lumbar pain and a 2-year history of right hip pain. His hip pain was worse when weight bearing or climbing stairs. He became extremely stiff after sitting for a brief period. Physical examination was most notable for an antalgic gait and severe restriction of rotation of his right hip. Radiographs revealed Paget's disease of the right hemipelvis with destruction of the acetabular cartilage of the right hip evidenced by medial joint space loss. The right proximal femur was spared. Serum alkaline phosphatase activity was four times normal. An initial course of calcitonin provided moderate pain relief for about 8 months. A nonsteroidal antiinflammatory agent was then added. Because of persistent symptoms, a total hip replacement (THR) was performed, resulting in complete pain relief and increased range of motion. His postoperative course was complicated by transfusion-associated hepatitis. Subsequently, D. H. developed acute gouty arthritis as well as nephrolithiasis secondary to a uric acid stone. He continues to do well 12 years after THR.

Hip

In the extremities, the femur and tibia are most frequently involved in Paget's disease. The deformity associated with femoral involvement is an outward bowing combined with coxa vara. Clinically, after years of involvement of the pelvis and femur, involvement of the hip joint, termed pagetic coxopathy, may result. The incidence of hip pain and what has been interpreted as degenerative joint disease in the published series of patients with Paget's ranges from 30% to 50%. Patients present with hip pain, characterized by a dull ache or stiffness that increases with weight bearing. Stiffness, particularly after a period of rest, is common. In a recent study review 25 of 50 patients with Paget's disease had symptomatic involvement of the hip joint.[3] Of these, 24 had Paget's disease involving the pelvis, femur, or both. Twelve of the 24 had both acetabular and femoral involvement. Pagetic involvement of the femur alone is rare and occurred in only 1 patient in this series. Acetabular involvement alone is more common and occurred in 11 of 24 patients. The most severe disease occurred in patients with both acetabular and femoral pagetic involvement. These findings were similar to those in the series reported by Franck et al.[1]

Roper[8] suggested on the basis of radiologic analysis that if hip joint space narrowing is medial and accompanied by acetabular protrusion, then Paget's disease is the cause. If the narrowing of the hip joint space is predominantly superior, then unrelated degenerative joint disease (DJD) is the "cause." (It is difficult to ascribe DJD as a cause, however, when pathogenesis is uncertain and the problem heterogeneous.) In some patients with acetabular Paget's disease alone, superior joint space narrowing can occur, but the problem is usually asymptomatic. In severe disease, acetabular protrusion is associated with both superior and medial joint space narrowing. In the series of Winfield and Stamp[3] it was noted that sclerosis, subarticular cyst formation, and osteophytosis were absent in their patients with Paget's disease and what was interpreted as "secondary" DJD.

Patients with symptomatic pagetic coxopathy should be treated for the Paget's disease, as discussed elsewhere in this volume. Those whose symptoms do not improve and who have progressive hip involvement clinically should be offered symptomatic relief with orthopedic devices, salicylates, or other nonsteroidal antiinflammatory medications. If hip pain is severe and persistent, patients should be referred for THR.

The results of THR for pagetic coxapathy have been reported from several centers.[9-12] McDonald and Sim[12] described 10-year follow up in 46 patients and shorter follow up in an additional 45. Overall, the results were noted as excellent in 74% using a standard score. The incidence of aseptic loosening in patients with Paget's disease was increased only slightly compared to that in patients undergoing THR without Paget's disease. The incidence of heterotopic bone formation in this series was high (37%), consistent with findings of other series of patients with Paget's disease. The patients who had marked heterotopic bone formation had slightly poorer scores on the clinical rating scales. In our experience, one patient developed disabling hip fusion secondary to heterotopic bone formation within 6 months of THR. Although Merkow and Lane[13] suggest that specific preoperative antipagetic therapy with calcitonin and/or bisphosphonates reduces surgical blood loss, no conclusion can be drawn as to whether this therapy will affect the rate of loosening of the prostheses or the degree of heterotopic bone formation.

A 72-year-old woman (E. M.), a retired traffic supervisor, had intermittent back and knee pain for approximately 20 years. E. M. noted that her left knee was larger than her right for about 20 years. Over the last 2 years E. M. noted an increase in severity of knee pain with minimal weight-bearing activity and stair climbing. Physical examination revealed an enlarged, boggy, and warm left knee held in 10-degree varus. Range of motion was decreased and mild crepitus was noted without instability. Radiographs revealed Paget's disease of distal femur with anterior bowing. Moderate medial and lateral joint space narrowing was evident (Figure 14.3). Serum alkaline phosphatase activity was approximately three times normal. E. M. was treated with two courses of disodium etidronate as well as sulindac with partial relief of pain. Glucocorticoid injection of the left knee provided temporary pain relief. Conservative management with a cane, knee cage, and intensive physical therapy resulted in moderate pain relief for approximately 6 months, delaying the need for surgical intervention. Because of increased pain, however, a total knee replacement was performed with excellent results. E. M. has required no further antipagetic therapy.

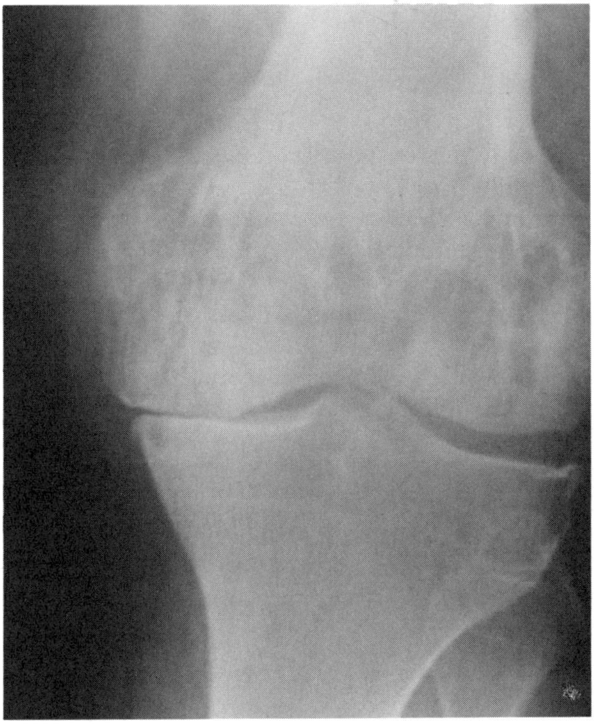

FIGURE 14.3. Radiographs of the left knee (E. M.) with extensive Paget's disease of the distal femur and severe medial joint space narrowing.

Knee

The incidence of knee pain in patients with Paget's disease varies from 11%[2] to 50%.[1] If Paget's disease involves the distal femur or proximal tibia and disease is adjacent to the joint, pain is likely to be present. Joint space narrowing is usually accompanied by pain. Osteophyte formation may be found. Initial therapy in patients with knee pain and associated Paget's disease adjacent to the knee joint should be directed at the Paget's disease. Decreased weight bearing is advised and nonsteroidal antiinflammatory medications should be administered. In patients with tibia vara and internal torsion of the tibial shaft secondary to Paget's disease with minimal loss of articular cartilage of the medial compartment of the knee, tibial osteotomy has resulted in pain relief and correction of the tibial deformity.[14] Total knee replacement may be indicated in more severe cases.[9] O'Driscoll and Hastings[15] reported one case of a patient who underwent arthrodesis of the knee after a tibial osteotomy failed to decrease the pain. Subsequently, 6 years after the surgical fusion, the patient exhibited increasing knee pain and was found to have extension of the Paget's disease from the femur to the tibia.

Back

The spine, especially the lumbosacral region, is a common site of Paget's disease. Involvement of the spine may result in neurologic compression, but more commonly pain is the associated clinical feature. One needs to be careful, however, in attributing back pain to Paget's disease. In one series, Altman and Collins[2] found back pain solely related to pagetic changes in only 7 patients. Forty-five patients had pain thought to be secondary to pagetic involvement combined with degenerative changes where distortion of the articular facets with juxtaposed pagetic bone was present. An additional 45 patients had lumbar pain unrelated to the pagetic process. In a later study, Altman et al[16] reviewed 25 patients with low back pain and severe Paget's disease. Only 3 of these individuals had pain attributable to Paget's disease alone. Suppressive therapy with disodium etidronate was beneficial in only 8 of 22 patients with Paget's and DJD of the lumbar spine. These observations illustrate how one must attempt to elucidate the cause of the pain and use physical therapy and/or nonsteroidal antiinflammatory agents when secondary DJD may be a contributing factor.

CONCLUSIONS

Paget's disease alone may be associated with pain of skeletal or articular origin. Crystal-induced arthritis, systemic inflammatory arthritis such as rheumatoid arthritis, psoriatic arthritis, systemic lupus erythematosus, dermatomyositis, and ankylosing spondylitis have been reported as coincidental occurrences in patients with Paget's disease. Gout or hyperuricemia may occur with an increased incidence in patients with severe Paget's disease. Pagetic involvement of subchondral bone in hip and knee joints that results in cartilage loss and articular deformity may cause severe pain. Orthopedic devices, salicylates, or other nonsteroidal antiinflammatory agents may be of value in these patients. A role for THR for pagetic coxopathy and tibial osteotomy for associated tibia vara and knee joint involvement has been established.

ACKNOWLEDGMENTS

We thank M. Angelo for preparation of the manuscript. Original work referred to here was supported by NIH grants AR-03564 and AR-07258.

REFERENCES

1. Franck WA, Bress NM, Singer FR, Krane SM: Rheumatic manifestations of Paget's disease of bone. *Am J Med* 1974;56:592–603.
2. Altman RD, Collins B: Musculoskeletal manifestations of Paget's disease of bone. *Arthritis Rheum* 1980;23:1121–1127.
3. Winfield J, Stamp TCB: Bone and joint symptoms in Paget's disease. *Ann Rheum Dis* 1984;43:769–773.
4. Lluberas-Acosta G, Hansell JR, Schumacher R Jr: Paget's disease of bone in patients with gout. *Arch Intern Med* 1986;146:2389–2392.
5. Alarcon GS, Ball GV, Goldfarb PM Jr: Systemic lupus erythematosus, gout, and Paget's disease. *Arthritis Rheum* 1983;26(2):238.
6. Leonard-Segal A, Johnson JJ, Nashel DJ: Coexistence of Paget's disease and dermatomyositis. *J Rheumatol* 1988;15:1565–1567.
7. Alarcon-Segovia D, Martinez-Cordero E: Ankylosing spondylitis and rheumatoid arthritis in a patient with Paget's disease. *Arch Intern Med* 1985;145:1915–1917.
8. Roper BA: Paget's disease involving the hip joint. *Clin Orthop* 1971;80:33–38.
9. Hadjipavlou A, Lander P, Srolovitz H: Pagetic arthritis: Pathophysiology and management. *Clin Orthop* 1986;208:15–19.
10. Merkow RL, Pellicci PM, Hely DP, Salvati EA: Total hip replacement for Paget's disease of the hip. *J Bone Joint Surg* 1984;66(A):752–758.
11. Milgram JW: Orthopedic management of Paget's disease of bone. *Contemp Orthop* 1985;10:64–70.
12. McDonald DJ, Sim FH: Total hip arthroplasty in Paget's disease. *J Bone Joint Surg* 1987;69(A):766–772.
13. Merkow RL, Lane JM: Current concepts of Paget's disease of bone. *Orthop Clin North Am* 1984;15:747–763.
14. Meyers MH, Singer F: Osteotomy for tibia vara in Paget's disease under cover of calcitonin. *J Bone Joint Surg* 1978;60(A):810–814.
15. O'Driscoll SW, Hastings DE: Extension of monostotic Paget disease from the femur to the tibia after arthrodesis of the knee. *J Bone Joint Surg* 1989;71(A):129–132.
16. Altman RD, Brown M, Gargano F: Low back pain in Paget's disease of bone. *Clin Orthop* 1987;217:152–161.

CHAPTER **15**

Surgery in Paget's Disease

Frederick S. Kaplan

INTRODUCTION

The orthopedic surgeon is often called on to help manage the complications of Paget's disease. These complications include severe bone pain, joint pain, skeletal deformity, pathologic fracture, and malignant degeneration. In this chapter, I will review the biologic basis of deformity in Paget's disease and then examine a few common problems likely to require the attention of an orthopedic surgeon.

THE BIOLOGIC BASIS OF DEFORMITY IN PAGET'S DISEASE

Living bone is never metabolically at rest.[1–6] It constantly remodels or rearranges its architectural microstructure along lines of mechanical stress. The relationship between applied load and bone morphology was first recognized by Galileo. In 1683, he noted a direct correlation between body weight and bone size. During the next two centuries, others observed that bone remodels, but Julius Wolff, a Berlin anatomist, was the first to link the two vital concepts. He noted that changes in bone mass accompanied changes in mechanical load, via the process of skeletal remodeling. In "The Law of Bone Transformation," published in 1892, Wolff explained, "Every change in the function of a bone is followed by certain definite changes in internal architecture and external conformation in accordance with mathematical laws." Stated more simply, "form follows function."

Although the mechanism by which bone cells transform mechanical or bioelectric signals into a useful biologic response remains enigmatic, Wolff's observations are as valid today as they were nearly a century ago.

Although the factors that control bone formation and resorption are not well understood, the two processes are exquisitely coupled in the adult skeleton under *normal* remodeling conditions so that net bone formation equals net bone resorption. In Paget's disease, this relationship is preserved, but at a much accelerated and chaotic rate. The ability of bone to withstand mechanical stress depends greatly on both its material and structural properties. The material properties of bone are determined by the inorganic and biochemical constituents of bone; the structural properties are determined primarily by the architectural arrangement of the bone material. The constituents of pagetic bone are similar to those of normal bone, but the arrangement of the bone tissue is vastly more chaotic in Paget's disease. This defect in bone architecture arises from defects in the bone cell metabolism at various stages in the natural history of Paget's disease.

Normal bone bends slightly when subjected to mechanical stress. But pagetic bone bends more than normal bone and may grossly deform. Normal bone continually remodels to minimize the strain or deformation that it experiences with mechanical stress. In Paget's disease, however, the bone remodeling process is often accelerated to a level that is detrimental to the bone's mechanical and structural needs. This results in bone that is haphazardly arranged, architecturally unsound, and less able than normal bone to withstand mechanical stress. This disorder of architectural remodeling may result in bone fractures, bone deformity, bone overgrowth, bone pain, joint incongruity, joint deformity, and even neurologic impairment from pressure on nerves or abnormal blood flow to nerves as they pass through neural foramina.

The structural abnormalities seen in Paget's disease arise as a result of a disorder in the rate of skeletal remodeling. The primary abnormality appears to be an increase in osteoclastic resorption of bone possibly related to a slow viral infection of the osteoclasts. Both the size and number of active osteoclasts are increased, as are the number of nuclei per cell. Through the process of coupling, increased bone resorption leads to a compensatory increase in bone formation. The rate of bone remodeling is greatly accelerated, resulting in a predominance of highly vascular, immature woven bone that is often structurally weak, and prone to deformities and pathologic fracture (Figure 15.1). When Paget's disease involves a long bone in the limbs, it nearly always involves the metaphyses. The abnormal Paget's bone often extends into the diaphysis and may involve the entire bone. It rarely affects the diaphysis exclusively. Metaphyseal involvement

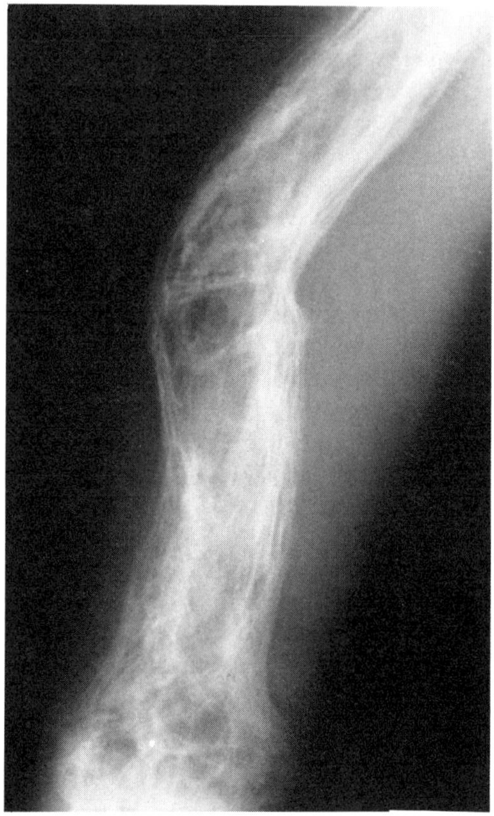

FIGURE 15.1. Anteroposterior roentgenogram demonstrating malunion of transverse (chalk-stick) fracture of midshaft of humerus affected with Paget's disease. Note enlargement of humerus, coarse trabecular structure, and contiguous lytic and sclerotic areas.

on one side of a diarthrodial joint may lead to bone enlargement, joint incongruity, and subsequent degenerative arthritis. When either component of the hip is affected, for example, in acetabular protrusion into the pelvis together with diarthrodial cartilage, destruction may result. A similar process may involve any diarthrodial joint whose contiguous bones are affected by Paget's disease. This process is most often symptomatic in the spine and lower limbs, where the additional factor of weight bearing may become a significant problem.

Painful fissure fractures and completed pathologic fractures (transverse or chalk-stick fractures) frequently occur in areas of high mechanical stress, particularly in the weight-bearing bones of the lower limbs. Fracture healing is often complicated, and delayed union and nonunion of bones are common. When a fracture heals through pagetic bone, the regenerated bone tissue is also pagetic. Complete immobilization of pagetic bone is best prevented, if possible, and all attempts at long-term preservation of function should prevail.

Indications for surgical intervention in Paget's disease are few; they include certain unstable fractures that are difficult to treat by nonoperative methods and severe arthritis that is refractory to treatment with antipagetic medication. Malalignment of the major weight-bearing bones of the lower limb may be treated with appropriate braces to prevent worsening of the deformity along with antipagetic medication to help retard the chaotic bone remodeling. Also, realignment of severe lower limb deformities may play some role in reestablishing normal weight-bearing relationships across synovial joints, thus leading to diminished mechanical stress on the joints and thus a likely delay in arthritic changes. This is true especially of malalignment affecting the knees and ankles. The judicious and intermittent use of canes and crutches may help considerably to relieve mechanical stress to bones and joints already overburdened and unable to redistribute weight-bearing loads effectively. Joint replacement may be indicated in end-stage joint disease if symptoms warrant.

THE ROLE OF THE ORTHOPEDIC SURGEON

In addition to surgical management, the orthopedic physician is often involved in the primary management of Paget's disease.[2,7–11] In some communities, the patient with asymptomatic Paget's disease (noted incidentally on roentgenograms or because of serum alkaline phosphatase elevation) may be referred to the orthopedic surgeon for further evaluation and guidance. In such a capacity, the orthopedic surgeon may be called on to render a definitive diagnosis or to participate in patient education. The orthopedic surgeon should be familiar with all aspects of Paget's disease management (medical and surgical), including resources available for patient education. Depending on the medical referral patterns of a particular community, the orthopedic surgeon may be required to participate in the medical management of patients with Paget's disease, or perhaps only in surgical management of late complications. The orthopedic physician should be acquainted with the full gamut of commonly used and available therapeutic modalities (Table 15.1).

FRACTURE MANAGEMENT IN PAGET'S DISEASE

Fractures are second only to bone pain as a complication of Paget's disease.[10–13] The presence of pain in pagetic bone should always raise suspicion of a pathologic fracture (Figure 15.2). Full roentgenographic evaluation should be obtained especially if there is a mechanical or weight-

TABLE 15.1 Therapeutic Modalities Available to the Orthopedic Surgeon

- Educational
  - American Academy of Orthopaedic Surgeons (AAOS)
  - The Paget's Disease Foundation
- Medical
  - Calcitonin
    - Salmon
    - Human
  - Bisphosphonates
    - EHDP
    - APD (investigational in United States)
  - Nonsteroidal antiinflammatory medication
- Physical Therapy
  - Ambulatory devices
    - Canes
    - Crutches
    - Walkers
  - Orthotics
  - Exercise programs
  - Transcutaneous nerve stimulation
- Surgical
  - Fracture fixation
    - Splinting-casting
    - Cast-bracing
    - Open reduction-internal fixation
  - Osteotomy for bone deformity associated with joint pain
  - Total joint replacement
    - Hip
    - Knee
    - Other
  - Ablative surgery secondary to Paget's sarcoma

bearing component to the bone pain. Increased metabolic activity in (and blood flow to) active pagetic bone poses added complications when fractures occur (Table 15.2), although none of the listed complications is specific to Paget's disease. However, the heightened risk of such complications in pagetic fractures suggests that special vigilance be taken in the management of such fractures. In addition to following basic principles of fracture management known to every orthopedic surgeon, special attention should be given to decreasing metabolic activity and blood flow in pagetic bone. Inhibitors of bone formation should be avoided when fracture healing is proceeding. Prolonged generalized immobilization or disuse should be assiduously prevented as it can further exacerbate osteopenia and provoke metabolic complications of hypercalcemia and hypercalciuria. Many of these principles are best realized with a course of calci-

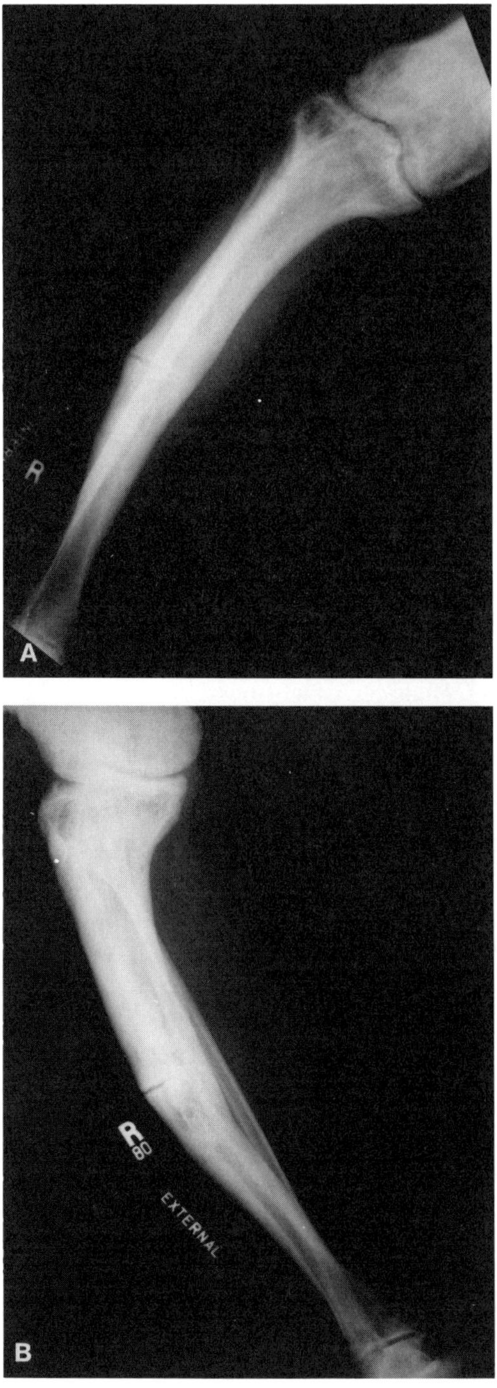

FIGURE 15.2. Anteroposterior and lateral roentgenogram of knee and leg. Note pagetic involvement of femur and tibia with sparing of fibula. Also note intensely sclerotic tibia with deformity and fissure fracture of midshaft of tibia. Patient responded symptomatically to calcitonin and functional cast bracing.

TABLE 15.2 Complications of Fractures in Pagetic Bone

Excessive bleeding
Compartment syndromes
Neurovascular compromise
Delayed union
Hardware failure
Nonunion
Malunion with increased deformity
Focal osteopenia of disuse
Hypercalcemia
Hypercalciuria

tonin, with the use of functional fracture bracing, and reliance on open reduction and internal fixation of fractures when absolutely necessary.

OSTEOTOMIES IN PAGET'S DISEASE

Osteotomy, or the surgical cutting of bone, may be part of a procedure to realign painful weight-bearing joints, especially the knee.[2,10,11,14] With the proper indications (of disabling mechanical weight-bearing pain of the knee or ankle unresponsive to adequate medical therapy) tibial osteotomy has proved to be a relatively safe and effective procedure. The operation should be performed only under full preoperative cover of calcitonin. When calcitonin is used to rule out bone pain as a cause of the disability and to minimize bleeding, complications are minimal. Tibial osteotomy is an effective surgical procedure to realign the knee and ankle, to minimize weight-bearing stress on the bones and ligaments, and to decrease pain and increase function (Figure 15.3).

TOTAL JOINT ARTHROPLASTY

Total joint arthroplasty has revolutionized the care of end-stage degenerative joint disease and has played a major role in alleviating severe joint pain associated with joint destruction from Paget's disease.[15–21] The indications

FIGURE 15.3. Posterior-anterior and lateral roentgenograms of leg. (A and B) Before osteotomy. (C and D) Immediately postoperatively, demonstrating osteotomy and internal fixation device. (E and F) Ten months later, demonstrating bony healing.

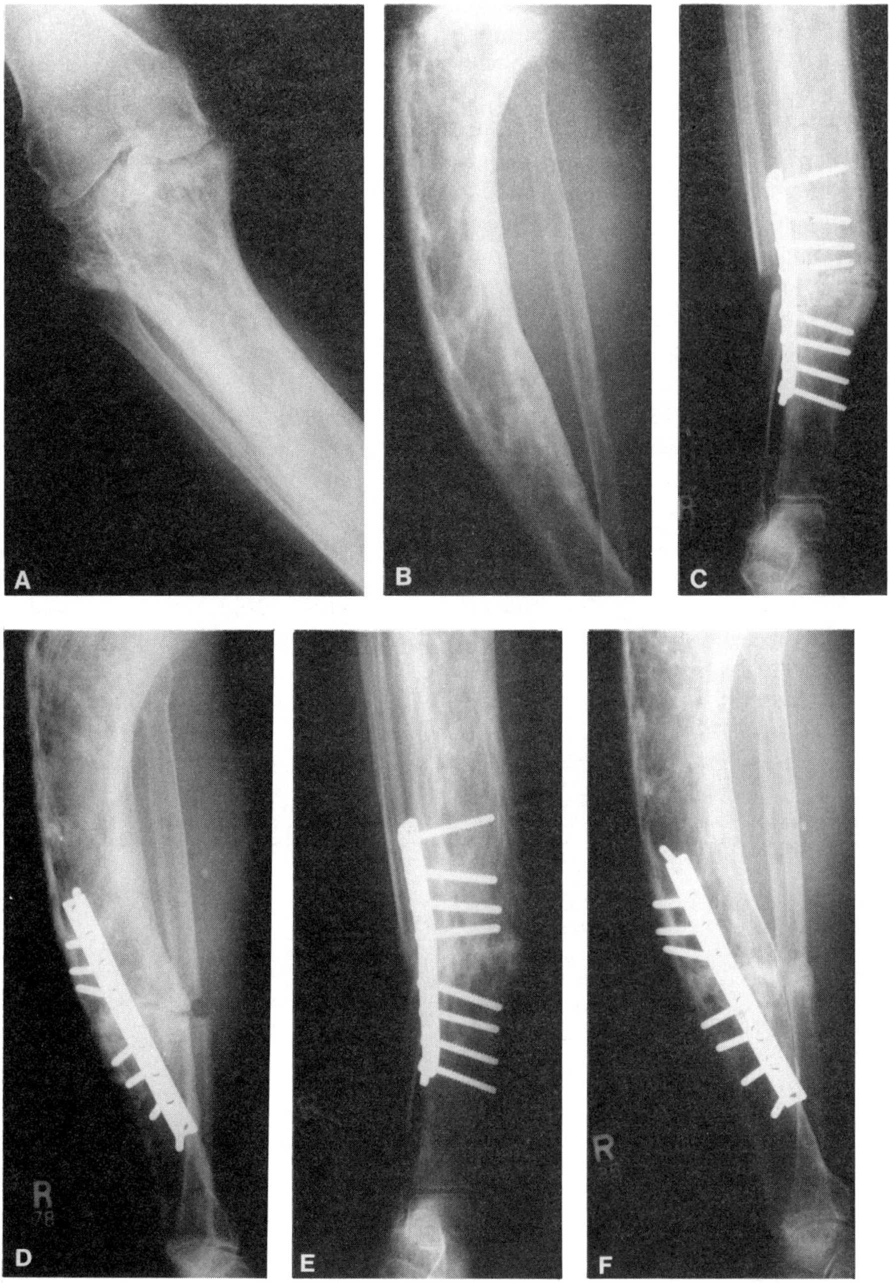
A
B
C
D
E
F

for total hip arthroplasty are severe residual functional limitation due to pain and presence of joint stiffness and deformity not alleviated by antipagetic medication. It is essential that the orthopedic surgeon distinguish "hip pain" as a chief complaint from mechanical pain emanating from the hip joint. Hip joint abnormality commonly refers pain to the groin and anterior thigh and occasionally to the knee, but rarely to the buttock region. Yet patients often complain of "hip pain" and point to the buttock or posterior thigh region. Pain in those regions often arises from abnormality in the lumbar and sacral areas, other common sites of involvement with Paget's disease. Another important consideration is whether the pain is osseous or articular in nature. Joint pain is often relieved by rest and aggravated by activity (especially if it is degenerative). In addition, it is often exacerbated by passive range of motion of the involved joint. The hip should specifically be examined for any painful flexion contractures, a common sign of intraarticular inflammation. A clinical trial of antipagetic medication often helps distinguish between bone pain and joint pain. Groin pain associated with Paget's disease may also be secondary to pagetic involvement of the pubis, stress fractures or pathologic fractures of the femoral neck, or associated visceral and/or neurologic involvement (Table 15.3; Figure 15.4). Further elucidation of a chief complaint of "hip pain" in Paget's disease should involve the use of nonsteroidal antiinflammatory medications and intraarticular injections with an anesthetic agent to distinguish osseous from intraarticular disease (Table 15.4), when necessary. The

TABLE 15.3 Differential Diagnosis of Groin Pain in Paget's Disease

- Bone pain from Paget's disease
  - Acetabulum
  - Femoral neck
  - Pubis
- Joint pain from pagetic arthritis
  - Hip joint
  - Symphysis pubis
- Stress fractures
  - Femoral neck
  - Ischiopubic ramus
- Associated visceral and/or neurologic involvement
  - Ureteral stones
  - Urinary tract infections
  - Hernias
  - Appendicitis
  - T-12 or L-1 radiculopathy from Paget's disease
- Malignant degeneration: Paget's sarcoma

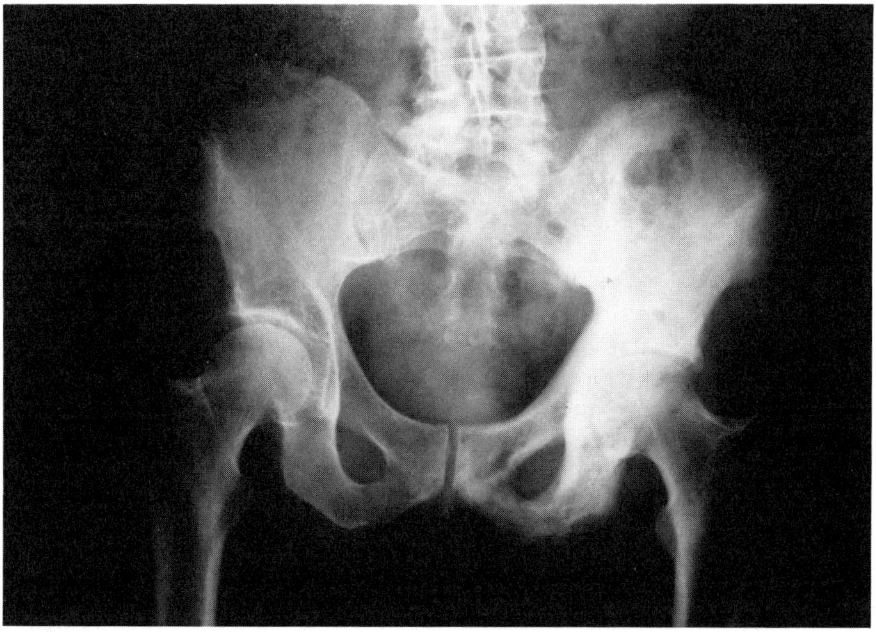

FIGURE 15.4. Anteroposterior roentgenogram of patient with pagetic involvement of hemipelvis and degenerative arthritis of sacroiliac and hip joint. Likely sources of groin pain: (**A**) Paget's disease of ilium. (**B**) Paget's disease of pubis. C, Secondary degenerative arthritis of hip.

orthopedic surgeon should also be aware of common rheumatic arthralgias and bursitides associated with Paget's disease (Table 15.5).

Once a decision has been made to proceed with total joint arthroplasty, a thorough preoperative evaluation should be undertaken and should include a complete medical evaluation. Any anticipated dental procedures such as tooth extraction or urologic procedures such as prostate surgery should be completed before total joint arthroplasty to minimize

TABLE 15.4 Evaluation of "Hip Pain" in Paget's Disease

Groin pain v. buttock pain
Range of motion of hip
Check for flexion contracture
Roentgenograms of pelvis, including hips
Antipagetic medication: bone pain v. joint pain
NSAIF: bone pain v. joint pain
Intraarticular injection with anesthetic agent

TABLE 15.5 Common Rheumatic Arthralgias Associated with Paget's Disease

Calcific periarthritis
Bursitis
Gout
Pseudogout
Polymyalgia rheumatica

risks of postoperative bacterial seeding of the endoprosthesis. The patient should be evaluated by a physical therapist, who can provide education about the rehabilitative process following discharge from the hospital, assess patient motivation as a necessary accompaniment to a successful therapeutic program, and anticipate any special rehabilitative needs that may arise after surgery. The patient should receive at least 6 weeks of antipagetic preoperative medication to decrease chaotic bone remodeling activity and minimize intraoperative bleeding. Autologous preoperative blood donation and banking should be considered. And finally, as in all total joint arthroplasties, perioperative prophylactic antibiotics should be administered systemically (Table 15.6).

Technical problems arising at the time of surgery and of potential concern to the operating surgeon include increased blood loss, osseous deformity, and sclerotic pagetic bone. Excessive blood loss can be reduced by judicious preoperative use of antipagetic medication. Special instrumentation needs should be considered if severe osseous deformity or sclerotic bone is anticipated. If osteotomies requiring bony healing (such as a trochanteric osteotomy for ease of exposure) are anticipated, then perioperative antipagetic medication should be restricted to those agents that do not directly interfere with osteoblastic activity.

Several large series in the literature have retrospectively evaluated

TABLE 15.6 Preoperative Management of Paget's Patient for Total Hip Arthroplasty

Thorough medical evaluation and management of Paget's disease
Dental and urologic evaluation
Physical therapy evaluation
Autologous blood donation
Perioperative antipagetic medication to decrease disease activity and minimize bleeding
Prophylactic antibiotics

additional long-term complications of total hip arthroplasty in Paget's disease. In addition to the 1% to 2% risk of major perioperative complications encountered in most large series of nonpagetic total hip arthroplasties, increased risk due to aseptic loosening, heterotopic bone formation, acetabular protrusion, or varus deformity of the femoral component needs to be considered in the patient with Paget's disease (Table 15.7).

Mechanical failure requiring reoperation has been cited at between 10% and 15% in several large series (Figure 15.5). Nevertheless, the results of total hip arthroplasty in patients with severe end-stage disabling pagetic arthritis of the hips have been encouraging and rated as good to excellent in 75% to 85% of patients on the basis of well-accepted functional evaluation scales. The incidence of associated pagetic problems that might affect the overall perceived success of the surgery has been rated at about 50% and may often be anticipated preoperatively. Although generalized guidelines are helpful in planning surgery and expediting perioperative evaluation, assiduous attention must be given to the extenuating factors in each case.

Although total hip arthroplasty has been evaluated in several large retrospective studies, similar data are not yet available for total knee arthroplasty nor for joint replacement in the upper limb in patients with Paget's disease. Numerous areas for prospective study have been identified.

Through the use of medical and physical therapy modalities available to all physicians and through the judicious choice of surgery in selected cases, the orthopedic surgeon is often able to preserve and restore function in this common disorder.

ACKNOWLEDGMENT

This work was supported in part by grants (R01-DK-32760-01, SCOR:1-P50-AR39226-01, and 5M01-RR00040) from the National Institutes of Health, and by a Fellowship in Aging from The Hartford Foundation.

TABLE 15.7 Major Complications of Total Hip Arthroplasty in Paget's Disease

Aseptic loosening
Radiographic (15%–30%)
Acetabular (15%)
Femoral (30%)
Clinically significant (15%)
Heterotopic bone
Radiographic (25%–55%)
Clinically significant (5%–8%)
Acetabular protrusion (25%–50%)
Varus deformity (5%–10%)
Mechanical failure requiring reoperation (10%–15%)

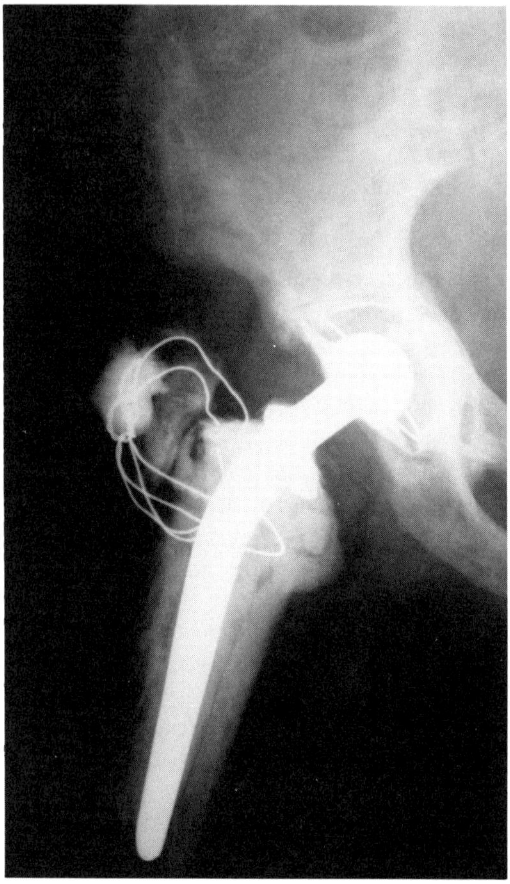

FIGURE 15.5. Anteroposterior roentgenogram of hip in patient with painful failed total hip arthroplasty. Note the following: (**A**) Pagetic involvement of pelvis and femur. (**B**) Nonunion of greater trochanteric osteotomy with broken fixation wires. (**C**) Acetabular protrusion. (**D**) Roentgenographic loosening of femoral and acetabular component. (**E**) Varus positioning of femoral component.

REFERENCES

1. Carter DR, Hayes WC: The compressive behavior of bone as a two-phase porous structure. *J Bone Joint Surg* 1977;59A:954–962.
2. Kaplan FS: Why there is deformity in Paget's disease and what can be done about it? *The Paget's Disease Foundation Inc. Fall 1987 Update.* 1987;9(1):4–5.
3. Parfitt AM: The coupling of bone formation to bone resorption: A critical analysis of the concept and of its relevance to the pathogenesis of osteoporosis. *Metab Bone Dis* 1982;4(1):1–6.

4. Reilly DT, Burstein AH: The mechanical properties of cortical bone. *J Bone Joint Surg* 1974;56A:1001–1022.
5. Rubin CT, Hausman MR: The cellular basis of Wolff's law: Transduction of physical stimuli to skeletal adaptation. *Rheum Dis Clin North Am* 1988;14:503–517.
6. Treharne RW: Review of Wolff's law and its proposed means of operation. *Orthop Rev* 1981;10(1):35–47.
7. Altman RD, Brown M, Gargano F: Low back pain in Paget's disease of bone. *Clin Orthop* 1987;217:152–161.
8. Dalinka MK, Aronchick JM, Haddad JG: Paget's disease: Symposium on Orthopaedic Radiology. *Orthop Clin North Am* 1983;14(1):3–19.
9. Douglas DL, Duckworth T, Kanis JA, et al: Spinal cord dysfunction in Paget's disease of bone: Has medical treatment a vascular basis? *J Bone Joint Surg* 1981;63B:495–503.
10. Haddad JG, Kaplan FS: Paget's disease of bone, in *The CIBA Collection of Medical Illustrations.* vol 8: *Musculoskeletal System.* Part I: *Anatomy, Physiology, and Metabolic Disorders*; Netter FH (illust). West Caldwell, NJ, Ciba-Geigy Corp, 1987; pp 236–238.
11. Siris ES, Canfield RE: Paget's disease of bone: Current concepts as to its nature and management. *Orthop Rev* 1982;11(12):43–49.
12. Dove J: Complete fractures of the femur in Paget's disease of bone. *J Bone Joint Surg* 1980;62B:12–17.
13. Johnston CC, Altman RD, Canfield RE, et al: Review of fracture experience during treatment of Paget's disease of bone with etidronate disodium (EHDP). *Clin Orthop* 1983;172:186–194.
14. Meyers MH, Singer FR: Osteotomy for tibia vara in Paget's disease under cover of calcitonin. *J Bone Joint Surg* 1978;60A:810–814.
15. Cameron HU: Total knee replacement in Paget's disease. *Orthop Rev* 1989;18(2): 206–208.
16. Franck WA, Bress NM, Singer F, Krane SM: Rheumatic manifestations of Paget's disease of bone. *Am J Med* 1974;56:592–603.
17. Hoppenfeld S: *Physical Examination of the Spine and Extremities.* Norwalk, CT, Appleton-Century-Crofts, 1976.
18. Lluberas-Acosta G, Hansell JR, Schumacher HR: Paget's disease of bone in patients with gout. *Arch Intern Med* 1986;146:2389–2392.
19. McDonald DJ, Sim FH: Total hip arthroplasty in Paget's disease: A follow-up note. *J Bone Joint Surg* 1987;69A:766–772.
20. Merkow RL, Pellicci PM, Hely DP, Salvat EA: Total hip replacement for Paget's disease of the hip. *J Bone Joint Surg* 1984;66A:752–758.
21. Stauffer RN, Sim FH: Total hip arthroplasty in Paget's disease of the hip. *J Bone Joint Surg* 1976;58(A):476–478.

Annotated Bibliography

Acknowledgment
This bibliography was prepared by Cheryl Harris, a member of the NAMSIC staff. It was produced for the National Institute of Arthritis and Musculoskeletal and Skin Diseases, under contract No. NO1-DK-7-2290.

PATIENT EDUCATION MATERIALS

1

Altman, R. D.

Osteoarthritis and Paget's disease. *Paget's Disease Foundation Update.* 1988;10(3):3. Available from Paget's Disease Foundation, Inc., 165 Cadman Plaza East, Brooklyn, NY 11201. (718) 596-1043. PRICE: $.50 for postage and handling.

This newsletter article discusses the occurrence of osteoarthritis in patients with Paget's disease. Osteoarthritis is a disease that starts as an abnormality of the joint surfaces. It progresses to involve the bone adjacent to the joint and is accompanied by thickening and inflammation of the sac around the joint (synovium). Osteoarthritis is most often asymptomatic but can be associated with pain, reduced function, and other overt signs of inflammation. Paget's disease can cause osteoarthritis by changing the bone around the joint. Occasionally, the combination of osteoarthritis and Paget's disease requires surgical consultation.

2

Arthritis Foundation

***Paget's disease.* (Arthritis Medical Information Services). Atlanta, Arthritis Foundation, 1987. Available from the Arthritis Foundation, P.O. Box 19000, Atlanta, GA 30326. (404) 872-7100. PRICE: Free.**

This brochure discusses the cause, symptoms, diagnosis, and treatment of Paget's disease. Paget's disease is a bone disorder in which bone formation is speeded up, changing the strength and shape of the bone. The parts of the skeleton most commonly affected include the pelvis, low back (lumbar spine), tailbone (sacrum), skull, and long bones in the legs (the femur or the tibia). Paget's disease usually centers in one or more areas of the skeleton and rarely spreads to other areas. The rest of the skeleton is normal. With early diagnosis and treatment, most people who have Paget's disease are able to lead active, independent lives.

2a

Bone, H. G.

New drugs in development for Paget's disease. *Paget's Disease Foundation Update* 1990;12(3):1, 4. Available as a reprint from Paget's Disease Foundation, Inc. 165 Camden Plaza East, Brooklyn, NY 11201. (718) 596-1043. PRICE: $1.00 for a set of reprints that includes this article.

This newsletter article identifies the two main classes of drugs used to treat Paget's disease: calcitonins and bisphosphonates. It also describes gallium nitrate, another agent that inhibits bone resorption. The article explains the disorder of the bone metabolism that occurs in Paget's disease and the action of calcitonins, bisphosphonates, and gallium nitrate to inhibit the disease process. Drug dosages and known side effects are also discussed.

3

Johnson, J. B.

Explanation of certain bone diseases, including Paget's. *Paget's Disease Foundation Update* 1988;10(1):3. Available from Paget's Disease Foundation, Inc. 165 Camden Plaza East, Brooklyn, NY 11201. (718) 596-1043. PRICE: $.50 for postage and handling.

This newsletter article describes the characteristics of metabolic bone diseases, with emphasis on Paget's disease (osteitis deformans), a metabolic bone disorder that appears to be initiated by increased bone resorption due to an increase in osteoclasts. The report also discusses the ways that metabolic bone diseases differ; the characteristics of osteoporosis, osteogenesis imperfecta, osteomalacia, and rickets; and bone hormones and their roles.

3a

Kaplan, F. S.

Surgical treatment of Paget's disease. *Paget's Disease Foundation Update* 1990;12(1):1, 3. Available from Paget's Disease Foundation, Inc. 165 Camden Plaza East, Brooklyn, NY 11201. (718) 596-1043. PRICE: $1.00 for a set of reprints that includes this article.

One of the most commonly asked questions of patients with Paget's disease is whether surgery will be needed. Surgery is rarely required but is considered when other methods prove less effective for relief of symptoms. This newsletter article discusses the three situations in which surgery is likely to be considered. These situations are (1) for fractures, (2) when arthritis occurs as a complication, or (3) when bone deformity affects lower limbs and weight-bearing bones. Surgical fixation of fractures may allow better healing. Total joint replacement surgery and cutting of bone (osteotomy) to realign painful weight-bearing joints are rarely necessary and are considered optional when symptoms warrant. The patient is advised to seek the advice of an orthopedic surgeon and to explore all options as well as potential risks when considering surgery.

4

Kaplan, F. S.

Why there is deformity in Paget's disease—and what can be done about it. *Paget's Disease Foundation Update* 1987;9(1):4–5. Available from Paget's Disease Foundation, Inc., 165 Camden Plaza East, Brooklyn, NY 11201. (718) 596-1043. PRICE: $.50 for postage and handling.

This newsletter article describes the pathologic process of Paget's disease and the way that bone formation is disturbed. Bones affected by Paget's disease may be structurally weak and prone to deformities and fractures. Possible therapies and mechanical aids and devices to help relieve bone stress are discussed.

4a

Lyles, K. W.

Exercise and Paget's disease of bone. *Paget's Disease Foundation Update* 1990;12(2):3. Available from Paget's Disease Foundation, Inc., 165 Cadman Plaza East, Brooklyn, NY 11201. (718) 596-1043. PRICE: $1.00 for a set of reprints that includes this article.

This newsletter article presents exercise guidelines for Paget's disease patients. The recommendation to undertake an exercise program should first come from a physician. Patients with Paget's disease involving the bones of the lower extremities may benefit from walking to strengthen hip and leg muscles. For those with pelvic involvement, weight-bearing exercises may be inappropriate, and exercises in water and range of motion exercises may be advised. In some instances, back pain can be treated with a program to improve posture, increase flexibility, and strengthen muscles. Improved functional ability and sense of well-being are among the potential benefits of an exercise program for patients.

5

McKinstry, D. W.

Researching the cause and treatment of Paget's disease of bone. *Research Resources Reporter* 1984;8(1):1–7. Available from Research Resources Information Center, 1601 Research Boulevard, Rockville, MD 20850. (301) 984-2870.

Paget's disease is a slowly progressive disorder in which normal bone is resorbed and replaced by abnormal bone. As many as 3 million Americans have Paget's disease, although many of these patients do not show symptoms and do not require any therapy. Research on the treatment and cause of Paget's disease is discussed. A promising lead is the discovery of imprints of a slow virus infection in practically all osteoclasts involved in Paget's disease. Genetics also may play a role in the causes of Paget's disease. The author discusses tests used to uncover Paget's disease and available therapeutic agents: calcitonins, diphosphonates (bisphosphonates) and rarely, mithramycine (plicamycin). Each is effective in relieving symptoms and decreasing biochemical markers of Paget's disease, with a subsequent partial restoration of the normal histologic structure of the bone.

6

Medical Times

Paget's disease. (Medical Times Patient Education Chart). *Medical Times* 1988;116(12):55–61. New York, Romaine Pierson Publishers, 4 pages. Available from Medical Times, 80 Shore Road, Port Washington, NY 11050.

This color-illustrated patient information brochure provides basic information on the symptoms and management of Paget's disease. A chart depicts the sites of the symptoms of Paget's disease and lists diagnostic tests and available drug therapies. A fact sheet that answers questions about the history of Paget's disease and its occurrence, prevalence, symptoms, and treatment is included. A 3-page article, explaining in more detail the history, diagnosis, symptoms, and treatment of Paget's disease, accompanies the brochure.

7

Monsell, E. M.

Hearing loss in Paget's disease. *Paget's Disease Foundation Update* 1989;11(2):3. Available from Paget's Disease Foundation, Inc., 165 Cadman Plaza East, Brooklyn, NY, 11201. (718) 596-1043. PRICE: $.50 for postage and handling.

This newsletter article describes hearing loss in patients with Paget's disease. Hearing loss in Paget's disease may be conductive, sensorineural, or both. The author recommends that persons with Paget's disease involving the skull undergo a baseline hearing test and evaluation. Although hearing loss cannot always be corrected with medication or surgery, most losses can be overcome with a hearing aid. An illustration is included.

8

National Institutes of Health

Understanding Paget's Disease. **Bethesda, MD, National Institutes of Health, 1985, 12 pages. Available from National Arthritis and Musculoskeletal and Skin Diseases Information Clearinghouse, Box AMS, Bethesda, MD 20892. (301) 468-3235. PRICE: Free.**

This booklet defines Paget's disease and describes the disease process through the initial, active, and inactive stages. Although the disease is usually symptom-free, any symptoms that are present may resemble other disorders such as arthritis. Diagnosis, treatment with drugs or orthopedic management, cause, and areas of research also are covered.

9

National Organization for Rare Disorders

Paget's Disease. **New Fairfield, CT, National Organization for Rare Disorders, 1987, 3 pages. Available from National Organization for Rare Disorders. NORD Literature Department, P.O. Box 8923, New Fairfield, CT 06812. (203) 746-6518. PRICE: $2.50 plus $0.50 postage and handling.**

This factsheet from the National Organization for Rare Disorders discusses Paget's disease, also known as formans, osteitis deformans, Pozzi's, congenital hyperphosphatasemia, hyperostosis corticalis deformans, or corticalis deformans. Paget's disease is a slowly progressive disease of the skeletal system characterized by abnormally rapid bone breakdown and formation, leading to the development of bones that are dense but fragile. It usually affects middle-aged and elderly people and most frequently occurs in the spine, skull, pelvis, thighs, and lower legs. Sources for additional information are provided.

10

Paget's Disease Foundation, Inc.

New Direction, New Hope. **Brooklyn, NY, Paget's Disease Foundation, Inc., 1987, 3 pages. Available from Paget's Disease Foundation, Inc., 165 Cadman Plaza East, Brooklyn, NY 11201. (718) 596-1043. PRICE: $.50 for postage and handling.**

This brochure for people with Paget's disease of bone, a chronic skeletal disorder that may result in enlarged and deformed bones, outlines the characteristics of this disease and treatment advances. Information also is included about the Paget's Disease Foundation and the services it provides.

11

Paget's Disease Foundation, Inc.

Questions and Answers about Paget's Disease of Bone. **Brooklyn, NY, Paget's Disease Foundation, Inc. 1990, 9 pages. Available from Paget's Disease Foundation, Inc., 165 Cadman Plaza East, Brooklyn, NY 11201. (718) 596-1043. PRICE: $1.00 for postage and handling.**

This brochure provides responses to 29 common questions concerning Paget's disease. Topics cover the nature of the disease and its possible causes, symptoms and diagnosis, treatment, prognosis, relationships among Paget's disease and other medical conditions, heredity, and effect of nutrition and exercise. References to other Paget's Disease Foundation brochures are also included.

12

Singer, F. R.

Who should provide medical care for the patient with Paget's disease? *Paget's Disease Foundation Update* 1989;11(1):3. Available from Paget's Disease Foundation, Inc., 165 Cadman Plaza East, Brooklyn, NY 11201. (718) 596-1043. PRICE: $.50 for postage and handling.

This newsletter article provides some guidelines for patients as to which physicians are most appropriate to provide care for the patient with Paget's disease. Care and consultation provided by primary care physicians, endocrinologists, rheumatologists, and surgical specialists such as orthopedic surgeons, neurosurgeons, and otolaryngologists are discussed.

13

Siris, E. S.

Paget's Disease in Families. *Paget's Disease Foundation Update* 1989;11(2):4–5. Available from Paget's Disease Foundation, Inc., 165 Cadman Plaza East, Brooklyn, NY 11201. (718) 596-1043. PRICE: $.50 for postage and handling.

The author discusses current research on the occurrence of Paget's disease within families. For a long time, doctors caring for Paget's disease have noticed that, in some cases, it seems to occur in more than one member of a family. In one study, 18% of patients had at least one other family member with the disorder. In the control group, which consisted of people the same age but who did not have Paget's disease, 3% of their blood relatives had Paget's disease. Although the information available strongly suggests that Paget's disease may be inherited, it has not yet been proved.

For those with Paget's disease in their family, the risk of developing the disease is still small. However, for those over 40, the author suggests a alkaline phosphatase blood test every 2 to 3 years.

14

USV Pharmaceutical Corporation

Simplifying Your Injections. **Tarrytown, NY, USV Pharmaceutical Corporation, 1988, 8 pages. Also available as a 14-minute VHS videotape. Available from Rorer Pharmaceuticals, 500 Virginia Drive, Ft. Washington, PA 19034. Attention: Calcimar Product Manager. PRICE: Single copies of the booklet and videotape free.**

This patient education booklet, also available in a videotape version, is a guide to the technique of administering Calcimar (calcitonin-salmon) injections. It provides detailed instructions with pictures for preparing the injection, filling the syringe, cleaning the injection site, and injection techniques, record keeping, and cleanup. A diagram of recommended injection sites is included.

15

Whyte, M. P.

Why does the doctor measure your blood alkaline phosphatase level? ***Paget's Disease Foundation Update*** **1988;10(2):3. Available from Paget's Disease Foundation, Inc., 165 Cadman Plaza East, Brooklyn, NY 11201. (718) 596-1043. PRICE: $.50 for postage and handling.**

This newsletter article describes the relationship between blood alkaline phosphatase levels and Paget's disease. Paget's disease is described as a disturbance in the process of bone buildup and breakdown. Cells that normally build up bone or try to repair the bone destruction in Paget's disease are rich in alkaline phosphatase. The increased presence is detectable in the blood.

PROFESSIONAL EDUCATION MATERIALS

General Medical Reviews

16

Altman, R. D.

Paget's disease of bone (osteitis deformans). ***Bull Rheum Dis*** **1984;34(3):1–8.**

Paget's disease can be defined as a structural abnormality whereby isolated areas of the skeleton undergo increased bone resorption resulting in subsequent deposition of bone that is disorganized, enlarged, and structurally weak. Eighty percent of people with Paget's disease are asymptomatic. When they are symptomatic, the clinical manifestations are defined by the complications of the disease: bone pain, deformity, fractures, secondary osteoarthritis, high cardiac output, sarcoma, skull symptoms, hearing loss, angioid streaks, neural compression, hyperparathyroidism, and hypercalcemia. When the disease is localized and asymptomatic, no therapy is required. Orthotics may correct symptoms related to flexion contractures. Orthopedic management includes correction of deformity, treatment of fractures, or orthopedic treatment of arthritis. Total hip arthroplasty has been very successful. Though there are no uniformly accepted indications for suppressive therapy of Paget's disease, proposed indications for medicinal therapy are listed; these include bone pain, paraparesis, hypercalcemia, osteolytic wedge of long bone, and need to prevent additional complications. (20 references)

17

Arnold, A.; Nagant de Deuxchaisnes, C.

Paget's disease of bone, in DeGroot LJ (ed): *Endocrinology*, ed. 2 Philadelphia, WB Saunders Co, 1989, pp 1208–1244. Available from WB Saunders, Curtis Center, Washington Square West, Philadelphia, PA 19106. 3 volumes. ISBN: 0721622224.

This book chapter reviews the incidence, cause, histology and pathophysiology, laboratory parameters, and radiographic findings in Paget's disease. Medical management is evaluated in depth. The aim of therapy and techniques to evaluate results are discussed. The pharmacodynamics and therapeutic uses of the calcitonins, diphosphonates (bisphosphonates), and mithramycin (plicamycin) are presented. The newer antiosteolytic agents are able to treat the major symptoms and complications of Paget's disease, including neurologic compression, cardiac failure, and the rare immobilization hypercalcemia. Some may prevent spontaneous fractures. Adequate monitoring of effect and side effects should be undertaken. Calcitonin, the most expensive agent, does not, however, require any monitoring for side effects. It is so far the only agent available that exerts a uniformly positive action on the focal bone balance, as shown by sequential radiologic analysis. Many tables, graphs, and radiographs are included. (310 references)

18

Avioli, L. V.

Paget's disease: State of the art. *Clin Therapeutics* 1987;9(6):567–576.

This technical review details the current understanding of the pathogenesis, diagnosis, and treatment of Paget's disease, an inflammatory bone disorder that results in crippling and gross distortion of skeletal anatomy. Pathologically, it is characterized by extensive vascularity, increased marrow fibrosis, and intense cellular activity with irregular areas of lamellar bone interspaced by poorly stained "cement" lines, the latter simulating a mosaic pattern. Other symptomatic features are described. Nonetheless, many people with Paget's disease are totally asymptomatic throughout the course of their disease. Elevated levels of serum alkaline phosphatase and urinary hydroxyproline can usually be correlated with the extent and activity of the disease, although normal levels of these markers have been found in some patients with early active disease detected by radioisotopic scintigraphic imaging. Until the last decade, treatment of Paget's disease was unsatisfactory; however, new agents such as calcitonin, mithramycin (plicamycin), and sodium etidronate have proved effective. Most cases have been observed in the United States, United Kingdom, Australia, France, and Germany, with about 750,000 people in England and Wales alone diagnosed with this disease. (41 references)

19

Bijvoet, O. L. M.; Vellenga, C. J.; Harinck, H. I. J.

Paget's disease of bones: Assessment, therapy and secondary prevention, in Kleerekoper M, Krane SM (eds): *Clinical Disorders of Bone and Mineral Metabolism: Proceedings of the Laurence and Dorothy Fallis International Symposium.* New York, Mary Ann Liebert, 1989, pp 525–542. Available from Mary Ann Liebert, Inc., 1651 Third Avenue, New York, NY 10128. (212) 289-2300.

Less than two decades ago no treatment was available for Paget's disease. The discovery of the therapeutic potential of calcitonin and bisphosphonates has changed this completely, and at present the possibility that pain, functional impairment, and disability are preventable emerges. This book chapter emphasizes that the goal of therapy is to evolve from a period in which the major aim is to suppress pagetic activity in symptomatic patients to one that aims at early treatment and prevention. This requires standards for diagnosis and ability to assess the likelihood that the disease will cause complications, as well as criteria for the evaluation of drug efficacy with respect to long-term preventive potential and safety and simplicity of treatment. The authors review the parameters of Paget's disease, noting its histology, pathogenesis, radiodiagnosis, biochemical implications, epidemiology, symptoms, and prognosis. The discussion on treatment includes short-term efficacy and the predictability and completeness of response and remission, including the importance of monitoring and complications of therapy. Several tables and graphs are included. (142 references)

19a

Dequeker, J.

Paget's disease in a painting by Quinten Metsys (Massys). *Br Med J* 1989;299(6715):1579–1581.

Works of art of different kinds may provide important evidence of the occurrence of rheumatic diseases before their recognition as established medical conditions. In 1882, Sir James Paget clearly described the lack of physical historical evidence of osteitis deformans in London. Yet lesions of the skull and clavicles in the painting, *A Grotesque Old Woman*, attributed to Quinten Metsys (1465–1530), suggest that osteitis deformans was not a new disease in the nineteenth century. The painting represents an old woman holding a rosebud. The face is accurately executed with deformations, disfigurement, and distortions, including a bulging area beneath the nose. A modern photograph of a woman with Paget's disease affecting maxillary bones presents several similar deformities. Statements made about the Metsys painting have claimed that the caricature was imagined rather than copied from real life. A drawing by Leonardo da Vinci was probably the source for the painting and points to the greater likelihood that the image represents pathologic features actually observed. The finding of pagetoid deformities in the Metsys painting raises questions as to whether the condition arose as recently as Paget believed. (13 references)

20

Excerpta Medica

***Paget's Disease of Bone: Comments by Eight Specialists.* Princeton, NJ, Excerpta Medica, 1988, 40 pages. Available from Norwich Eaton Pharmaceuticals, Inc., 17 Eaton Avenue, Norwich, NY 13815. (607) 335-2111. PRICE: Single copies free.**

This publication, which is based on responses to a brief questionnaire, provides an in-depth discussion of current knowledge of Paget's disease. It presents an overview of the cause and disease process of Paget's disease, presenting symptoms, diagnostic signs, and relevant laboratory and roentgenographic procedures. A discussion of appropriate drug therapy follows, with emphasis on analgesic versus antipagetic therapy and use of etidronate disodium, calcitonin, and plicamycin. Photos and charts are included. (6 references)

21

Freeman, D. A.

Paget's disease of bone. ***Am J Med Sci*** **1988;295(2):144–158.**

Paget's disease is a relatively common bone disease. This review presents recommended treatments and their background. Basic bone cell biology, biochemistry, and pathology are presented, as are speculations about possible causes of this disease. The section on treatment of Paget's disease discusses calcitonin and diphosphonates (bisphosphonates) and reviews the mechanism of action of the drugs, clinical studies of their effectiveness, and advantages and disadvantages of each. The review article concludes with specific treatment recommendations for each of the six clinical settings in which treatment of Paget's disease is justified. (110 references)

22

Gross, J. S.

Paget's disease of bone, ***Physician Assist*** **1988;12(2):94–95, 99–103, 133 passim.**

Paget's disease affects approximately 2.5 million people in the United States and is a cause of significant morbidity. Patients can exhibit myriad of clinical findings—pain, headache, and hearing impairment are common complaints—reflecting varying degrees of organ system dysfunction. However, more than 90% of patients are asymptomatic, the disease being discovered when elevated alkaline phosphatase levels or radiographic study changes are found incidentally. The spine, skull, pelvis, and long bones are most commonly involved. Measurements of serum alkaline phosphatase and urinary hydroxyproline are used to assess disease severity. Proper diagnosis and therapy can alleviate pain, minimize morbidity, and maintain skeleton function. Antipagetic medications used are calcitonin and etidronate disodium. (34 references)

23
Hadjipavlou, A.; Lander, P.; Srolovitz, H.
Pagetic arthritis: Pathophysiology and management. *Clin Orthop* 1986;(208):15–19.

A review of the records of 112 patients demonstrates modern concepts of pathogenesis and treatment of Paget's disease. Medical treatment for pain from pagetic arthritis should initially be aimed at modulation of bone blood flow. Patients, even those with impressive arthritic reactions, can respond dramatically. Pain persists in patients with end-stage destruction of articular cartilage and/or stress microfractures. Patients with deformity without joint space loss may be candidates for osteotomy. Advanced cartilage destruction is treated by total arthroplasty and continuation of antipagetic therapy after surgery, possibly to reduce the incidence of component loosening. Articular cartilage erosion and subchondral bone destruction are attributable to the disease process. Vascular invasion and joint surface collapse are associated with cartilage thinning and sequestration. (7 references)

24
Haering, S. J.; Smelts, D. S.
Paget's disease of bone. *Can Nurse* 1985;81(9):36–38.

This article reviews the clinical symptoms, epidemiology, cause, diagnosis, and therapy of Paget's disease, with emphasis on nursing care and assessment. A case study of a patient with Paget's disease is presented to illustrate the progression of the disease. The nursing care plan used with this patient is discussed. A list and description of complications of Paget's disease are included. (5 references)

25
Hahn, B.; Dishart, P. W.; Feldman, F.
***Differential Diagnosis of Low Back Pain in the Aging Patient.* (audiovisual). Norwich, NY, Norwich Eaton Pharmaceuticals, 1987. ¾-inch or ½-inch VHS videocassette (29 minutes). Available from Norwich Eaton Pharmaceuticals, Inc., 17 Eaton Avenue, Norwich, NY 13815-0231. (607) 335-2247. Catalog Number D1962.**

In this videotape, leading practitioners discuss the differential diagnosis and management of cases of osteoporosis and Paget's disease. Case studies include reviews of the patient's medical history, physical examinations, laboratory tests, and radiographs. The diagnostic process also involves a musculoskeletal radiologist who analyzes the different lesions on the various radiographs. After the differential diagnosis, the need for therapy is emphasized and various treatment regimens are explained.

26

Jacobs, T. P.

Diagnosis and management of Paget's disease. *Compr Ther* 1986;12(3):30–34.

Paget's disease is a relatively common problem among the aging populations of the United States and several other Western countries. Although its cause is still unknown, several lines of evidence point to an acquired, possibly viral, agent that affects the osteoclasts of susceptible persons. Although most patients with Paget's disease have no symptoms, a minority of those who experience pain, fractures, deformity, or other complications require management. Specific treatment of the disease process with diphosphonates (bisphosphonates) and/or calcitonin is available and is usually effective. Primary physicians caring for the elderly will be required to consider initiation of these and other therapies increasingly often as detection and public awareness of this disease continue to increase. (16 references)

27

Jacobs, T. P.; Siris, E. S.

Paget's disease: A common problem of the aging skeleton. *Geriatr Med Today* 1984;3(12):7 pages.

Paget's disease of bone is a frequently seen skeletal disease in the elderly. Because most of these patients are asymptomatic, the disease is often detected after roentgenography or blood tests performed for unrelated conditions. Others have pain that is not easily differentiated from pain associated with osteoarthritis or other mechanical or inflammatory conditions, and a smaller group experience symptoms clearly related to Paget's disease. The authors discuss the various clinical presentations of Paget's disease of bone, as well as patient management, including drug therapy and surgical intervention for symptomatic patients. (21 references)

28

Kattapuram, S. V.; DeLuca, S. A.

Paget's disease. *Am Fam Physician* 1986;34(5):121–126.

This illustrated report describes the radiographic and clinical features of Paget's disease, in which accelerated osteoclastic activity progresses, causing bone resorption. Pictures of the skull, long bones, spine, and pelvis illustrate these features. Radiographic evidence of increased density or sclerosis of bone may be seen in both the active and inactive stages of the disease. The report also discusses the use of scintigraphy in diagnosis, complications occurring in Paget's disease (fractures, sarcomas), and treatment with calcitonin and diphosphonates (bisphosphonates) (etidronate). (3 references)

29

Krane, S. M.

Paget's disease of bone, In *Primer on the Rheumatic Diseases*, ed 9. Atlanta, GA, Arthritis Foundation, 1988, pp 261–262. Available from the Arthritis Foundation, 1314 Spring Street, N.W., Atlanta, GA 30309. (404) 872-7100.

This book chapter discusses current knowledge on the cause, disease process, diagnosis, symptoms, possible complications, and therapy of Paget's disease. The pagetic process is reviewed, along with radiographic signs. (7 references)

30

Krane, S. M.

Paget's disease of bone, *Calcif Tissue Int* 1986;38(6):309–317.

This detailed editorial report summarizes and discusses the presentations and findings of a 1985 workshop of experts on Paget's disease of bone, held at the National Institutes of Health. The theme of the workshop was to stimulate ideas that might lead to further understanding of the pathways and controls involved in the pagetic process, the causative factors in Paget's disease, local growth factors, and regulators and inhibitors that affect bone formation. The status of therapeutic approaches using calcitonin, diphosphonates (bisphosphonates), and alternative untested drugs (antiviral agents, nonglucocorticoid steroids, interferons) also is discussed. (0 references)

31

Krozy, R. E.

Paget's disease: Implications for home nursing. *Home Health Care Nurse* 1987;5(2):32–33, 36–39.

Paget's disease of the bone is a chronic, destructive process in which there are excessive bone resorption and replacement with new bone that is weak, fibrotic, highly vascular, irregular, and larger than normal. Many people with Paget's disease are asymptomatic, and the disease is often discovered accidentally when the individual is being examined via blood test or radiograph for some other problem. The majority of people with extensive disease can manage independently and do not need to be hospitalized. However, they may require instruction about the disease and self-care, which may include instruction in injection technique. When the disease interferes with the individual's ability to perform the activities of daily living because of pain or mobility restrictions, home care from a visiting nurse and use of auxiliary help may be needed. With early diagnosis and proper treatment, however, the prognosis can be quite favorable. Although each individual responds differently to treatment, the disease is essentially incurable. Nursing interventions are discussed, and the role of the nurse is presented in terms of monitoring progress, teaching proper health management, identifying and securing resources, and providing emotional support. (11 references)

32

Lander, P. H.; Hadjipavlou, A. G.

A dynamic classification of Paget's disease. *J Bone Joint Surg* 1986;68(3):431–438.

A new dynamic classification of Paget's disease is proposed, incorporating both the radiographic phases of bone remodeling and the scintigraphic findings. Osteolytic, mixed, and osteoblastic phases are associated with increased scintigraphic activity, whereas the osteosclerotic phase of remodeling is associated with normal or diminished activity and an osteoblastic radiographic appearance. Abnormal modeling of bone leading to deformity is produced by accelerated apposition or absorption at the periosteal and endosteal envelopes of the bone. In 112 patients with symptoms of Paget's disease, 527 lesions were classified. The most frequent remodeling phase was the mixed one, and the most common modeling state was bone expansion with endosteal and periosteal apposition. Of 88 patients treated medically, 12 had lesions that progressed to increased bone formation without a change in modeling, and the active lesions in 7 patients became inactive. Prolonged treatment with disodium etidronate led to progressive osteopenia in 11 patients. (37 references)

33

Merkow, R. L.; Lane, J. M.

Current concepts of Paget's disease of bone. *Orthop Clin North Am* 1984;15(4):747–763.

Paget's disease of bone is a process of increased bone remodeling, resulting in architecturally abnormal bone. The disease may affect any area of the skeleton. Paget's disease may present wide variation in the clinical and radiographic picture. Symptoms depend on the site of disease and the extent of skeletal involvement. The two major therapeutic agents available for medical treatment are calcitonin and diphosphonate (bisphosphonate). Surgical intervention in Paget's disease is indicated for (1) selected fractures, (2) severe disabling arthritis, and (3) extreme bowing deformities causing malalignment of weight-bearing joints. (16 references)

34

Merkow, R. L.; Lane, J. M.

Metabolic bone disease and Paget's disease in the elderly: II. Paget's disease. *Clin Rheum Dis* 1986;12(1):70–96. Also reprinted in Sculco, T. P., (ed.): *Orthopaedic Care of the Geriatric Patient.* St. Louis, CV Mosby, 1985, pp 253–268. Available from CV Mosby Co., 1130 Westline Industrial Drive, St. Louis, MO 63146. (800) 325-4177. ISBN: 0801644038.

This article describes Paget's disease of bone as a process of increased bone remodeling. Paget's disease is more common than once thought: the incidence rate in certain populations is 3% to 4% in middle-aged patients and 10% to 15% in the elderly. The cause is unknown, although recent evidence appears to support a virus as an important factor. Radiographic findings include the "mosaic" pattern, which results from new bone formation. The most common complaints in patients with Paget's disease are pain, skeletal deformity, changes in skin temperature, pathologic fractures, neurocompression, arthritis, and symptoms resulting from vascular shunting. Systemic, metabolic, and rheumatoid manifestations have been noted, as well as hypercalcemia, hypercalciuria, hyperuricemia, apathy, lethargy, and cardiovascular complications or malignant degeneration. Surgical intervention is indicated for selected fractures; severe, disabling arthritis, and extreme bowing deformities that may cause poor alignment of weight-bearing joints. Several charts, tables, and radiographs are included. (14 references)

34a

Merkow, R. L.; Lane, J. M.

Paget's disease of bone. *Endocrinol Metab Clin North Am* 1990;19(1):177–204. *Orthop Clin North Am* 1990;21(1):171–189.

Paget's disease of bone is defined as a process of increased bone remodeling; the primary event is increased resorption (osteoclastic activity), followed by subsequent reactive bone formation (osteoblastic activity). It is usually asymmetric and may be asymptomatic. The cause is unknown, but recent evidence appears to support the theory that a virus is an important factor. It may present wide variation in the clinical and radiographic picture. The most frequent sites of involvement include the spine, femora, cranium, pelvis, and sternum. The most common complaints are pain, skeletal deformity, and change in skin temperature. Pathologic fractures may be the presenting manifestations or complications in a patient with known Paget's disease. They occur most frequently in the long weight-bearing bones of the lower extremities such as the femoral neck and subtrochanteric and tibial regions. The two major therapeutic agents available for treatment are calcitonins (porcine, salmon, or human) and diphosphonates (bisphosphonates). The aim of such therapy is to control the metabolic activity of the disease, to normalize the biochemical parameters, and to improve the symptoms. Fortunately, tumors are rare; early diagnosis may give rise to more effective palliation, if not a significant cure rate. (32 references)

35

Merrick, M. V.; Merrick, J. M.

Observations on the natural history of Paget's disease. *Clin Radiol* 1985;36(2):169–174.

Whole-body skeletal scintigraphy was performed in 4,700 adult patients from southeast Scotland. In 3,831 with proven or suspected malignant disease, the prevalence of osteitis deformans in men is 0.006 in those aged 15 to 54 years, 0.026 in the age group 55 to 84 years, and 0.24 over the age of 84 years. The corresponding figures in women are 0.002, 0.021, and 0.15, respectively. Previous estimates of prevalence should be increased by at least 25% to account for peripheral and monostotic disease, which is more common than hitherto recognized. The increase in prevalence with age may not be linear. Possible associations with environmental and genetic factors that would account for such a distribution are considered. It is suggested that the conventional distinction between "active" and "burned-out" Paget's disease may be incorrect. (28 references)

36

Meunier, P. J.; Russell, G.

***Paget's Disease of Bone.* (audiovisual). Norwich, NY, Norwich Eaton Pharmaceuticals, 1983. 16-mm film or ½-inch VHS videocassette (27 minutes), color, sound. Available from Norwich Eaton Pharmaceuticals, Inc., 17 Eaton Avenue, Norwich, NY 13815-0231. (607) 335-2247. Catalog Number D1962.**

This audiovisual presentation discusses various aspects of Paget's disease of bone, noting that there may be as many as 2 million patients with this disease in the United States. The presentation provides an in-depth discussion of the cause, diagnosis, and state-of-the-art treatment of this disease. The presentation is designed to enhance the awareness and understanding of the process of this disease.

37
Norwich Eaton Pharmaceuticals
Paget's Disease of Bone. **(audiovisual). Norwich, NY, Norwich Eaton Pharmaceuticals, 1983. 60 color slides with written text. Available from Norwich Eaton Pharmaceuticals, Inc., 17 Eaton Avenue, Norwich, NY 13815-0231. (607) 335-2247. Catalog Number D1618.**

This slide series covers various aspects of Paget's disease of the bone, pointing out that the incidence of this disease has been estimated at 3% of the general population over age 40 and noting that the prevalence of this disease increases with age and that it is more common in individuals of western European origin. This presentation illustrates and discusses the presenting signs and symptoms, diagnosis, and treatment of Paget's disease of the bone. (0 references)

38
Pharmacy Times
3 million Americans are affected by Paget's disease of bone. ***Pharmacy Times*** **1988;54(1):47–48, 52.**

This article provides a general overview of Paget's disease symptoms and available treatment, including orthopedic management and prognosis. (0 references)

39
Resnick, D.
Paget disease of bone: Current status and a look back to 1943 and earlier. ***AJR*** **1988;150(2):249–256.**

This retrospective review summarizes and discusses advances made in the understanding of the nature of Paget's disease of bone from the early days of its recognition by Sir James Paget in 1877 to the present. Attention is given to its cause, skeletal distribution and extent, natural history and effect of therapy, and complications. Reference is made throughout the review to the work of Paget. The article includes scintigraphs and X-rays to illustrate the characteristics and progressive stages of the disease. Information is provided on the pathophysiology and potential musculoskeletal consequences of the disease, including osseous deformities, fractures, neoplasms, soft-tissue masses, osteomyelitis, crystal deposition, and possible neurologic abnormalities. (72 references)

40

Rosenthal, M. J., et al.

Paget's disease of bone in older patients: UCLA Grand Rounds. *J Am Geriatr Soc* 1989;37(7):639–650.

Although cases of Paget's disease have been found on study of remains dating back to Neanderthal humans, the widespread occurrence of the disease is rare before the age of 40 and the prevalence increases with advancing age. From 1% to 3% of the American population over the age of 65 is affected, with frequency rising to 10% above age 80. Hence, this is a disease estimated primarily to affect the elderly person. Although many patients are asymptomatic, the complications of Paget's disease can be devastating. In this UCLA Grand Rounds, several case histories of Paget's disease patients are presented. Pathogenesis, clinical presentation, complications, and diagnosis are discussed. Approaches to therapy, which include follow-up, reassurance, and explanation to asymptomatic patients, are reviewed. Appropriate therapy for symptomatic patients includes assessment, counseling, rehabilitation, pain management, drug therapy, and possibly surgery. (99 references)

41

Ross, D. G.

Paget's disease. *Orthop Nursing* 1984;3(3):41–44.

This article reviews current findings about the cause, pathophysiology, and clinical diagnosis of osteitis deformans. The author presents a diagnostic overview of commonly affected areas of the body and radiographic and laboratory findings. Medications used to treat Paget's disease and their possible effects are discussed. (6 references)

42

Shapiro, J. R.

Paget's disease of bone, in *Current Concepts of Bone Fragility.* Published Proceedings in the 12th Applied Basic Science Course, Ottawa, Canada, 1985. New York, Springer-Verlag, 1986, pp 227–235. Available from Springer-Verlag, 175 Fifth Avenue, 19th floor, New York, NY 10010. (800) 526-7254.

This paper discusses the course of Paget's disease, including spontaneous flares and remissions, and the treatment options. The author poses to physicians several issues and questions dealing with the clinical problems of Paget's disease, including the meaning of familial clustering and its possible viral cause; whether a biopsy should be used to confirm the diagnosis; which pharmacotherapy should be used and for how long; how much back or joint pain is due to osteoarthritis and how much is the result of the pagetic process; and when joint replacement for spinal compression is indicated. (34 references)

43

Singer, F. R.

Paget's disease of bone, in Raisz L, Martin EJ (eds.): *Clinical Endocrinology of Calcium Metabolism.* New York, Marcel Dekker, 1988, pp 369–402. Available from Marcel Dekker, 270 Madison Avenue, New York, NY 10016. (800) 228-1160.

This book chapter presents an overview of the history, prevalence, and epidemiology of Paget's disease. The author discusses the disease and possible causes, reviewing the evidence for hormonal, vascular, autoimmune, neoplastic, metabolic, and virologic causes. Clinical manifestations and skeletal distribution of Paget's are discussed, along with available diagnostic technologies, which include roentgenograms, computerized tomography, radioisotope scanning, and laboratory measurement of alkaline phosphatase, urinary hydroxyproline, and osteocalcin levels. Therapeutic intervention for Paget's disease, including the indications for therapy, is discussed. Relief of bone pain is cited as the most common indication for treatment. Pain relief can be achieved in a high percentage of patients. The author discusses the administration, dosage, and comparative efficacies of available pharmacologic agents and provides guidelines for surgical intervention. (80 references)

44

Singer, F. R.

Paget's disease of bone, in Kelley WN, et al (eds): *Textbook of Rheumatology*, ed 2, Philadelphia, WB Saunders, 1985, p 1676–1687. Available from WB Saunders Co., Curtis Center, Independence Square West, Philadelphia, PA 19106-3399. ISBN: 0721653626. PRICE: $195.00.

This chapter provides an overview of Paget's disease. It addresses signs and symptoms, clinical biochemistry, radiographic evaluation, bone disease, complications, pathogenesis, and treatment. Drug therapy and elective surgery are discussed. (27 references)

45
Siris, E. S.
Diagnosis and treatment of Paget's disease of bone. ***Compr Ther*** **1983;9(9):47–53.**

This paper summarizes and discusses the characteristics, clinical presentation, diagnosis, and treatment of patients with Paget's disease of bone. This disease is a localized disorder of bone remodeling that characteristically occurs in middle-aged and elderly patients. Specific attention is given to the use of three drugs (calcitonin, diphosphonates [bisphosphonates], and mithramycin [plicamycin]) for therapy. (9 references)

46
Strewler, G. J.
Paget's disease of bone. ***West J Med*** **1984;140(5):763–768.**

This article discusses improvements in the treatment of Paget's disease of bone. Specific attention is given to the clinical features of this disease; its rheumatologic, metabolic, and neoplastic complications; indications for therapy; and treatment with calcitonin (a peptide hormone), etidronate (a diphosphonate; bisphosphonate) and mithramycin (plicamycin; a cytotoxic antibiotic). Long-term subcutaneous dosing with calcitonin has been shown to produce excellent results in patients, significantly decreasing pain; etidronate has produced prolonged remission of symptoms and biochemical hypercalcemia in malignancy; however, although the clinical responses to mithramycin (plicamycin) have been profound, the drug can present considerable toxicity to the liver, kidney, and bone marrow. It is acknowledged that, despite these advances, the treatment of Paget's disease is in its infancy. (29 references)

47
Wallach, S.
Chronic joint pain; Arthritis or osteitis? ***Hosp Pract*** **1985;20(11A):29–39.**

The author presents a case involving a 53-year-old man, who complained of chronic pain in the shoulder and buttocks, with a recent onset of pain in the upper shin accompanied by swelling and heat sensation. The findings on the patient's physical examination and laboratory and radiographic studies were reviewed, and a diagnosis of Paget's disease was made. The author discusses the complications of Paget's disease, including neurologic and cardiovascular manifestations. Specific therapeutic agents and criteria for their use are discussed. (7 references)

48

Wallach, S.

Paget's disease of bone, in Calkins E, Davis PJ, Ford AB (eds): *The Practice of Geriatrics.* Philadelphia, WB Saunders, 1986, pp 431–440. Available from W. B. Saunders Co., Curtis Center, Washington Square West, Philadelphia, PA 19106. ISBN: 0721623298.

This textbook chapter discusses the demographics, pathogenesis, clinical features, laboratory and imaging features, differential diagnosis, and management of Paget's disease. The musculoskeletal manifestations include pain, deformities and fractures, and possible malignancy. The neurologic complications of Paget's disease include optic atrophy, deafness, tinnitus, facial sensory loss, and other symptoms of cranial nerve, medulla, and cerebellum involvement; peripheral neuropathies; and carpal tunnel syndromes. Cardiovascular complications derive from several factors; they include increase in blood flow, calcification, and atherosclerosis. Indications for treatment of Paget's disease are described, and benefits and specific characteristics of therapies are discussed. The author concludes with a summary of the impact of Paget's disease on the patient and family, emphasizing that although life-style adjustments and psychological support may be necessary, the majority of pagetic patients appear to enjoy a normal family life. (14 references)

49

Weisz, G. M.

Changing aspects of clinical syndrome of Paget's disease. *Orthop Rev* 1987;16(5):334–340.

A group of 29 patients with symptomatic Paget's disease of bone was studied. As a result of this study, the author concludes that (1) familial incidence of Paget's disease is not uncommon and should be investigated, (2) lumbar symptomatology is prominent, and (3) malignancies are not uncommon and should be investigated. (33 references)

50

Yates, A. J.

Paget's disease of bone. *Bailliere's Clin Endocrinol Metab* 1988;2(1):267–285.

Paget's disease is a common bone disorder of presumed viral cause, which, in a minority of patients, may produce severe symptoms. Both calcitonin and the diphosphonates (bisphosphonates) have specific antipagetic effects. Newer diphosphonates, unlike etidronate, do not impair mineralization, and when they become available they will be the drugs of choice. Until that time, both calcitonin and etidronate continue to be useful in the management of this disorder. (46 references)

51

Zajac, A. J.; Phillips, P. E.

Paget's disease of bone: Clinical features and treatment. *Clin Exp Rheumatol* 1985;3(1)75–88.

Paget's disease of bone is often discovered incidentally but can have extensive metabolic and local mechanical complications. Treatment is not required for all patients and should only be undertaken for certain indications and with a clear understanding of the three types of drugs available. Bone pain unmanageable with analgesics and pathologic fractures are the most common indications for treatment; neurologic symptoms, hypercalcemia, and congestive heart failure are less frequent indications. Calcitonin or mithramycin (plicamycin) is used for the more urgent indications, and calcitonin or the diphosphonate (bisphosphonate) etidronate sodium (EHDP) for the more chronic ones. The drugs are generally efficacious and well tolerated. (47 references)

Etiology

52

Barker, D. J. P.; Detheridge, F. M.

Dogs and Paget's disease. *Lancet* 1985;2(8466):1245.

The authors comment on a previously published paper on dogs and Paget's disease and describe their own case-controlled studies. Their results show a small but not significant difference between the case and the control individuals. There were no differences in exposures to other household pets, including cats and birds. Although laboratory evidence supporting the canine distemper hypothesis has been sought in the past, it has not been found. (3 references)

53

Basle, M. F., et al.

Measles virus RNA detected in Paget's disease bone tissue by in situ hybridization. *J Gen Virol* 1986;67(Pt 5):907–913.

Morphologic and immunocytologic studies have demonstrated the presence of paramyxovirus antigens in Paget's bone disease tissue and, in particular, antigens related to measles virus and respiratory syncytial virus. To examine the relationship between measles virus and Paget's bone disease, this study used in situ hybridization and a cloned measles virus DNA probe specific for the nucleocapsid protein to detect and locate measles virus RNA sequences in Paget's bone tissue. In five patients with the disease, measles virus RNA sequences were detected not only in 80% to 90% of the multinucleated osteoclasts where there is morphologic and immunocytologic evidence of measles virus activity but also in 30% to 40% of mononucleated bone cells, mainly osteoblasts, osteocytes, fibroblasts, and lymphomonocytes. In contrast, no hybridization was observed in bone tissue from three control patients without signs of Paget's bone disease. These results indicate that the host cell range for measles virus in Paget's disease is more widespread than has been supposed. They also demonstrate the usefulness of the in situ hybridization method to detect viral genetic information in cells where viral antigenic activity is not detectable. These observations further support the hypothesis that measles virus is involved in the pathogenesis of Paget's bone disease. (27 references)

54

Basle, M. F., et al.

On the trail of paramyxoviruses in Paget's disease of bone. *Clin Orthop* 1987;(217):9–15.

The ultrastructural discovery of microcylindric inclusions in the nuclei and cytoplasm of osteoclasts in tissue affected by Paget's disease of bone has created a new approach to studying the cause of the disease. The morphologic similarity of the inclusions to viral structures has stimulated further studies involving immunocytologic techniques and in situ hybridization. Polyclonal antibodies reveal the presence of paramyxovirus antigens, measles virus, and respiratory syncytial virus in pagetic osteoclasts. Monoclonal and monospecific polyclonal antibodies demonstrate paramyxovirus antigens of measles virus, simian virus (SV5), and human parainfluenza virus (PF3). In situ hybridization carried out with a ^{3}H-labeled DNA probe specific for the measles nucleocapsid protein detects measles virus nucleotide sequences in the nuclei and cytoplasm of pagetic osteoclasts, confirming ultrastructural and immunocytologic findings. Surprisingly, the tritiated probe also hybridizes with a large proportion of mononucleated cells: osteoblasts, osteocytes, fibroblasts, and lymphocytes. This suggests a very wide host cell range for measles virus genomic information, which, however, would appear to undergo translation only in osteoclasts. The cause-effect relation between the viral information contained by diseased bone cells and Paget's disease of bone remains to be established. (44 references)

55

Breanndan-Moore, S.; Hoffman, D. L.

Absence of HLA linkage in a family with osteitis deformans (Paget's disease of bone). ***Tissue Antigens.*** **1988;31(2):69–70.**

HLA genotyping was carried out on two generations of a family with familial osteitis deformans. No evidence of major histocompatibility linkage of the disease could be demonstrated. (4 references)

56

Harvey, L.

Viral aetiology of Paget's disease of bone: A review. ***J R Soc Med*** **1984;77(11):943–948.**

It is now widely accepted that Paget's disease is, pathogenetically, an example of a primary osteoclast dysfunction. This report summarizes the results of studies that have focused on characterizing this osteoclast abnormality, discusses earlier theories for the pathogenesis of this disease, and outlines epidemiologic features and current evidence of the disease relevant to the proposed viral cause. Hard scientific evidence or proof of a viral cause has been hampered by the lack of a suitable animal or laboratory model for the disease; however, there are several areas of support for the viral hypothesis. The criticisms of a viral etiopathogenesis for Paget's disease are likewise identified and assessed. It is concluded that the increasing sophistication in the application of techniques already in use should help to confirm or refute the viral etiopathogenetic theory. (34 references)

56a

Holdaway, I. M., et al.

Previous pet ownership and Paget's disease. ***Bone Mineral*** **1990;8(1):53–58.**

The relationship between pet ownership and Paget's disease of bone was investigated in 112 patients who were matched with a similar number of community-based control individuals. There was a significantly increased frequency of dog ownership by patients with Paget's disease less than 60 years. Multivariate logistic regression analysis revealed that there was a significant age-related increase in risk of Paget's disease associated with past or present ownership of either dogs or cats, with younger patients' having the greatest risk. These results suggest that slow virus infection of osteoclasts by paramyxoviruses acquired from pets may contribute to the development of Paget's disease in the younger patient. (12 references)

57

Lagier, R.

Sudeck-type dystrophy in Paget's disease of bone: An anatomico-radiological approach. *Clin Rheumatol* 1985;4(1):62–67.

Anatomicoradiologic study of a humerus affected by Paget's disease and an unhealed fracture makes it possible to demonstrate the uneven development of the disease according to local conditions. The possible role of a bone dystrophy similar to that in Sudeck's disease that might, along with a slow virus infection, be involved in the development of Paget's disease is discussed. The discussion is based on the present case and on two previous studies as well as on data found in the literature. (32 references)

58

Mills, B. G.; Singer, F. R.

Critical evaluation of viral antigen data in Paget's disease of bone. *Clin Orthop* 1987;(217):16–25.

This study evaluates previous viral antigen data obtained from fixed tissue sections and cells grown in culture from bone affected by Paget's disease. Presence of antigens to both respiratory syncytial virus (RSV) and measles virus (MV) in the same osteoclasts of ten patients could not be explained on the basis of any previously known cross reactivity. Therefore, possible causes for these observations were sought. Monoclonal antibodies to viral proteins of RSV and MV were used to label proteins. Polyclonal antibodies that were monospecific and were produced exclusively in non-human species were used to rule out nonspecific reaction with human proteins. Antivimentin antibody was used to test the possibility of cross reactivity with a cytoskeletal protein, as a second antibody F(ab′)2 conjugated to fluorescein was used to rule out nonspecific reactivity with Fc receptors. Electron microscopy was used to evaluate bone cell cultures derived from Paget's bone compared with Paget's osteoclasts. Results showed that the pattern of monoclonal viral antibody labeling followed different causes in different patients. Nonspecific reactivity was ruled out by significant negative and positive controls. Cross reactivity with vimentin could not account for the positive immunofluorescence results because of an entirely different pattern of fluorescence in the same samples of live and fixed cells after colchemid treatment. It was concluded that specific viral antigens are present in osteoclasts and in cells grown from pagetic bone and that the present data are compatible with the possibility that Paget's disease of bone is a slow virus infection.

59

Mirra, J. M.

Pathogenesis of Paget's disease based on viral etiology. *Clin Orthop* 1987;(217):162–170.

It has been slightly over 100 years since Sir James Paget's classic descriptions of "osteitis deformans" first appeared. He described the middle to late stages of the disease in patients with the chronic, debilitating, rare, and polyostotic forms of the disease. It is now known that the milder forms are quite common, particularly in those of Anglo-Saxon ancestry. Paget believed the condition to be a chronic inflammation of unknown cause because of its asymmetrical skeletal distribution and chronicity and the gross appearance of the bones. With regard to the possible cause of Paget's disease of bone, nothing worthy of note had been discovered until 1974, when viruslike inclusions were reported within the osteoclasts of all Paget's disease patients. In the ensuing decade, a great deal more circumstantial evidence from electron microscopic and immunologic studies supported the view that Paget's disease represents a slow virus infection. This article deals with the possible to probable viral cause of Paget's disease with respect to its pathogenesis and its potential for eventual eradication. For many years Paget's disease was considered a disease almost exclusively confined to adulthood. Evidence now suggests that "familial chronic hyperphosphatasemia" represents the childhood form of Paget's disease. (29 references)

60

O'Driscoll, J. B.; Anderson, D. C.

Past pets and Paget's disease. *Lancet* 1985;2(8461):919–921.

There is strong morphologic evidence that Paget's disease is caused by a chronic focal paramyxovirus infection of osteoclasts, but the source of this virus and the reason for the wide variation in the incidence of the disease are unknown. The infection may be zoonotic, with a domestic animal as the usual host. Past exposure to pets was studied in 50 patients with Paget's disease and 50 age- and sex-matched control subjects with diabetes mellitus. Dog ownership was significantly more common in the patients than in the control subjects (odds ratios at different ages varied between 4 and 8). Forty-four of the Paget's patients and 30 of the control subjects had had dogs before the time of diagnosis of Paget's disease (or the equivalent age in the control subjects). Exposure to domestic cats was identical in both groups (26 each), and there was no significant difference in exposure to budgerigars. This suggests that a canine virus (possibly canine distemper) might be the primary infective agent, although other factors probably contribute to the particularly high incidence in the northwest of England. (21 references)

61

Otis, L. L.; Terezhalmy, G. T.; Glass, B. J.

Paget's disease of bone: Etiological theories and report of a case. *J Oral Med* 1986;41(4):214–219, 273.

This paper presents a case study together with some interesting theories concerning the cause and management of Paget's disease of bone, often diagnosed in people of European extraction. It is suggested that this disease may be involved in the progression to osteosarcoma. The paper presents a review of the literature in this area and discusses the biochemical nature and pathogenesis of the disease. Attention is given to epidemiologic findings, clinical features, oral and dental manifestations, radiographic features, laboratory findings, microscopic features, diagnosis versus differential diagnosis, and drug therapy. The importance of radiographic examination in the early diagnosis of sarcomatous transformation and of periodic clinical and radiographic examination is emphasized. (48 references)

62

Pippard, C.

***Aetiology of Paget's Disease of Bone: Proceedings of a Meeting Held on 2nd December 1983 at the Medical Research Council Environmental Epidemiology Unit.* Southampton, England, Southampton General Hospital, 1984. 35 pages. Available from Southampton General Hospital, Southampton, England S09 4XY. ISBN: 0903730103.**

This British publication documents the conference held in December 1983 to discuss the virus hypothesis for the cause of Paget's disease in light of epidemiologic findings and new knowledge of bone structure, physiology, and disease. Specific topics covered include the epidemiology, time trends, familial occurrence, and geography of Paget's disease; biology and morphology of Paget's disease; virology of Paget's disease, including animal models; and characteristics of the respiratory syncytical (RS) virus. (85 references)

63

Pringle, C. R.; Wilkie, M. L.; Elliott, R. M.

A survey of respiratory syncytial virus and parainfluenza virus type 3 neutralizing and immunoprecipitating antibodies in relation to Paget disease. *J Med Virol* 1986;17(4):377–386.

The cause of Paget's disease of bone has not been established, but certain features have suggested involvement of a parainfluenzalike virus. To seek further evidence of the possible role of paramyxoviruses in Paget's disease, the authors surveyed the presence of neutralizing and immunoprecipitating antibodies to both respiratory syncytial virus and parainfluenza virus type 3 in the sera of patients attending a bone disease clinic. These two viruses were implicated by the sporadic observation of viral antigen in individual nuclei of osteoclasts in Paget's disease bone lesions. A total of 315 samples was obtained from 177 patients attending the clinic during 1 year. Thirty-six of the patients had confirmed Paget's disease and the remainder other conditions. All sera possessed neutralizing activity to both viruses. The mean titers for each virus were similar in patents with Paget's disease and in those with other conditions whether matched or not. In the case of respiratory syncytial virus the neutralizing titers were distributed more closely to the mean in the Paget's group and showed little variation in repeat samples taken over periods of up to 1 year, in contrast with the greater variability of the control group. The antigenic specificity of 20 age- and sex-matched sera from each group was examined by immunoprecipitation. No significant differences were observed between Paget's and non-Paget's patients. These results do not provide confirmation of involvement of either virus in Paget's disease, but the serologic data suggest that persistent infection with respiratory syncytial virus can occur. (26 references)

64

Siris, E. S.; Kelsey, J. L.; Flaster, E.; Parker, S.

Paget's disease of bone and previous pet ownership in the United States: Dogs exonerated. *Int J Epidemiol* 1990;19(2):455–458.

Paget's disease of bone is currently believed to be the result of a paramyxovirus infection of osteoclasts. A recent study reporting an increased exposure to dogs during childhood and adolescence in a small series of cases from the northwest of England proposed that a canine virus, possibly distemper, might be the primary infectious agent. To study this hypothesis further, the authors examined prior dog and cat ownership from childhood through adulthood in 433 individuals with Paget's disease and an equal number of matched control subjects living in the United States. They found no differences in prior pet ownership. The authors conclude that past dog or cat ownership is not a risk factor for the development of Paget's disease. (16 references)

Pathophysiology and Diagnosis

65

Baran, G. A.; McDonald, D. J.; Sundram, M.

Radiologic case study. Monostotic Paget's disease in the sacrum. *Orthopedics* 1989;12(5):750–751, 754–756.

This case study discusses the radiologic diagnosis of Paget's disease confined to the sacrum. Knowledge of the radiologic and scintigraphic features of Paget's disease should allay fears of a metastatic process and obviate unnecessary biopsy. (6 references)

66

Buxbaum, J. N.; Kammerman, S.

Immunoglobulin abnormalities in Paget's disease of bone. *Clin Exp Immunol* 1984;56(1):200–204.

Several patients with Paget's disease have been reported to have monoclonal IgM proteins in their serum. The authors systematically studied 26 patients with Paget's disease severe enough to require diphosphonate (bisphosphonate) therapy. Five of these patients were found to have isolated elevations of serum IgM that were well outside the normal range for their age, sex, and race. An additional patient had elevations of both IgG and IgM. These individuals seem to represent a subset of Paget's disease patients. They do not differ from the remainder of the group with respect to severity or extent of disease, response to therapy, presence of intercurrent disease, or age. They do have a different male/female ratio. These observations suggest that some patients with Paget's disease may have disordered immune regulation or that they may be undergoing a primary response to an agent involved in the cause of pathogenesis of the disease. (18 references)

66a

Chaudhuri, T. K.; Fink, S.

Radionuclide imaging in osteitis deformans. *Am J Physiol Imaging* 1990;5(1):42–45.

New knowledge of osteoclastic function and new treatments to reduce osteolytic activity have combined to yield new degrees of biochemical control over the increased rate of bone resorption and formation that characterizes osteitis deformans. The authors briefly outline current concepts and provide an example of the role that radionuclide imaging can play in delineating the skeletal areas involved in this disease. (36 references)

67

Connolly, J. F.

Pathologic fractures. ***Emerg Med*****, 1984;16(11):61–63, 67, 68, 71 passim.**

This journal article describes the characteristics of a variety of causes of bone fractures and dislocation that occur in people, emphasizing the importance of careful diagnosis to prevent complications that can result from using an unwary or uninformed treatment approach. One of these causes, Paget's disease, is the second most common disease of bone formation after osteoporosis. It begins as a localized area of bone resorption, progressing through rapidly alternating cycles of bone formation and resorption. The femur is the most common site for pathologic fractures associated with Paget's disease. Clinical aspects, complications, and treatment are illustrated and discussed. Other causes of bone fractures include osteogenesis imperfecta, congenital pseudoarthrosis, cortical defects, bone cysts, eosinophilic granuloma, osteoclastoma, primary bone malignancies, and metastatic malignancy. (17 references)

68

Delmas, P. D., et al.

Serum bone GLA-protein is not a sensitive marker of bone turnover in Paget's disease of bone. ***Calcif Tissue Int*** **1986;38(1):60–61.**

Serum bone GLA-protein (sBGP) was measured in 32 patients with untreated Paget's disease of bone. Despite clinical and biologic symptoms of active disease in all patients, sBGP was normal in 13/32 patients (41%). There was a striking discrepancy between the modern increase of sBGP above normal values (11.4 ± 4.5 versus 6.0 ± 2.1 ng/mL) and the marked increase of both serum alkaline phosphatase (sAP) and urinary hydroxyproline (uOHP). sBGP was weakly correlated with sAP ($R = 0.50$, $P < 0.01$), uOHP ($R = 0.48$, $P < 0.01$), and extension of the disease ($R = 0.48$, $P < 0.01$). We conclude that sBGP is not a sensitive marker of bone turnover in patients with Paget's disease of bone and should be interpreted with caution in this condition. (10 references)

69

Fallon, M. D.; Schwamm, H. A.

Paget's disease of bone: An update on the pathogenesis, pathophysiology, and treatment of osteitis deformans. ***Pathol Annu*** **1989;24(p 1):115–159.**

In this review article, the authors discuss recent advances regarding the cause, pathophysiology, and treatment of Paget's disease. Because the presentation of Paget's disease of bone is diverse, the surgical pathologist may encounter problems in the differential diagnosis from a variety of clinical sources. Therefore, the authors present the radiologic and pathologic diagnostic features of Paget's disease. Tables, charts, radiographs, and slide illustrations are included. (26 references)

70

Foldes, J.; Shamir, S.; Kidroni, G.; Menczel, J.

Vitamin D in Paget's disease of bone. ***Clin Orthop*** **1989;(243):275–279.**

The role of vitamin D metabolism in Paget's disease of bone has not been well defined. Serum levels of the main, circulating vitamin D metabolites were measured in 23 patients with Paget's disease. Values of 25(OH)D3 and 24,25(OH)2D3 were increased in 11 (48%) patients. Markedly elevated levels (930298 pg/mL) were found in 5 patients. In a subgroup of patients with high 1,25(OH)2D3, the mean serum alkaline phosphatase activity was insignificantly higher and serum calcium level, phosphorus level, and kidney function were the same as in a subgroup with normal 1,25(OH)2D3. 1,25(OH)2D3 Levels were not affected by treatment with either calcitonin or etidronate disodium. Serum 1,25(OH)2D3 levels may be increased in a subset of patients with Paget's disease of bone. (10 references)

71

Gainey, J. C., et al.

Gait analysis of patients who have Paget disease. ***J Bone Joint Surg*** **1989;71(4):568–579.**

Eighteen patients who had Paget's disease were evaluated in a gait-analysis laboratory. The results were compared with those of ten healthy age-matched control subjects in order to quantitate the biomechanical changes and to describe the specific patterns of walking that occur secondary to bowing of a lower extremity. Kinetic and kinematic data were acquired by using infrared video cameras and force platforms; electromyographic data were obtained by using surface electrodes. Velocity and cadence were decreased, and stride time and double-limb support time were increased in the patients who had Paget's disease compared to those of the control subjects. Frequently, the knee of the limb that was affected by Paget's disease was flexed during stance and flexed less during swing. When the involved knee was in varus angulation, it also had an increased adduction moment, which may be related to the bowing deformity. Although the patterns of ground-reaction force were similar in the patients and the control subjects, the magnitudes of forces were reduced in the patients. Phasic muscle activity was similar in the two groups. (10 references)

72

Greenfield, G. B.

Paget's disease (osteitis deformans), in: *Radiology of Bone Diseases*, ed 4. Philadelphia, JP Lippincott, Co, pp 110–141. Available from Lippincott, East Washington Square, Philadelphia, PA 19105. (215) 238-4200.

This book section discusses the use of roentgenology to diagnose Paget's disease and identify and assess the pagetic process. Radiologically, four stages of Paget's disease can be discerned: (1) the destructive stage, (2) the combined phase, (3) the sclerotic phase, and (4) malignant change. The author reviews these phases throughout the anatomy: skull, spine, pelvis, ribs, long bones, joints, and hands. Thirty-six radiographs and CT scans are included. (24 references)

73

Guillard-Cumming, D. F., et al.

Abnormal vitamin D metabolism in Paget's disease of bone. *Clin Endocrinol (Oxf)* 1985;22(4):559–566.

The authors have studied several biochemical indexes of bone turnover and vitamin D metabolism in 32 untreated patients with Paget's disease and in 32 age-matched control subjects. Patients with Paget's disease, as expected, were characterized by high bone turnover, as judged by alkaline phosphatase and urinary excretion of hydroxyproline. Serum values of 24,25-dihydroxyvitamin D3 [24,25(OH)2D3] and ratio of 24,25(OH)2D3 to 25-OHD were significantly lower in patients than in control subjects. Serum concentrations of 1,25(OH)2D3 were normal in Paget's disease. The distribution of values for 24,25(OH)2D3 was log normal. On the basis of the normal range computed from control subjects, patients were divided into those with low and those with normal values for 24,25(OH)2D3. Disease activity, as judged by biochemical indexes, was significantly higher in the patients with the lower values of 24,25(OH)2D3. The authors conclude that Paget's disease is characterized by low circulating concentrations of 24,25(OH)2D3, particularly in patients with more extensive or severe disease. (22 references)

74

Harinck, H. I., et al.

Relation between signs and symptoms in Paget's disease of bone. *Q J Med* 1986;58(226):133–151.

The relation between signs and symptoms of Paget's disease of bone was studied in 180 patients consecutively submitted for treatment. In these patients, 826 lesions were identified by scintigraphy. The intensity of scintigraphic uptake was correlated with long-term calcium uptake in bone. The frequency distribution of lesions over the patients was compatible with a 65% chance of local disease once the patient had been exposed to an extraneous agent. The spatial distribution within a skeleton was related to the local density of the osteoclast population. The particular frequency distribution resulted in a log-normal distribution diagram for anatomic spread. Within lesions, increases in numbers of osteoclasts and osteoblasts were proportional, and these too had a log-normal distribution. Increases of alkaline phosphatase levels and hydroxyproline excretion were closely related and reflected anatomic spread on the one hand and local activity on the other. They were also closely correlated with overall calcium fluxes. It was shown that alkaline phosphatase is the more sensitive and hydroxyproline the more accurate of the biochemical signs. Maximum values, corresponding to total skeletal disease, were approximately 25 times the upper limit of normal. Equilibrium between bone formation and resorption was not always maintained. There were, indeed, wide variations of urinary calcium, which were significantly related to the difference between bone formation and resorption, but the extracellular calcium homeostasis was generally maintained. This may explain the frequent occurrence of normocalcemic and hypercalcemic hyperparathyroidism. The hypercalciuria constitutes an additional risk for urolithiasis in men. The most frequent complaint was pain (86%). Extent of lesions was important, but a major decisive factor was the specific nature of the bone affected. The findings allowed assessment of the relative importance of the various signs, symptoms, and locations as criteria of disease severity and as indications for treatment. (50 references)

75

Healy, J. H.; Lane, J. M.

Bone metabolism, in Fitzgerald, R.H., Jr., (ed): *Orthopaedic Knowledge Update II.* Park Ridge, IL, American Academy of Orthopaedic Surgeons, 1987, pp 19–34. Available from the American Academy of Orthopaedic Surgeons, 222 South Prospect, Park Ridge, IL 60068-4058. (312) 823-7186.

This chapter of a home study syllabus for orthopedic surgeons covers the aspects of cell biology, physiology, and endocrinology that govern bone and calcium metabolism. Paget's disease is discussed in terms of these processes. Drug therapy that acts to decrease osteoclast resorption of bone is reviewed. (41 references)

75a

Khetarpal, U.; Schuknecht, H. F.

In search of pathologic correlates for hearing loss and vertigo in Paget's disease: A clinical and histopathologic study of 26 temporal bones. *Ann Otol Rhinol Laryngol* 1990;(Suppl 145);1–16.

Mixed sensorineural and conductive hearing loss is a common clinical manifestation of Paget's disease of the temporal bone, and although there are numerous clinical and pathologic reports on the condition, none has identified a consistent pathologic explanation for the hearing loss. Histologic studies on 26 temporal bones exhibiting Paget's disease from 16 persons, of whom 7 had had audiometric testing, were performed. Contrary to common opinion, conductive hearing loss is not caused by ossicular fixation; in fact, no cause could be found in the seven ears with documented conductive hearing losses. Although the sensorineural hearing losses were greater than normal for age, the study could not identify cochlear disorders that could be attributed to Paget's disease. The authors concluded that the hearing losses in Paget's disease are caused by changes in bone density, mass, and form that serve to dampen the finely tuned motion mechanics of the middle and inner ears. (58 references)

76

Krane, S. M.; Simon, L. S.

Metabolic consequences of bone turnover in Paget's disease of bone. *Clin Orthop* 1987;(217):26–36.

High rates of bone resorption, bone formation, and marrow fibrosis are characteristic of Paget's disease of bone. This excessive bone turnover is reflected by increased fluxes of calcium ions out of and into the skeleton. The rates of these fluxes are so highly geared to each other that calcium balances are close to zero in the absence of fracture or significant immobilization. An increased turnover of bone matrix also is made evident by increased urinary excretion of collagen breakdown products (oligopeptides of hydroxyproline, hydroxylysine, and hydroxylysine glycosides) as well as products (peptides of higher molecular weight) related to collagen synthesis. Increased circulatory levels of procollagen extension fragments reflect increased synthesis of type I collagen (bone matrix) and type III collagen (marrow fibrosis). Increased levels of bone gamma-carboxyglutamic acid-protein presumably primarily reflect bone matrix synthesis but bone resorption as well. When bone resorption is suppressed pharmacologically, the abnormal levels of these markers of matrix turnover and oteoblastic activity (alkaline phosphate) also decrease, presumably as a result of coupling of resorption and formation. (54 references)

77

Levine, R. B., et al.

Paget disease: Unusual radiographic manifestations. ***CRC Crit Rev Diagn Imaging*** **1986;25(3):209–232.**

Paget's disease (osteitis deformans) is not a difficult diagnosis when presented with typical radiographic features. However, an atypical appearance or an unusual location can be a diagnostic challenge. This review emphasizes the less common presentations, with their diagnostic clues. The authors also consider such complications as malignant degeneration, fracture, and coexistent systemic disease, which can obscure the underlying Paget's disease. The cause, pathogenesis, and effects on bone structure and function attributed to Paget disease are updated. (58 references)

78

Maldague, B.; Malghem, J.

Dynamic radiologic patterns of Paget's disease of bone. ***Clin Orthop*** **1987;(217):126–151.**

Within the diaphyseal cortex, the primary resorption phase of Paget's disease is often limited either to the endosteum or the central layers of the cortex. This results in primary resorption fronts that are usually discrete, both radiologically and scintigraphically. The subsequent activation of the subperiosteal cortex may be delayed, leading to secondary expanding fronts associated with subperiosteal new bone formation. Sequential radiographs of 19 untreated patients followed 6.4 ± 1.2 years showed that the mean extension rate of the lesions within cortical bone was 8 ± 0.5 mm/yr per advancing front. This extension rate showed no significant change in 15 patients treated with calcitonin (CT) and/or ethane-1-hydroxy-1, 1-diphosphonate (bisphosphonate) (EHDP) but was significantly decreased in 14 patients treated with 3-amino-1-hydroxypropilidene-1,1-diphosphonate (bisphosphonate) (APD). The increased remodeling rate of pagetic bone magnifies the radiologic changes due to mechanical, dystrophic, and metabolic interferences. Thus, a sclerotic pattern of the disease may rapidly change into a mixed or even a lyric pattern under the influence of any rarefying factor. Conversely, lytic pagetic bone may transform into dense bone through the administration of antiosteoclastic medications such as CT and APD. The reconstructive action of any new therapeutic regimen should be monitored radiologically. (70 references)

79

Meunier, P. J., et al.

Skeletal distribution and biochemical parameters of Paget's disease. *Clin Orthop* 1987;(217):37–44.

Quantitative bone scans were performed with ^{99m}Tc-EHDP in 170 untreated pagetic patients (93 men, 77 women; mean age, 65.4 years). The distribution of 863 pagetic skeletal locations was analyzed. Bone scans demonstrated 8.3% more pagetic sites than roentgenograms. The extent of Paget's disease was evaluated in each patient by a scintigraphic skeletal index. This index correlated with serum alkaline phosphatase (SAP) and urinary hydroxyproline (HyPro) levels and with hypocalcemic acute response to calcitonin. The correlation of SAP with an index of activity (extent index adjusted by uptake ratios) was better than with the nonadjusted index. Only 30.6% of pagetic sites were responsible for clinical symptoms. No correlation between age and skeletal index of the disease was found. (20 references)

80

Moser, R. P., Jr., et al.

Paget disease of the anterior tibial tubercle. *Radiology* 1987;164(1):211–214.

A study was made of 13 cases of biopsy-proven Paget's disease in which the disease involved the anterior tibial tubercle with extension into the metaphysis and diaphysis, but without apparent involvement of the proximal tibial epiphysis. Case data were obtained from archives containing more than 350 cases of Paget's disease. Age, sex, symptoms, serum alkaline phosphatase level, and histologic and radiographic appearance of the lesions were evaluated. Patients were young at clinical presentation, averaging 36 years of age. In five of six patients the alkaline phosphatase level was normal. The proximal extent of the disease was the anterior tibial tubercle rather than the proximal epiphysis. Radiographic patterns ranged from predominantly lytic to mixed lytic and blastic to predominantly blastic, and the lesion was marginated by a flame-shaped configuration. The radiographic appearance of Paget's disease of the anterior tibial tubercle is characteristic and should be sufficient to suggest the diagnosis and preclude biopsy. (11 references)

81

Nuti, R., et al.

Total body and regional bone mineral analysis by dual-photon absorptiometry in Paget's disease of bone. ***Bone Mineral*** **1988;3(4):359–367.**

Total body density (TBD), total body bone mineral (TBBM), and bone mineral content of major anatomic skeletal areas were measured in 66 patients with Paget's disease of bone (54 polyostotic; 12 monostotic; 38 men; 28 women; 38 to 88 years) by dual-photon absorptiometry (^{153}Gd). TBD was elevated in 23 men and 3 women with Paget's disease; a statistically significant correlation was found between elevated values of TBD and a widespread extent of the disease. The mean value of TBBM was higher in pagetic men; in pagetic women it was similar to that in normal subjects. The separate analysis of anatomic areas allowed the researchers to appreciate increased values of bone mineral content in head, trunk, spine, pelvis, and arms. Moreover, in 28 patients with easily detectable pagetic lesions of long bones, 38 specific regions of interest (ROI) were evaluated; pagetic areas showed significantly higher values of bone density and bone mineral content than contralateral uninvolved areas. (35 references)

82

Papapoulos, S. E., et al.

Serum osteocalcin in Paget's disease of bone: Basal concentrations and response to bisphosphonate treatment. ***J Clin Endocrinol Metab*** **1987;65(1):89–94.**

Serum osteocalcin concentrations were measured in 42 patients with Paget's disease of bone and elevated serum alkaline phosphatase (AP) levels. High serum osteocalcin levels were found in only 22 patients. Serum osteocalcin was significantly correlated with urinary hydroxyproline excretion ($R = 0.747$; $P < 0.001$) and, to a lesser extent, with serum AP levels ($R = 0.483$; $P < 0.01$). In 23 patients who were followed during treatment with intravenous (3-amino-1-hydroxypropylidene) 1,1-bisphosphonate (APD) for 10 days, a dissociation among these three biochemical parameters was found. Urinary hydroxyproline excretion fell significantly ($P < 0.001$); serum AP levels decreased, but not significantly; and serum osteocalcin concentrations increased progressively ($P < 0.001$). This increase was greater when initial levels were lower than expected for the activity of the disease. The rise in serum osteocalcin correlated significantly with the concomitant increase in serum 1,25-dihydroxyvitamin D concentrations. Three months after initiation of treatment, all three parameters—urinary hydroxyproline (OHP) excretion, serum AP, and serum osteocalcin levels—were near or within the normal range. These results indicate that serum osteocalcin is not a clinically useful parameter for assessment of the activity of Paget's disease. Its basal concentrations lag behind those expected from the activity of the disease, suggesting defective osteocalcin production. It appears that the functions of osteocalcin and AP as well as their initial expression by the osteoblasts are different and that this difference may be important for the quality of bone formed in Paget's disease. APD can modulate the release of osteocalcin, possibly through stimulation of 1,25-dihydroxyvitamin D production, although other factors may be involved. (36 references)

83

Proops, D.; Bayley, D.; Hawke, M.

Paget's disease and the temporal bone—a clinical and histopathological review of six temporal bones. *J Otolaryngol* 1985;14(1):20–29.

Paget's disease of bone occurs more commonly in the elderly and has been reported to involve the temporal bone in 30% of those afflicted. The clinical and histopathologic features of six temporal bones from three patients with this disease were reported and the relevant literature reviewed. The effect of Paget's disease on the middle ear structures was more variable than its extension into the otic capsule. Pagetic involvement of the otic capsule was observed in five temporal bones. One patient had bilateral asymptomatic neurofibromas in the eighth cranial nerve. The potential mechanisms responsible for the conductive deafness, sensorineural deafness, and vestibular dysfunction associated with Paget's disease are discussed. (27 references)

84

Som, P. M., et al.

Paget disease of the calvaria and facial bones with an osteosarcoma of the maxilla: CT and MR findings. *J Comput Assist Tomogr* 1987;11(5):887–890.

Findings from computed axial tomography (CAT) and magnetic resonance imaging (MRI) of Paget's disease of the calvaria and facial bones are described and compared with one another. The sites of dense, woven bone, myeloid marrow, and background pagetic matrix can be clearly identified. A rare case of Paget's sarcoma (osteogenic sarcoma) of the facial bones is also presented. The distinction between this sarcoma and the Paget's bone was clearer on CAT than on MRI. This presumably is because the bone is directly seen on CAT and only indirectly imaged on MRI. (8 references)

85

Swartz, J. D., et al.

High resolution computed tomography: VI. Craniofacial Paget's disease and fibrous dysplasia. *Head Neck Surg* 1985;8(1):40–47.

This report focuses on the use of computerized axial tomography to diagnose, characterize, and contrast craniofacial Paget's disease and fibrous dysplasia. In Paget's disease, the calvaria is most commonly involved, often in addition to the skull base, including the temporal bone. As opposed to the exuberant facial changes in fibrous dysplasia, extensive alterations in the facial bones with Paget's disease are infrequent; however, maxillary involvement (and, to a lesser extent, mandibular involvement) is occasionally encountered. A total of 29 illustrations are included, together with descriptive information. (6 references)

86

Taylor, W. H.

Low serum magnesium concentration in Paget's disease of bone (osteitis deformans). *Ann Clin Biochem* 1985;22(Pt 6):591–595.

Approximately 25% of patients having Paget's disease of bone have a low serum magnesium concentration (below 0.74 mmol/L). Metabolic balance studies of 12 normomagnesemic and 7 hypomagnesemic subjects show that the latter have a significantly more positive balance and significantly higher net absorption of magnesium than the former. The urinary output of the two groups did not differ significantly. The serum magnesium and alkaline phosphatase (log) concentrations were significantly negatively correlated, as were the serum magnesium and daily urinary hydroxyproline (log) output. Low serum magnesium concentrations are thus associated with highly active Paget's disease; they do not arise from increased urinary loss nor from a lowered net absorption of magnesium, but probably from increased uptake by bone. The balance data show that to prevent negative magnesium balance, the magnesium intake in Paget's disease should be at least 8.0 mmol/d. (5 references)

87

Vellenga, C. J.; Bijvoet, O. L.; Pauwels, E. K.

Bone scintigraphy and radiology in Paget's disease of bone: A review. *Am J Physiol Imaging* 1988;3(3):154–168.

Because effective treatment of Paget's disease is now feasible, knowledge of the possibilities of diagnostic imaging, especially the changes in these images induced by treatment, has become essential. Some forms of treatment may lead to radiographic improvement, indicating that the macroscopic bone texture is changing; radiologic imaging, however, is painstaking and liable to technical errors. Different information is derived from the bone scintigram, which is a good monitor of the local bone metabolism and often a sensitive means of identifying lesions. Some parts of the skeleton appear to be affected more often than others, and the likelihood that a bone is involved depends on its size and the proportion of bone marrow. Local scintigraphic uptake appears to correlate with the grade of radiologic deformation and the frequency of pain; the total skeletal uptake correlates with the severity of the biochemical abnormalities. Evidently, the metabolic activity of a lesion plays a major role in the occurrence of deformation and the development of pain. Lesions not visible on the radiograph (about 15%) usually show low uptake and are asymptomatic. During successful treatment the scintigram findings improve impressively, but in remission 20% of the original uptake is retained as a result of persistent structural abnormalities. Recurrence is accompanied by deterioration of the scintigram result. Radiology and scintigraphy offer valuable additional information that confirms and supports the clinical and biochemical evaluation. (73 references)

88

Vellenga, C. J.; Pauwels, E. K.; Bijvoet, O. L.

Some characteristics of local scintigraphic and radiologic patterns of Paget's disease of bone (osteitis deformans). *Diagn Imaging Clin Med* 1985;54(5):273–281.

This illustrated report describes some of the characteristic local scintigraphic and radiographic abnormalities observed in Paget's disease of bone (osteitis deformans). Three specific areas are addressed: the distinction between osteolysis and sclerosis, the correlation between local scintigraphic and radiographic patterns, and similarities of the scintigraphic and radiographic demarcation zones. Scintigrams and radiographic patterns are shown for the skull and long bones in seven figures. Other areas also discussed and illustrated include the pelvis, hips, and whole body. This paper addresses additional features of radiographic and scintigraphic patterns that have been either omitted or only casually cited previously. (37 references)

89

Vellenga, C. J., et al.

Untreated Paget disease of bone studied by scintigraphy. *Radiology* 1984;153(3):799–805.

The authors determined that the concentration of radioactivity in a lesion of Paget's disease correlates with the grade of radiologic deformation and the frequency of pain; the total skeletal uptake correlates with the severity of the biochemical abnormalities. The major determinant of uptake in untreated lesions is abnormal metabolic activity, and in lesions in remission it is structural deformation of mineralized tissue. It is likely that the metabolic activity, and possibly also the rate of progression of the individual lesions, will differ among individual patients and that metabolic activity determines the amount of deformation and the chance of pain. Lesions not visible on the radiograph usually show only low uptake of ^{99m}Tc-Sn-EHDP; the majority of these lesions are asymptomatic and reflect low activity of the disease. Radiologic differentiation of sclerotic and osteolytic lesions does not reflect differences in scintigraphic uptake, metabolic activity, or pain. (30 references)

90

Wilder-Smith, C. H.; Raue, F.; Holz-Gottswinter, G.; Ziegler, R.

Procollagen-III peptide serum levels in Paget's disease of the bone. *Klin Wochenschr* 1987;65(4):174–178.

A commercially available radioimmunoassay kit was used to determine amino-terminal procollagen-III peptide (pNcoll III) serum levels in patients with Paget's disease of the bone and in control subjects. In patients with Paget's disease, pNcoll III concentrations were significantly elevated. They decreased to varying degrees under chronic therapy with human and salmon calcitonin, disodium ethane 1-hydroxy 1,1-diphosphonate (bisphosphonate) (EHDP), or a combination therapy of EHDP and human calcitonin. The results were compared with the effect on traditional biochemical markers of disease activity: serum alkaline phosphatase and urinary hydroxyproline excretion, both of which reacted more acutely to the various therapies than pNcoll III, although pretreatment correlations were close. The most probable source of pNcoll III is not the pagetic bone per se but the vascular, fibrous connective tissue replacing normal bone marrow. (19 references)

91

Wilkinson, M. R., et al.

Serum osteocalcin concentrations in Paget's disease of bone. ***Arch Intern Med*** **1986;146(2):268–271.**

Total body scintiscans, serum alkaline phosphatase estimations, and serum osteocalcin radioimmunoassays were performed in 49 consecutive patients with Paget's disease of bone. Eleven were receiving calcitonin (salmon synthetic) at the time of the study. The serum alkaline phosphatase activities were elevated in all but 1 patient, with the highest value almost 50 times the upper limit of the reference range. Serum osteocalcin concentrations were elevated in 53% of patients and normal in the rest. The highest serum osteocalcin value was 4.2 times the upper limit of the reference range. The correlation coefficient between the extent of skeletal involvement and serum osteocalcin level was 0.70; that between skeletal involvement and serum alkaline phosphatase level was 0.55. In spite of the better correlation between bone scintiscans and serum osteocalcin level, osteocalcin measurements are diagnostically less useful than serum alkaline phosphatase estimations in patients with Paget's disease of bone. (22 references)

92

Winfield, J.; Stamp, T. C.

Bone and joint symptoms in Paget's disease. ***Ann Rheum Dis*** **1984;43(6):769–773.**

Fifty patients with Paget's disease of bone were reviewed with regard to the basis of their symptoms and the long-term results of treatment. Twenty-four patients (48%) had pain localized within bone; 17 (34%) had symptoms of degenerative joint disease. Three patients had bone pain and arthritis, and the remaining 6 had fractures, ataxia, or painless deformity. Symptomatic osteoarthritis of the hip (OA) developed in 25 patients (50%);

approximately half developed radiologic changes identical to those of idiopathic OA. Among the other patients those with coxa vara tended to show medial (rather than superior) joint space narrowing and severe Paget's disease on both sides of the joint. Arthritic pain, stiffness, and reduced mobility in other joints (knee, ankle, and wrist) were associated clinically with bone deformity adjacent to the affected joint and radiologically with distorted articular surfaces and narrowed joint spaces; sclerosis, subarticular cyst formation, and osteophytosis were usually absent. Fifteen patients were treated with calcitonin for bone pain alone; all claimed long-term "good-to-complete" relief. By contrast, none of the 14 with arthritic symptoms responded to calcitonin when assessed retrospectively. Results of surgical and other medical treatment were analyzed. Careful clinical evaluation is a prerequisite for optimal treatment in Paget's disease. (11 references)

93

Zlatkin, M. B., et al.

Paget disease of the spine: CT with clinical correlation. ***Radiology*** **1986;160(1):155–159.**

Thirty-six patients with pagetic involvement of the spine were evaluated clinically and by computed axial tomography (CAT). Pagetic phase, modeling expansion, degree and site of spinal stenosis, and pagetic facet joint arthropathy were recorded for each involved vertebral segment. CAT demonstrated spinal stenosis in 20 patients, 11 of whom exhibited spinal stenosis on plain films. Twenty-one patients had symptoms of neck or back pain, with associated neurologic dysfunction in 13. Spinal stenosis was present in 81% of the symptomatic patients and 20% of the asymptomatic patients. Severe pagetic facet arthropathy was present in 17 of the symptomatic patients. The authors conclude that spinal stenosis is an important cause of vertebral pain and neurologic dysfunction. (25 references)

Epidemiology

94

Barker, D. J.

The epidemiology of Paget's disease of bone. ***Br Med Bull*** **1984;40(4):396–400.**

This paper summarizes and discusses mortality data and the geographical prevalence of Paget's disease of bone (osteitis deformans), whose cause is unknown. Most of the paper focuses on a summary and comparison of the prevalence of the disease, principally based on radiologic surveys, in Western Europe, Britain, North American, Australia, and New Zealand. It is concluded that the epidemiologic studies on Paget's disease, despite its remarkable differences in geographical prevalence (for example, its comparative rarity in Scandinavia and Ireland relative to British towns and its extreme rarity in Africa despite similar prevalence rates in American blacks and whites), do not of themselves lead to specific etiologic hypotheses. Suggested causative factors for Paget's disease are discussed; however, none has shown unequivocal evidence for clear cause nor exhibited a direct correlation with epidemiologic findings. (22 references)

95

Bloom, R. A.; Libson, E.; Blank, P.; Nubani, N.

Prevalence of Paget's disease of bone in hospital patients in Jerusalem: An epidemiologic study. *Isr J Med Sci* 1985;21(12):954–956.

Epidemiologic studies have revealed the widely varied prevalence of Paget's disease of bone. The highest rates have been found in parts of England. The disease has been reported rarely in Jews, and no previous studies of prevalence have been performed in the Middle East or Asia. In the present study an age- and sex-adjusted rate of 1% was found among Jews, which is similar to that in many Southern European populations. No case of Paget's disease of bone was found among Arabs in this study. (9 references)

96

Guyer, P. B.; Chamberlain, A. T.

Paget's disease of bone in South Africa. *Clin Radiol* 1988;39(1):51–52.

A survey of Paget's disease of bone in Johannesburg, South Africa, has revealed a prevalence rate of 2.4 % in whites aged 55 years and over, which is similar to that of some centers in Europe; it has also revealed a high prevalence rate of 1.3% among blacks. These findings are discussed in relation to recent concepts o the pathogenesis of Paget's disease. (7 references)

97

Polednak, A. P.

Rates of Paget's disease of bone among hospital discharges, by age and sex. *J Am Geriatr Soc* 1987;35(6):550–553.

Paget's disease of bone (PDB) is of particular public health interest in view of the increasing proportion of elderly persons in Western populations. Data were analyzed on 1,078 hospital discharges with PDB as the principal diagnosis among New York state residents from 1980 to 1983. Rates of PDB per 100,000 total hospitalizations and per 100,000 total population increased with age in both sexes. These rates were not higher in men than in women except in older age groups. Population rates were similar in blacks and whites except for higher rates among blacks in the group 80 years and older. Average length of hospital stay was also significantly longer for blacks in this oldest age group. (19 references)

98

Sofaer, J. A.; Holloway, S. M.; Emery, A. E.

A family study of Paget's disease of bone. *J Epidemiol Community Health* 1983;37(3):226–231.

Familial aggregation of Paget's disease of bone occurs occasionally, and an exclusively genetic cause has been proposed in the past. On the other hand, epidemiologic surveys point to an important environmental contribution, and evidence to suggest that the disease may be caused by a slow virus infection is accumulating. Analysis of 407 family history questionnaires completed by patients with Paget's disease confirmed the familial nature of the disease. Overall, the findings were consistent with the hypothesis that Paget's disease is caused by infection with a common and widespread virus superimposed on genetic variation for susceptibility and perhaps severity of the disease. (33 references)

Complications

99

Altman, R. D.; Brown, M.; Gargano, F.

Low back pain in Paget's disease of bone. *Clin Orthop* 1987;(217):152–161.

Clinical and laboratory evaluation with bone scan, radiography, and computerized axial tomography were performed on 25 patients with severe Paget's disease of bone and low back pain. Back pain was classified as caused by Paget's disease in only 3 patients. The remaining 22 patients had coexistent Paget's disease and osteoarthritis. There was difficulty localizing the cause of back pain in those patients with coexistent Paget's disease and osteoarthritis, even when the disease appears to precipitate osteoarthritis and several low back syndromes. Suppressive therapy with disodium etidronate (EHDP) for Paget's disease was beneficial in 8 of 22 patients (36%) with identifiable osteoarthritis. It is suggested that EHDP and perhaps other suppressive agents for Paget's disease receive limited use in patients with back pain unless a defined pagetic lesion appears related to the clinical syndrome in the absence of identifiable osteoarthritis. (34 references)

100

Arnalich, F., et al.

Cardiac size and function in Paget's disease of bone. ***Int J Cardiol*** **1984;5(4):491–505.**

The authors performed noninvasive assessment of cardiac size and function by clinical criteria, standard electrocardiography, chest radiography; systolic time intervals, and echocardiography in 27 patients with Paget's disease of bone and in 20 control subjects. The patients were divided into two groups on the basis of the degree of skeletal involvement (less than 15% in group I and greater than 15% in group II). No differences in heart size parameters of left ventricular performance were noted between group I and controls. Cardiomegaly, increased left ventricular diastolic dimension, and increased left ventricular mass indicative of ventricular hypertrophy were found in group II compared to control subjects. In addition, patients with more extensive skeletal involvement had signs of depressed myocardial contractility, increased left ventricular volumes in diastole an systole, and enlarged stroke volume, with no differences in echographic cardiac output compared to that of group I and controls. The findings show an above-normal incidence of cardiac enlargement and disturbed left ventricular performance in patients with Paget's disease and osseous lesions in more than 15% of the skeleton. The clinical implications of the altered cardiac function in patients with Paget's disease are briefly discussed. (32 references)

101

Ashman, S.; Lever, S.; Weiss, M.

Osteogenic sarcoma and Paget's disease of the mandible: Review of the literature and case report. ***J Md State Dental Assoc*** **1986;29(2):53–55.**

Increased incidence of osteogenic sarcoma developing in pagetic bone has been mentioned throughout the literature. Despite this reported increase in malignant change, there have been very few cases of osteogenic sarcoma arising from the mandible. This article reports a case of osteosarcoma in pagetoid mandible. This article reports a case of osteosarcoma in pagetoid mandible and reviews the past literature, emphasizing diagnosis, symptoms, and treatment outcomes. (13 references)

102

Baraka, M. E.

Rate of progression of hearing loss in Paget's disease. *J Laryngol Otol* 1984;98(6):573–575.

A number of studies have indicated that patients with Paget's disease of the skull frequently have hearing impairment, which may be quite severe and may also be progressive. Recent studies have suggested that as many as 60% of the normal population over the age of 70 years have a hearing impairment sufficient to handicap them in normal conversation. The intent of this study is to clarify whether or not the hearing loss in patients with Paget's disease of the temporal bone can be explained on the grounds of age alone or whether it is directly attributable to the disease process. The results of this study indicate that the rate of progression of hearing loss is generally faster in patients with Paget's disease. (6 references)

103

Barnett, F.; Elfenbein, L.

Paget's disease of the mandible: A review and report of a case. *Endodont Dent Traumatol* 1985;1(1):39–42.

Paget's disease is a chronic progressive disease of bone of unknown cause. Jaw involvement is seen in approximately 17% of cases, and usually it is the maxilla that is involved. This paper reports a case of Paget's disease involving the mandible and reviews the literature on the features and symptoms of this disorder. (25 references)

103a

Bidner, S.; Finnegan, M.

Femoral fractures in Paget's disease. *J Orthop Trauma* 1989;3(4):317–322.

Since the original description of osteitis deformans, the treatment of femoral fractures occurring in this disease process has been difficult. A retrospective study of 35 fractures treated over an 8-year period was undertaken to identify the factors that influenced the results. The fractures were classified according to four fracture patterns: subcapital, intertrochanteric, subtrochanteric, and shaft. Chart and radiographic analyses were then performed. The results identified subtrochanteric fracture, occurring in a somewhat younger population, as the problem fracture. The other three fracture groups did well with standard methods of treatment. Uncemented arthroplasties were not successful; this outcome correlates with the known bone physiology of this age group and this disease process. (15 references)

104

Chakravorty, N. K.

Neurological complications of Paget's disease of bone. ***Br J Clin Pract*** **1985;39(9):335–338.**

This paper covers neurologic complications resulting from Paget's disease. Headache, epilepsy, dementia, vasilar invagination, hydrocephalus, dysphasia, and dysarthria are discussed. Information on cranial nerve involvement and spinal cord dysfunction if presented. Physicians responsible for the care of patients of Western European extraction are likely to encounter individuals suffering from this disease as people continue to live longer. Availability of effective drugs and development of advanced neurosurgical techniques have enabled clinicians to provide satisfactory treatment to patients with neurologic complications. (21 references)

105

Ellis, G. L.; Connole, P. W.

Diffuse mandibular enlargement. ***J Am Dent Assoc*** **1985;111(4):630–632.**

Paget's disease of the jaw has the following characteristics: slow progression of jaw enlargement; bilateral jaw involvement; often polyostotic, but not generalized, skeletal disease; diffuse, irregular radiopaque areas of the jaw; elevated serum alkaline phosphatase level; and a biopsy specimen showing thick, irregular bone trabeculae with a mosaic pattern of reversal lines and numerous osteoblasts and osteoclasts in a fibrovascular stroma. Management of a patient with Paget's disease of bone usually is carried out by treating the symptoms of the disease as they arise. Bone can be removed for aesthetic reasons when necessary. (4 references)

106

Ellis, G. L.; Connole, P. W.

Diffuse mandibular enlargement caused by osteitis deformans. ***Ear Nose Throat J*** **1985;64(10):466–472.**

Paget's disease of bone, or osteitis deformans, is one of the more common disorders affecting bone. Although any bone site can be affected, isolated presentations may occur in the craniofacial skeleton. Paget's disease of the mandible has the following characteristics: (1) slow progression of mandibular enlargement; (2) bilateral mandibular involvement; (3) often polyostotic, but not generalized skeletal disease; (4) diffuse irregular radiopacities of mandible; (5) elevated serum alkaline phosphatase; and (6) a biopsy specimen showing thick, irregular bone trabeculae with a mosaic pattern of reversal lines and numerous osteoblasts and osteoclasts in a fibrovascular stroma. Management is symptomatic and bone can be removed if necessary. (14 references)

107

Eretto, P., et al.

Optic neuropathy in Paget's disease. ***Am J Ophthalmol*** **1984;97(4):505–510.**

Of 22 patients (18 men and 4 women ranging in age from 50 to 89 years) with radiographic and clinical evidence of Paget's disease, 9 had visual field defects. All 9 had arcuate scotomas, and 5 of the 9 had generalized constriction. The visual field changes were asymptomatic in 6 of 9 patients and progressive in 2 patients. Only 2 patients had radiographic evidence of optic canal constriction by bony impingement. There was no objective improvement in the optic neuropathy in the 3 patients treated with synthetic salmon calcitonin. This data suggested that the optic neuropathy of Paget's disease cannot be explained solely on the basis of bony compression, and the cause of optic neuropathy in patients with normal optic canals remains unknown. (21 references)

108

Haibach, H.; Farrell, C.; Dittrich, F. J.

Neoplasms arising in Paget's disease of bone: A study of 82 cases. ***Am J Clin Pathol*** **1985;83(5):594–600.**

This article reviews 82 cases of neoplasms in patients with Paget's disease of bone recorded in the Mid-America Bone Tumor Registry between 1958 and 1983. There were 77 osteosarcomas, 3 fibrosarcomas, 1 chondrosarcoma, and 1 giant cell tumor. The men/women ratio was 2:1. The age distribution was as follows: less than 51 years, 18%; 51 to 60 years, 29%; 61 to 70 years, 36%; and greater than 70 years, 17%. The femur was involved by tumor in 22%, the humerus in 21%, the pelvis in 21%, the calvarium in 12%, the tibia in 10%, and other bones in 15% of the cases. There were 48% survivors after 1 year, 17% after 2 years, and 5% after 3 and 5 years; 2 additional patients with tumors lived for more than 7 and 11 years. Radiographs available for simultaneous study in 43 cases revealed predominant tumor patterns that were mixed in 69%, osteoblastic in 21%, and osteolytic in 10%. Other radiographic data and the clinical and histopathologic data are in agreement with those of five earlier major studies. Although the prognosis of neoplasms arising in Paget's disease generally is not good, a small fraction of long-term survivors after aggressive therapy makes this complication a challenge for timely radiographic diagnosis and histopathologic confirmation. (22 references)

109

Huvos, A. G.; Butler, A.; Bretsky, S. S.

Osteogenic sarcoma associated with Paget's disease of bone: A clinicopathologic study of 65 patients. *Cancer* 1983;52(8):1489–1495.

Among 1,177 osteogenic sarcoma cases diagnosed and treated at Memorial Hospital, 65 (5.5%) were associated with either monostotic or polyostotic Paget's disease. The overall median age was 64 years (range, 39 to 82 years). In those patients older than 40 years of age, the frequency of sarcomatous transformation rose to 27%. There were slightly more men (55%) than women. The most common skeletal sites were the pelvic bones (34%), the humerus (22%), the femur (19%), and the craniofacial bones (14%). Unrelenting pain and tender swelling were the most common presenting symptoms (85%), with pathologic fracture in 14 (22%) patients. In two thirds of the cases, the radiographic presentation was that of a lytic destructive lesion; in the other it showed a sclerotic, mixed, or permeative character. In almost one half of the cases, the histologic appearance of the osteogenic sarcomas was either fibrohistiocytomatous or osteoblastic. In spite of radical surgical amputations, only 3 patients survived longer than 5 years. The prognosis of Paget's sarcoma is significantly less favorable than that of osteogenic sarcoma arising de novo in patients of comparable age. (47 references)

110

Lluberas-Acosta, G.; Hansell, J. R.; Schumacher, H. R., Jr.

Paget's disease of bone in patients with gout. *Arch Intern Med* 1986;146(12):2389–2392.

In a study designed to evaluate the radionuclide images in patients with gout, 6 (23%) of the 26 patients had clear evidence of Paget's disease of bone by technetium-99m-medronate imaging. A reference population consisting of 333 technetium-99m-medronate bone scans ordered for other reasons was reviewed, and only 7 scans (2.1%) had evidence of Paget's disease. This difference was found to be highly significant. All cases of

Paget's disease were confirmed by independent radiologic evaluation. The authors conclude that there is a significant association between Paget's disease and gout, the basis for which is not yet known. (8 references)

111

Milgram, J. W.; Ryan, W. G.

Skeletal deformities of Paget's disease of bone. *Contemp Orthop* 1985;10(3):64–70.

Although Paget's disease of bone may seem to be a relatively static process to most physicians who follow such patients for short periods of time, this unusual bone disease can remain active for three decades or more. It can lead to significant progressive deformity of the affected areas of the skeleton with secondary dysfunctions of adjacent nerves and joints. Deformities of the head include cranial vault enlargement; headaches; cranial nerve compression syndromes, which are commonly auditory but may affect the optic or trigeminal nerves; and maxillary involvement that can result in malocclusion and cosmetic deformities. Paget's disease rarely affects the cervical spine, but the osteopenia associated with early active disease may cause a collapse in height of an affected vertebra. Deformities of the pelvis can be common, as are deformities of the long bones of the arm and forearm, femur, and tibia. With the availability of therapeutic agents that can suppress, but not eradicate, the active disease process, there are implications that the deformities associated with Paget's disease in different sites of the body may possibly be prevented. Several illustrations, slides, and radiographs are included. (5 references)

112

Seret, P., et al.

Sarcomatous degeneration in Paget's bone disease. *J Cancer Res Clin Oncol* 1987;113(4):392–399.

The authors report 12 cases (8 men and 4 women) of sarcomatous degeneration in Paget's bone disease, with an average age of 72.3 years. Sarcomatous degeneration occurred often in polyostotic Paget's disease, and osteitis deformans was seen in 4 cases. Femur and pelvis were the bones most affected. Pain was a constant feature, whereas tumefaction and fracture were less common. Osteolytic lesions were more frequent than condensed or mixed lesions, and radiologic signs of malignancy were usually found. Seven cases were histologically classified as osteogenic sarcoma and 3 cases as fibrosarcoma. Electron microscopy was performed on two osteogenic sarcomas and in one case revealed microcylindrical inclusions in pagetic osteoclasts and in multinucleated giant tumor cells, but none in mononucleated tumor cells. The average survival time for the patients in this study was only 4.5 months. (37 references)

113

Siris, E. S., et al.

Parathyroid function in Paget's disease of bone. *J Bone Mineral Res* 1989;4(1):75–79.

In order to determine the prevalence of secondary hyperparathyroidism in patients with Paget's disease of bone, the authors measured serum parathyroid hormone levels (aminoterminal assay) in 39 patients with a wide range of pagetic activity. All patients had normal serum calcium levels. A total of 30 patients either were untreated or had received no treatment for 6 months or longer when studied; the other 9 were receiving either salmon calcitonin (3) or EHDP (6). The findings showed that in 7 of the 39 patients (18%) parathyroid hormone levels were increased above normal. These were among the most severely affected individuals, as manifested by the degree of elevation of three pagetic biochemical indexes: serum alkaline phosphatase, plasma bone GLA protein, and 24-hour urinary hydroxyproline/creatinine ratios. Levels of 25-hydroxyvitamin D3 and 1,25-dihydroxyvitamin D3 were normal. The relationships between parathyroid hormone and each of the three pagetic indexes as well as serum calcium for the entire group of 39 patients were also studied. Parathyroid hormone values did not correlate with serum calcium measurements ($R = -0.241$, $P =$ NS) but did correlate significantly with serum alkaline phosphatase ($R = 0.496$, $P < 0.001$), plasma bone GLA protein ($R = 0.537$, $P < 0.001$) and urinary hydroxyproline ($R = 0.450$, $P < 0.011$). The authors conclude that relative or absolute increases in parathyroid hormone may occur in moderately active Paget's disease, possibly in the setting of greater calcium demands during periods of increased pagetic new bone formation. This may be of pathophysiologic importance, since higher concentrations of parathyroid hormone may drive responsive pagetic osteoclasts to levels of bone-resorbing activity that exceed their intrinsically augmented states, contributing to the metabolic expression of Paget's disease. (27 references)

114

Smith, J.; Botet, J. F.; Yeh, S. D.

Bone sarcomas in Paget's disease: A study of 85 patients. *Radiology* 1984;152(3):583–590.

This is a comprehensive review of 85 patients who had been sarcoma associated with Paget's disease and who were seen at Memorial Sloan-Kettering Cancer Center between 1927 and 1982. There was an almost equal distribution of tumors in the axial and appendicular skeletons. The pelvis, humerus, femur, and skull were the tumor sites in 80% of cases. The tumors were bulky, large soft tissue masses. Lytic lesions were more common than sclerotic lesions. Mixed lytic and sclerotic lesions were much less common than either single type. Periosteal reaction was uncommon and found in less than 7%. Methylene diphosphonate (bisphosphonate) scans of the bone often showed a cold area that was associated with marked increase in uptake on the gallium scan. Angiography, which was performed in 13 patients, was useful, but computerized axial tomography (CAT) was much more helpful in showing the soft tissue mass as well as the extent of bony disease. Only 3 patients in this study survived for 5 years. Present chemotherapy protocols were disappointing in the treatment of this highly lethal tumor. (34 references)

115

Sofaer, J. A.

Dental extractions in Paget's disease of bone. *Int J Oral Surg* 1984;13(2):79–84.

The results of a postal questionnaire completed by 360 patients with Paget's disease of bone, on behalf of themselves and their unaffected spouses, suggest that dental practitioners have some awareness of the potential problems associated with extractions for patients with Paget's disease. Nevertheless, patients with Paget's disease still experience greater difficulty with extraction and more postextraction complications than do those without Paget's disease. (14 references)

116

Strickberger, S. A.; Schulman, S. P.; Hutchins, G. M.

Association of Paget's disease of bone with calcific aortic valve disease. *Am J Med* 1987;82(5):953–956.

To test the hypothesis that Paget's disease of bone is associated with a greater incidence of calcific aortic valve disease, a computer-generated list of all autopsy subjects from the Johns Hopkins Hospital in whom Paget's disease was diagnosed ($n = 92$) was obtained. The severity of Paget's disease and cardiac valvular lesions was graded on a scale of 0 to 3, with 3 as the most severe. Two control cases were obtained for each case of Paget's disease. Each was the case either immediately before or after the Paget's case and was matched for age, race, sex, and extent of autopsy. The incidences of moderate (10.9%) and severe (5.4%) calcific aortic valve disease were both fourfold greater than in the control group (chi-square analysis, $P < 0.01$ and $P < 0.05$, respectively). Additionally, the frequency of advancing grades of calcific aortic valve disease was greater in more advanced stages of Paget's disease. In fact, there was a dose-response effect of Paget's disease on calcific aortic valve disease (trend analysis for proportion, $P < 0.01$). These data therefore support the hypothesis that Paget's disease is associated with calcific aortic valve disease in a dose-response manner. (18 references)

117

Wallach, S.

Neurological and cardiovascular complications of Paget's disease. *Geriatr Med Today* 1986;5(1):38–46.

Although Paget's disease is typically characterized by pain, deformity, and other skeletal abnormalities, it may be complicated by secondary neurologic and cardiovascular sequelae that can produce additional disability and complicate management. Fortunately, early diagnosis combined with effective suppressive therapy for Paget's disease can reverse most of these complications partially or completely and may obviate the need for neurosurgery. The physician must therefore be alert to the diagnosis of both Paget's disease and the associated complications. (0 references)

118

Weisz, G. M.

Lumbar canal stenosis in Paget's disease: The staging of the clinical syndrome, its diagnosis, and treatment. *Clin Orthop* 1986;(206):223–227.

The lumbar syndrome of Paget's disease is classified according to its severity, clinical findings, biochemical factors, and radiologic pattern. Pagetoid spinal stenosis may occur in three stages as a progressive clinical syndrome. Several diagnostic procedures, including computerized axial tomography, are analyzed to introduce the concept of spinal reserve capacity. Treatment with calcitonin is recommended at the appropriate stages of the syndrome. (25 references)

Therapy

119

Adami, S., et al.

Treatment of Paget's disease of bone with intravenous 4-amino-1-hydroxybutylidene-1,1-bisphosphonate. ***Calcif Tissue Int*** **1986;39(4):226–229.**

4-Amino-1-hydroxybutylidene-1,1-bisphosphonate (AHButBP) was given intravenously (2.5 to 25 mg/d for 4 days) to 14 patients with Paget's disease of bone, 5 of whom had been treated with dichloromethylidene bisphosphonate (Cl_2MBP) 32 months earlier. In the 9 patients who had not been treated previously with bisphosphonates, the short course of AHButBP induced a suppression of serum alkaline phosphatase and urinary hydroxyproline values down to 30% of initial values. The biochemical suppression of the disease was sustained for 2 to 18 months, and the time to relapse was correlated with the logarithm of the dose ($P < 0.001$). In the 5 patients previously treated for Paget's disease, an apparent resistance to treatment with AHButBP was observed. However, in these patients both serum alkaline phosphatase and urinary hydroxyproline fell to or even below the nadir values that had previously been achieved with Cl_2MBP, irrespective of the degree of relapse. Thus the degree of suppression of Paget's disease of bone, achievable after treatment with bisphosphonates, seems to be constant for each patient, such that normal levels of serum alkaline phosphatase and urinary hydroxyproline cannot usually be attained in patients with extremely active disease. (13 references)

120

Altman, R. D.

Paget's disease of bone, in Conn HF (ed): ***Current Therapy: Latest Approved Methods of Treatment for the Practicing Physician.*** **Philadelphia, WB Saunders, 1988, pp 507–510. Available from WB Saunders, Co., West Washington Square, Philadelphia, PA 19105. ISBN: 0721624294.**

This book section reviews treatment and goals of therapy. Since 80% of patients with Paget's disease are elderly and without clinical findings or complications, there should be a definite objective for therapy. Complications of Paget's disease are outlined, and mechanical aids and devices to help correct symptoms are discussed. Indications for medicinal therapy are reviewed, and the use of antiinflammatory drugs, calcitonin, diphosphonates (bisphosphonates), and plicamycin is discussed. (0 references)

121

Altman, R. D.; Collins-Yudiskas, B.

Synthetic human calcitonin in refractory Paget's disease of bone. *Arch Intern Med* 1987;147(7):1305–1308.

Fourteen patients with symptomatic and active Paget's disease of the bone who had demonstrated resistance to parenteral synthetic salmon calcitonin, oral disodium etidronate, or both in combination were treated with parenteral synthetic human calcitonin. Eleven patients (79%) demonstrated clinical and chemical improvement for up to 5 years. Two patients received additional benefit with combined synthetic human calcitonin and etidronate disodium. (23 references)

122

Altman, R. D.

Long-term follow-up of therapy with intermittent etidronate disodium in Paget's disease of bone. *Am J Med* 1985;79(5):583–590.

A long-term trial of etidronate disodium therapy in 93 patients with Paget's disease of bone yielded generally favorable results. Treatment or retreatment was initiated for symptomatic Paget's disease with elevated serum alkaline phosphatase and urinary hydroxyproline values. Improvement occurred in 60% of patients even in the presence of secondary osteoarthritis. There appeared to be three types of responses: (1) patients with prolonged clinical and chemical improvement after a single course of therapy (40%), who tended to have less active disease as determined on the basis of initial alkaline phosphatase and hydroxyproline values, with suppression to normal in 76% of patients after etidronate disodium therapy; (2) patients with response to retreatment (45%), who had modest disease as indicated by alkaline phosphatase and hydroxyproline values and required retreatment less often than once a year; and (3) patients with response to retreatment but eventual development of resistance to etidronate disodium (15%) who demonstrated the most severe disease in terms of clinical findings and on the basis of alkaline phosphatase and hydroxyproline values. In this last group, resistance to etidronate disodium (5 mg/kg/d) was common and early, and patients received etidronate disodium more often than one course per year; alkaline phosphatase response was transient, often of less than 3 months' duration. (30 references)

123

Atkins, R. M., et al.

Aminohexane diphosphonate in the treatment of Paget's disease of bone. *J Bone Mineral Res* 1987;2(4):273–279.

The author studied the effects of intravenous and oral administration of aminohexane diphosphonate (AHDP) in 42 patients with active Paget's disease of bone. Both oral (400 mg/d for 1 month) and intravenous (25 mg or 50 mg/d for 5 days) treatment induced marked suppression of biochemical indexes of disease activity. Urinary excretion of hydroxyproline fell to 39% and 42% of pretreatment values (for oral and intravenous treatments, respectively) and was followed by a similar decrease in the serum activity of alkaline phosphatase. In both groups of patients, disease activity remained suppressed for the 6 months of follow-up, and pain improved in 34 of 37 patients who had bone pain attributed to Paget's disease. Results of both biopsies indicated that osteoblast and osteoclast numbers decreased with no adverse effects on mineralization. Neither regimen was associated with significant side effects. The authors concluded that short courses of AHDP provide a promising treatment for the long-term control of Paget's disease. (28 references)

123a

Audran, M., et al.

Treatment of Paget's disease of bone with (4-chloro-phenyl) thiomethylene bisphosphonate. *Clin Rheumatol* 1989;8(1):71–79.

Introduction of the antiosteoclastic drugs calcitonin and etidronate has profoundly changed the treatment of active Paget's disease of bone. Nevertheless, the use of these drugs is limited in some patients by side effects or by resistance to therapy. The results of an open, nonrandomized study with a new bisphosphonate, (chloro-4 phenyl) thiomethylene bisphosphonate (Cl-TMBP), given orally to 35 patients with active Paget's disease of bone are reported. At two different dosages this new bisphosphonate induces a significant decrease in disease activity. Fourteen patients receiving a mean dosage of 5 mg/kg/d showed a significant reduction of serum alkaline phosphatase levels to 43% of pretherapeutic values while hydroxyproline/creatinine ratio decreased to 43% of baseline. A second group of 21 patients receiving a mean dosage of 11 mg/kg/d exhibited a similar response: serum alkaline phosphatase activity was reduced to 42% of initial values while hydroxyproline/creatinine ratio fell to 48% of baseline. This was accompanied by a reduction in radionuclide uptake in pagetic areas. A prolonged beneficial effect was observed in most patients. In patients receiving the highest dosage significant reduction in serum calcium and rise in parathyroid hormone were observed. Otherwise no clinical or biologic side effects occurred throughout the study. (24 references)

124

Broberg, M. A.; Cass, J. R.

Total knee arthroplasty in Paget's disease of the knee. ***J Arthroplasty* 1986;1(2):139–142.**

Seven patients with Paget's disease of the knee underwent total knee arthroplasty; they accounted for 0.1% of the population who underwent knee arthroplasty at one institution. The results continued to be satisfactory for up to 12 years of follow-up. Two patients had radiographic evidence of loosening, but neither required repeat surgery. (3 references)

125

Cameron, H. U.

Total knee replacement in Paget's disease. ***Orthop Rev* 1989;18(2):206–208.**

The common sites for Paget's disease, at least in a Canadian population, are the pelvis (45.4%), vertebrae (22%), femur (10%), tibiae (3.6%), and patellae (0.2%). Paget's disease occasionally gives rise to arthritic changes in a joint adjacent to the lesion, although the precise mechanism is uncertain. Disturbance of the subchondral bone due to hyperemia and overload due to increasing deformity have been cited as possible reasons. There is concern that joint replacement with cemented components would result in rapid loosening caused by increased bone turnover; however, it has yet to prove a major problem. So far no reports have appeared in the literature on the effects of Paget's disease on knee replacement, specifically the effects of the porous tissue ingrowth-type components that are now in common use. This paper discusses two patients with Paget's disease who had knee replacement of this type. They have been followed for 2 years and both have done well to date. It appears that ingrowth-type implants can be used in the presence of Paget's disease. (12 references)

126

Canfield, R. E.; Siris, E. S.

Paget's disease of bone, in *Current Therapy in Endocrinology and Metabolism,* ed 3. Toronto, BC Decker, 1988, pp 388–393. Available from B. C. Decker, 320 Walnut Street, Philadelphia, PA 19106. (215) 625-0001. ISBN: 1556640854.

This book chapter presents an overview of therapeutic goals and interventions for Paget's disease. The presence of symptoms referrable to Paget's disease constitutes the primary indication for therapy. Specific pharmacologic agents available for treatment include calcitonin, diphosphonates (bisphosphonates), and mithramycin (plicamycin). Other treatment modalities include antiinflammatory agents to relieve pain due to mild-to-moderate hip, knee, or ankle joint dysfunction, spinal stenosis, and lumbar or sacral involvement. Severe joint dysfunction at the hip or knee may respond only to joint replacement. Osteotomies of severely bowed limbs may be performed on those patients who have major gait disturbances or severe pain produced by stresses from the malalignment of the bone. Neurosurgical intervention may be required to relieve progressive spinal cord or root compression. (5 references)

127

Caniggia, A., et al.

Effect of a long-term treatment with the aminosuberic analog of eel calcitonin on osteocalcin in Paget's disease. *Panminerva Med* 1987;29(1):1–5.

This study was performed in 40 patients with Paget's disease of bone to evaluate the effect of the aminosuberic analogue of eel calcitonin (carbocalcitonin [carbo-CT]) on serum osteocalcin. Carbo-CT was administered parenterally at the dose of 40 MRC U every other day; the treatment lasted 4 to 12 months. The administration of carbo-CT was devoid of any untoward effect. Thirty-two of 40 pagetic patients were responsive to the calcitonin treatment in terms of serum alkaline phosphatase and 24-hour urinary excretion of hydroxyproline. In these patients a statistically significant diminution of serum osteocalcin was noticed; it paralleled decreases in serum alkaline phosphatase and urinary hydroxyproline. These results confirm the significance of serum BGP as a marker of bone turnover in Paget's disease and indicate that carbo-CT is effective in the treatment of this pathologic condition. (16 references)

127a

Cantrill, J. A.; Anderson, D. C.

Treatment of Paget's disease of bone. *Clin Endocrinol (Oxf)* 1990;32(4):507–518.

This article reviews treatment advances in Paget's disease. Before the late 1960s there were no modifying treatments for Paget's disease. Antiinflammatory or analgesic therapy has little if any effect on the underlying disease process. Two major types of agents now available to suppress disease activity are calcitonins and bisphosphonates (formerly called diphosphonates). The significant action of calcitonin on bone is to inhibit bone resorption directly by reducing osteoclastic activity. Pain relief usually begins after 2 to 6 weeks of therapy with a maximum response at 6 to 12 months. The plateau phenomenon in which a certain serum alkaline phosphatase level persists regardless of calcitonin dosage or type occurs in most patients. Because of the unacceptable incidence of side effects and the relative rarity of the desired response, the attention of more recent research has turned to five bisphosphonates: EHDP, Cl_2MDP, APD, AHDP, and AHButBP. Increasing evidence indicates that bisphosphonates, especially APD, lead to dramatic healing of bone with marked reduction in bone turnover. Because of unsatisfactory effects on mineralization, EHDP is unlikely to continue to be justifiably used. The safety and efficacy of the newer bisphosphonates have yet to be confirmed. (70 references)

128

Cantrill, J. A.; Buckler, H. M.; Anderson, D. C.

Low dose intravenous 3-amino-1-hydroxypropylidene-1,1-bisphosphonate (APD) for the treatment of Paget's disease of bone. ***Ann Rheum Dis*** **1986;45(12):1012–1018.**

Twenty patients with severe symptomatic Paget's disease were treated with a series of 15-mg intravenous infusions of 3-amino-1-hydroxypropylidene-1,1-bisphosphonate (APD). A regimen of either 5 consecutive days of treatment (regimen 1) or a course of 12 weekly infusions was administered (regimen 2). In five cases regimen 2 followed regimen 1 after a 3-month interval. Alkaline phosphatase levels fell in all patients and returned to the normal range in 12. All but 1 of the patients obtained symptomatic improvement. The median fall in alkaline phosphatase activity was 63%. Eight patients observed a transient increase in bone pain starting about 24 hours after the first infusion. Intravenous APD was well tolerated and appears to be an effective treatment for Paget's disease; this route of administration prevents the problem of poor and unpredictable gastrointestinal absorption seen when a bisphosphonate is given orally. The optimal dose and duration of APD therapy, frequency of relapse, requirement for further courses, and merits relative to those of other second-generation bisphosphonates remain to be established. (19 references)

129

Coulton, L. A.; Preston, C. J.; Couch, M.; Kanis, J. A.

An evaluation of serum osteocalcin in Paget's disease of bone and its response to diphosphonate treatment. ***Arthritis Rheum*** **1988;31(9):1142–1147.**

The author found that serum bone gamma-carboxyglutamic-acid-containing protein (BGP) (osteocalcin) had lower sensitivity and specificity for measurement of disease activity in Paget's disease of bone than other biochemical measures of disease activity. The administration of diphosphonates (bisphosphonates) induced suppression of urinary hydroxyproline excretion and subsequent decrease in alkaline phosphatase values, but no consistent change in BGP values. Serum BGP measurements have limited value as a screening test for Paget's disease or for monitoring treatment of the disorder. (15 references)

130

Delmas, P. D.; Chapuy, M. C.; Edouard, C.; Meunier, P. J.

Beneficial effects of aminohexane diphosphonate in patients with Paget's disease of bone resistant to sodium etidronate. *Am J Med* 1987;83(2)276–282.

Clinical and biochemical resistance to sodium etidronate therapy is not rare in patients with severe Paget's disease of bone, especially after several courses of treatment. Sixteen patients with Paget's disease of bone and well-documented resistance to sodium etidronate were treated with a new diphosphonate (bisphosphonate), aminohexane diphosphonate, given orally for 3 months at a daily dose of 400 mg. This patient group comprised a selected population of patients with very active disease, as shown by a mean 20-fold increase of serum alkaline phosphatase levels before aminohexane diphosphonate therapy. Aminohexane diphosphonate induced a striking reduction of serum alkaline phosphatase and urinary hydroxyproline levels sustained for up to 18 months after withdrawal of treatment. Two patients had a relapse 14 to 16 months after treatment and received a second course of aminohexane diphosphonate with the same efficacy. This was accompanied by marked clinical improvement, reduction of the radioisotope uptake by pagetic bones, and radiologic healing of osteolytic lesions in some cases. Iliac crest biopsy specimens taken after tetracycline double-labeling showed no impairment of bone mineralization. No clinical or biochemical adverse effects have been observed. (24 references)

131

Dewis, P.; Prasad, B. K.; Anderson, D. C.; Willets, S.

Clinical experience with the use of two diphosphonates in the treatment of Paget's disease. *Ann Rheum Dis* 1985;44(1):34–38.

The effects of EHDP 20 mg/kg/d) and APD (4.5 mg/kg/d) given for 3 months to patients with severe symptomatic Paget's disease have been compared in an open trial of 17 patients. Both drugs were equally effective in producing a prompt reduction in pair scores, urine hydroxyproline, and serum alkaline phosphatase levels. The remission was maintained for a variable period after cessation of treatment. Both drugs were well tolerated, and a 1-month course of either drug was not effective. Comparison with published responses from previous studies indicates that EHDP given at this dose as a relatively short course is more effective than a lower dose for a longer period of time; the present study does not suggest that APD has significant advantages. (13 references)

132

Dodd, G. W., et al.

Radiological assessment of Paget's disease of bone after treatment with the bisphosphonates EHDP and APD. *Br J Radiol* 1987;60(717):849–860.

The effects of therapy on the osteolytic bone lesions of Paget's disease were assessed from serial bone radiographs. Changes in the rate of progression of lytic "wedge" lesions were measured, and alterations in the texture of lytic "blade" lesions were graded on an empirical scale. Useful matching by using standard radiographs was possible, although special care was needed to prevent artifacts from suboptimal positioning, magnification, and variation in exposure. Serial radiographs were obtained of 57 lytic blade lesions in 54 patients receiving treatment with the bisphosphonate 1-hydroxyethylidene-1, 1-bisphosphonate (EHDP) and of 20 lesions in 20 patients treated with oral or intravenous 3-amino-1-hydroxypropylidene-1, 1-bisphosphonate (APD). Treatment with EHDP was associated with a significant deterioration in bone texture in 50% of lytic blade lesions and with healing in only 20%. Deterioration was accompanied by an increase in local bone pain in 17% of these patients. In contrast, significant healing was observed in 17 of 20 lytic lesions (8 wedge, 9 blade) within 6 months of beginning a course of intravenous or oral APD. In four of eight patients the progression of a lytic tibial wedge was arrested, and in the remaining four the direction of wedge movement was reversed. In two patients the wedge had almost completely "filled in," making measurement difficult. Bone healing was usually accompanied by pain relief, reduction in skin temperature, and rapid suppression of the urine hydroxyproline (uHP) into the normal range. However, in four patients who received intravenous APD, repair of lytic bone lesions was observed despite persisting elevation of uHP. These improvements with APD were sustained at 12 months, although in one patient whose biochemical indexes were restored to normal the resorption front showed further progression, despite initial temporary reversal. The trends apparent in these short-term studies were also seen in four patients in whom wedge velocities were measured over periods of 6 to 10 years. These results confirm that after treatment of Paget's disease, bone healing or deterioration can be accurately assessed from serial standard radiographs. (25 references)

133

El-Sammaa, M.; Linthicum, F. H., Jr.; House, H. P.; House, J. W.

Calcitonin as treatment for hearing loss in Paget's disease. ***Am J Otol*** **1986;7(4):241–243.**

Progressive hearing loss is a potential complication of Paget's disease, a metabolic disorder of accelerated bone formation and resorption. Calcitonin (Calcimar) is a recently introduced synthetic hormone used as a systemic treatment. Some studies have shown it to halt the progression of hearing loss. This is the first study of the effects of calcitonin on hearing loss in a large number of patients with continuous use of the drug and long-term follow-up. It confirms that the drug is effective. We conducted chart reviews to compare the degree of hearing loss over time in 45 patients. Twenty-six patients had been taking salmon calcitonin for 5 to 8 years to date, and 19 have received no treatment. Hearing loss was recorded at the initial examination (trial 1), 1 to 4 years later (trial 2), and then 1 to 5 years after the second evaluation (trial 3). Statistical analyses show a strong relationship between treatment and rate of hearing loss. The average hearing loss in the control group progressed from 47 dB in the first trial to 59 dB in the second trial to 75 dB in the third trial. Average hearing loss in the treated group remained at 47 dB over time. The difference in hearing loss over time between the two groups was less than 1 dB for the treated group and more than 28 dB for the control group. Results thus clearly show that calcitonin is effective in halting the progression of hearing loss in Paget's disease. (21 references)

134

Gagel, R. F.; Logan, C.; Mallette, L. E.

Treatment of Paget's disease of bone with salmon calcitonin nasal spray. ***J Am Geriatr Soc*** **1988;36(11):1010–1014.**

Subcutaneous daily or twice-daily administration of synthetic salmon calcitonin is an effective form of therapy for Paget's disease, but the requirement for parenteral injection deters geriatric patients from using the drug. This study compares a new intranasal preparation of salmon calcitonin with the subcutaneous version of the drug in 18 patients with Paget's disease using two different protocols. In the first protocol, 15 patients not previously treated with salmon calcitonin were given the agent for 3 months by either the intranasal or the subcutaneous route. Seven patients treated with intranasal calcitonin had a mean fall in the serum alkaline phosphatase of 33% over a 3-month period compared to a fall of 40% in the subcutaneously treated group; the difference between the two treatment groups was not statistically significant. In the second protocol, three patients previously stabilized on subcutaneous calcitonin were switched to the nasal spray with no subsequent change in alkaline phosphatase values during 6 months of treatment. These results demonstrate that intranasal salmon calcitonin is effective in lowering the serum alkaline phosphatase in Paget's disease. Ease of administration and patient acceptance make intranasal calcitonin a reasonable alternative for geriatric patients. (15 references)

135

Gibbs, C. J.; Aaron, J. E.; Peacock, M.

Osteomalacia in Paget's disease treated with short term, high dose sodium etidronate. *Br Med J* 1986;292(6530):1227–1229.

Eleven patients with Paget's disease treated with sodium etidronate (20 mg/kg/d) for 2 and 4 weeks showed significant reductions in plasma alkaline phosphatase activity and urinary hydroxyproline excretion, both of which are biochemical markers of bone turnover. After 4 weeks of treatment, however, histologic examination of iliac crest biopsy samples showed that despite a rapid reduction in bone resorption there was an appreciable mineralization defect; even after only 2 weeks' treatment the abnormalities in bone formation persisted for up to 10 weeks. The adverse effects of sodium etidronate on mineralization cannot be dissociated from its beneficial effect on resorption even when it is given for short periods. (14 references)

136

Gray, R. E., et al.

Duration of effect of oral diphosphonate therapy in Paget's disease of bone. *Q J Med* 1987;64(245):755–767.

The effects of the diphosphonates (bisphosphonates) etidronate and clodronate were studied in 144 patients with Paget's disease. All five programs of treatment tested induced a similar suppression of disease activity as judged by serum alkaline phosphatase concentrations, but the proportion of patients responding and the duration of responses differed significantly between programs. The proportion responding to etidronate 5 to 10 mg/kg/d for 6 months was less than for other regimens, and the most sustained response was after treatment with clodronate 1,600 mg/d for 6 months. More complete biochemical suppression was associated with the more prolonged responses irrespective of the regimen used. (47 references)

137

Hadjipavlou, A. G.; Lander, P. H.; Enker, I.

Paget's disease of bone: Orthopedic management, in *Current Concepts of Bone Fragility*. Published Proceedings of the 12th Applied Basic Science Course, Ottawa, Canada, 1985. New York, Springer-Verlag, 1986, pp 237–262. Available from Springer-Verlag, 175 Fifth Avenue, 19th floor, New York, NY 10010. (800) 526-7254.

Conservative medical therapy for Paget's disease is the mainstay of management, with surgery reserved for specific indications. This paper concentrates on the criteria for failure of medical treatment, indications for concurrent and/or subsequent surgical treatment, and monitoring of lesions for potential complications, such as malignant transformation and fractures. The authors review the literature on malignant transformations in Paget's disease. The development of sarcoma is the most serious complication of Paget's disease, and survival rates are low. They also discuss literature on the time of bone union in pagetic fractures. Therapeutic options for back pain and spinal stenosis are presented. Charts, tables, and radiographs are included. (65 references)

138

Harinck, H. I.; Bijvoet, O. L.; Blanksma, H. J.; Dahlinghaus-Nienhuys, P. J.

Efficacious management with aminobisphosphonate (APD) in Paget's disease of bone. *Clin Orthop* April 1987;217:79–98.

The effects of treatment with aminobisphosphonate (APD) were studied in a large and well-defined group of patients with Paget's disease over a period of 7 years. Particular attention was given to the pharmacology of the drug, methods of assessment of efficacy, and quality and long-term persistence of the treatment results. These studied are compared to previously reported studies on bisphosphonates (P-C-Ps). The data suggest that the efficacy of P-C-Ps in Paget's disease results from a physiologic adaptation of all cellular processes involved in bone metabolism to a primary inhibition of bone resorption. The prolonged persistence of remissions may indicate that this is associated with disappearance rather than suppression of pathogenic material. If the low specific toxicity of the new generations of P-C-Ps is confirmed, it will be possible to induce complete and prolonged remissions through short oral or parenteral treatment courses that are associated with minimal side effects. Early institution of treatment in selected patients may prevent the development of deformity, fracture, and pain. (92 references)

139

Harinck, H. I., et al.

Paget's disease of bone: Early and late responses to three different modes of treatment with aminohydroxypropylidene bisphosphonate (APD). ***Br Med J*** **1987;295(6609):1301–1305.**

Early and late responses to treatment with either oral (600 mg/d) or intravenous (20 mg/d) (3-amino-1-hydroxypropylidene)-1,1-bisphosphonate (aminohydroxypropylidene bisphosphonate: APD) were studied in 142 patients with Paget's disease of bone who had not previously been treated with bisphosphonate. The efficacy of three therapeutic regimens was compared: (1) oral aminohydroxypropylidene bisphosphonate given continuously until 6 months after the serum alkaline phosphatase activity had returned to normal (long-term); (2) oral aminohydroxypropylidene bisphosphonate given until urinary hydroxyproline excretion had returned to normal (short-term); (3) intravenous aminohydroxypropylidene bisphosphonate for 10 days. With either oral or intravenous treatment the decrease in urinary hydroxyproline excretion was rapid and always preceded the fall in serum alkaline phosphatase activity. Normal urinary hydroxyproline excretion is essential for return of the serum alkaline phosphatase activity to normal. Complete biochemical remission, defined as return of the serum alkaline phosphatase activity to normal, was obtained in 129 patients (91%). The median duration of remission as assessed by actuarial analysis was 2.7 years. This study found no difference in the long term among the three modes of treatment, suggesting that for most patients with Paget's disease a short course of intravenous aminohydroxypropylidene bisphosphonate produces long-lasting, complete remission without need for maintenance treatment. (23 references)

140

Heath, D. A.

Treating Paget's disease. ***Br Med J*** **1987;294(6579):1048–1050.**

This report describes and compares the use of calcitonin to that of etidronate for treating Paget's disease of bone, with the latter drug favored over the former. Other drugs that currently are unavailable are discussed for future use as well as indications for drug therapy. (22 references)

141

Hosking, D. J.

Paget's disease of bone: An update on Management. *Drugs* 1985;30(2):156–173.

The essential requirement for effective treatment of Paget's disease of bone is that the characteristic abnormality of bone remodeling be predictably corrected without significant side effects. Although the ideal agent is not currently available, appropriate use of the calcitonins or diphosphonates (bisphosphonates) goes a long way to achieving this goal. Calcitonin (50 to 100 MRC units subcutaneously daily or three times weekly) generally reduces bone turnover by approximately 50% within 6 months. However, very active disease is not controlled and bone turnover generally increases once treatment is withdrawn. Calcitonin has no significant side effects, although some patients develop antibody-mediated resistance to the exogenous calcitonin species. An advantage of calcitonin is that there is radiographic evidence of a return to normal bone remodeling during treatment. Although a number of diphosphonates (now more correctly termed bisphosphonates) are available for experimental use, only the first-generation compound, disodium etidronate (EHDP), is commercially available. It too reduces bone turnover by about 50% within 6 months when given in a dose of 5 mg/kg/d. Unlike calcitonin, it results in more sustained control of bone turnover with the additional advantage that it can be given by mouth. Although larger doses are more effective in controlling very active disease, there is a real risk of causing defective bone mineralization, which may result in the development of atraumatic long bone fractures or diffuse bone pains. Combinations of calcitonin and disodium etidronate in conventional dosage seem to produce an additive suppressant effect on bone turnover and may be indicated for more active disease. Advances in treatment are progressing rapidly, and it seems likely that in the next few years the introduction of new agents for the control of Paget's disease will more nearly approach the ideal goal of treatment. (126 references)

142

Kanis, J. A., et al.

Comparative effects of an antiviral drug, inosiplex, and diphosphonates in Paget's disease of bone. *Bone* 1985;6:69–72.

The effects of the antiviral drug inosiplex were assessed in four patients with Paget's disease of bone. Treatment for 6 months did not suppress disease activity as judged by serum alkaline phosphatase level and hydroxyprolinuria, and viral inclusions persisted in the one patient from whom a bone biopsy specimen was taken. These results contrasted markedly with the suppressive effects of diphosphonate (bisphosphonate) treatment in these same patients. (15 references)

143

Kanis, J. A., et al.

Effects of intravenous etidronate disodium on skeletal and calcium metabolism. ***Am J Med*** **1987;82(2A):55–70.**

The induction of hypercalcemia in malignant disease is almost invariably associated with increased bone resorption. However, tumor-induced changes in bone formation and renal tubular resorption of calcium are also important factors that induce hypercalcemia in some patients. In addition, alterations in calcium fluxes to and from the extracellular fluid secondary to hypercalcemia are important in maintaining or aggravating the hypercalcemic effects of increased bone resorption. These factors significantly affect the responses to treatment of hypercalcemia with inhibitors of bone resorption. This study examined the relative importance of these factors and the effects of intravenous etidronate disodium (etidronate) in neoplastic bone disease with and without hypercalcemia and in Paget's disease of bone. It is concluded that intravenous etidronate is an effective inhibitor of bone resorption, which accounts in large measure for its effects on serum calcium concentrations. These studies of etidronate in hypercalcemia suggest that the response is sustained for several weeks. (99 references)

144

Kanis, J. A.; Gray, R. E.

Long-term follow-up observations on treatment in Paget's disease of bone. ***Clin Orthop*** **1987;(217):99–125.**

The development of specific inhibitors of bone resorption has revolutionized the treatment of Paget's disease. The diphosphonates (bisphonates), the calcitonins, and mithramycin (plicamycin) are capable of inducing marked suppression of disease activity for prolonged periods as judged by biochemical, kinetic, and histologic techniques. Whereas the effects of the calcitonins and mithramycin persist only for the duration of treatment, diphosphonate treatment consistently produces a reduction of disease activity for many months or even years after cessation of treatment. The question whether the long-term control of the disease activity confers significant clinical advantages to the patient arises. Relief of bone pain, spinal neurologic syndromes, immobilization hypercalcemia, and high-output cardiac failure are related to the degree of biochemical control attained by treatment. New bone formed during treatment is lamellar, and radiologic progression of disease is favorably modified. It is not yet known whether long-term treatment decreases bone enlargement and deformity or reduces the risk of fracture. (169 references)

145

Kanis, J. A.

Monitoring the treatment of Paget's disease with etidronate: Editorial. ***Calcif Tissue Int*** **1984;36(6):629–631.**

This editorial argues that, although etidronate (a phosphonate drug [ethane-1-hydroxy-1, 1-bisphosphonate]) has been used with some success for many years for the treatment of Paget's disease, there is no consensus concerning the optimal dose or duration of treatment. Because of potential complications from the drug (bone mineralization impairment, bone pain, risk of fracture, and apparent osteolysis), patients treated with etidronate should be carefully monitored. Particular emphasis is placed on the minimum level of dose required. The editorial concludes that appropriate titration of dose may provide a more flexible treatment strategy that prevents unwanted effects while increasing the potential for benefits in Paget's disease patients. (23 references)

146

Levy, F., et al.

Formation of neutralizing antibodies during intranasal synthetic salmon calcitonin treatment of Paget's disease. ***J Clin Endocrinol Metab*** **1988;67(3):541–545.**

Nine patients with Paget's disease were treated with 200 U/d (15 nmol/d) synthetic salmon calcitonin (sCT) intranasally for 12 months. Five had received intramuscular or intranasal sCT therapy for 1 to 4 years up to 0.5 to 5 years before this study. Low-titer antibodies to sCT were detected in the serum of three of these five patients, but not in the four patients who had not received prior sCT therapy. After 2 months of intranasal sCT administration, four of the former group, but none of the latter group, had antibodies to sCT. After 12 months of treatment, antibodies to sCT were found in all patients who had received sCT earlier and in three of the four patients who had not. The half-maximal inhibition of [^{125}I]sCT binding ranged from 44 to 284 pmol/L sCT. In a cultured human breast cancer cell line (T47D) cAMP production was stimulated by sCT (EC_{50}, 70 pmol/L).

cAMP production stimulated by sCT (5 pmol/L) was reduced to 6% to 20% of the control value in the presence of serum from patients that inhibited [^{125}I]sCT binding by more than 50% in a dilution of 1:50 or greater. In patients with lower-titer antibodies cAMP production was not inhibited. Serum alkaline phosphatase activity was transiently lowered to 79 ± 6% (±SE) of basal levels in the patients who had earlier received sCT ($P > 0.1$); sustained reduction to between 66 ± 2% and 84 ± 6% of basal levels ($P < 0.05$) occurred in the patients who had not been treated with sCT previously. In conclusion, reexposure to sCT of five patients with Paget's disease caused secondary antibody responses and clinical resistance. (25 references)

146a

Ludkowski, P.; Wilson-MacDonald, J.

Total arthroplasty in Paget's disease of the hip: A clinical review and review of the literature. *Clin Orthop* 1990;255:160–167.

The results of a study of 30 Paget's disease patients with 37 affected hips treated with total hip arthroplasty (THA) for symptomatic coxarthrosis were compared with the results of previously reported series. Metabolic activity of the disease subsequent to surgery seemed to have no effect on the clinical outcome during 7.8 years of follow-up study; location of the disease (acetabulum only, femur only, or both) or presence of protrusio acetabuli alone also had no effect. For the femur, failure rates were similar for prostheses implanted in either pagetic or nonpagetic bone. Good results can be anticipated for patients with Paget's disease treated with cemented THA. (23 references)

147

Mautalen, C. A.; Gonzalez, D.; Ghiringhelli, G.

Efficacy of the bisphosphonate APD in the control of Paget's bone disease. *Bone* 1985;6(6):429–432.

Fifty-four patients with Paget's disease of bone were treated with the bisphosphonate APD. Twenty-six patients had not previously received treatment for Paget's disease, and 28 had been treated before with EHDP alone or in combination with calcitonin. APD was given orally in a mean dose of 500 mg daily (congruent to 6.8 mg/kg of body weight) for 4 to 12 months. Bone pain diminished or disappeared in 34 of 39 patients with symptoms. A very significant diminution of the biochemical indexes of bone turnover was observed in all patients, but the responses were faster in patients who had not previously received treatment for Paget's disease. After 4 months of treatment the serum levels of alkaline phosphatase of previously untreated patients diminished from 58.8 ± 8.0 to 20.0 ± 3.9 KA units ($P < 0.001$) and urinary excretion of hydroxyproline diminished from 108.6 ± 16.9 to 42.4 ± 8.3 mg/24 h ($P < 0.001$). In 23 of 26 previously untreated patients the biochemical indexes decreased to the normal range (complete response). A reduction of 50% or more without reaching the normal range was observed in the other 3 patients (partial response). Actuarial analysis of the duration of the effect 12 months after stopping APD disclosed that 63% of patients who had achieved a complete response but only 23% of those with a partial response were in biochemical remission. A second course of APD was administered to 11 patients. The results were as effective during the second as the first course in 9 patients, whereas 2 patients had no response to retreatment. (17 references)

148

McDonald, D. J.; Sim, F. H.

Total hip arthroplasty in Paget's disease: A follow-up note. ***J Bone Joint Surg* [*Am*] 1987;69(5):766–772.**

In 80 patients with Paget's disease of the hip who were seen between 1969 and 1982, symptomatic coxarthrosis led to total hip arthroplasty in 91 hips. The long-term clinical and radiographic results were analyzed by use of the Mayo Clinic hip-scoring system. The cases of the 46 patients (52 hips) who had been operated on before 1975 were analyzed 10 years after the arthroplasty. In this group, the incidence of aseptic loosening that required revision was approximately 15%; radiographic evidence of loosening was evident in approximately 30% of the femoral components and approximately 14% of the acetabular components. Actuarial analysis comparing these 46 patients with our overall experience of total hip arthroplasty during the same period in 7,222 hips of patients who did not have Paget's disease revealed an increase of slight statistical significance in the incidence of revision for aseptic loosening in the patients who had Paget's disease. However, the overall result was good or excellent 74% of these patients, suggesting that replacement of the hip using cemented components remains an acceptable form of treatment for degenerative coxarthrosis secondary to Paget's disease. (19 references)

149

Melick, R. A.

Treatment of Paget's disease of bone. ***Med J Aust* 1985;143(9):394–397.**

This report summarizes and discusses indications for treatment of Paget's disease of bone and available therapeutic agents and their use. The use, benefits, treatment duration, and potential side effects of calcitonin, diphosphonates (bisphosphonates) (etidronate), and mithramycin (plicamycin) are described. Present therapies do not cure this disease or control it completely but only reduce bone cell activity. It is hoped that future agents may allow early treatment aimed at preventing deformity and deafness. (26 references)

150

Merkow, R. L.; Pellicci, P. M.; Hely, D. P.; Salvati, E. A.

Total hip replacement for Paget's disease of the hip. ***J Bone Joint Surg [Am]*** **1984;66(5):752–758.**

The authors reviewed their experiences with total hip replacement for coxarthrosis due to Paget's disease. The clinical and radiographic results in 21 patients who had a total hip replacement between October 1972 and February 1982 were analyzed. The ages of the patients averaged 68.6 years (range: 57 to 80 years) and there were 12 women and 9 men. The follow-up averaged 5 years 2 months (range: 2 years to 11 years 4 months). A good to excellent result was achieved in 18 patients. Of the other 3 patients, 2 required a revision operation at 2.5 and 5 years postoperatively for symptomatic mechanical loosening of the femoral component. The remaining patient had only a fair result because of disease activity. Special problems that we encountered included varus deformity of the proximal end of the femur predisposing to varus placement of the femoral component, protrusio acetabuli, increased blood loss, sclerotic bone that made reaming difficult, and heterotopic ossification. (17 references)

151

Meunier, P. J., et al.

Intravenous disodium etidronate therapy in Paget's disease of bone and hypercalcemia of malignancy: Effects on biochemical parameters and bone histomorphometry. ***Am J Med*** **1987;82(2A):71–78.**

Nineteen patients with Paget's disease and 4 patients with hypercalcemia of malignancy underwent hypocalcemic therapy with etidronate disodium (etidronate) administered intravenously. The dosage for patients with Paget's disease was 4.3 mg/kg/d, infused on each of 7 consecutive days. Nine of the 19 patients also received oral etidronate 5 mg/kg/d for 3 months after administration of intravenous therapy. Etidronate administered orally sustained the decreases in urinary hydroxyproline produced by the infusions, whereas levels returned to pretreatment values in most patients receiving only the intravenously administered drug. Serum alkaline phosphatase levels were not reduced in the 10 patients receiving only intravenously administered etidronate, but they declined by approximately 50% in the 9 patients who received the additional orally administered etidronate. Transiliac-crest bone biopsy specimens obtained 3 months after intravenous therapy revealed a regular lamellar structure, compared with the characteristic woven pattern of pagetic bone. In all 4 patients with hypercalcemia of malignancy, normocalcemia was achieved by the tenth day of treatment using a dosage of 4.3 mg/kg/d. Oral etidronate therapy was beneficial in maintaining normocalcemia. (24 references)

151a

Muff, R., et al.

Efficacy of intranasal human calcitonin in patients with Paget's disease refractory to salmon calcitonin. *Am J Med.* 1990;89(2):181–184.

A cause for the resistance to intranasal salmon calcitonin (sCT) therapy in patients with Paget's disease is the occurrence of neutralizing antibodies to sCT. As a result, a new formulation of intranasal human calcitonin (hCT) was developed and the efficacy investigated in patients treated earlier with sCT. Twelve patients with Paget's disease were treated twice daily for 6 months with 1 mg synthetic hCT administered intranasally. A new formulation of intranasal hCT effectively lowered serum calcium levels, alkaline phosphatase concentrations, and urinary hydroxyproline excretion in patients with Paget's disease, some of whom were previously resistant to intranasal sCT because of neutralizing antibodies. (25 references)

152

Muir, H. G.; Schabort, I.; Hough, F. S.

Influence of disodium etidronate on Paget's disease of bone. *S Afr Med J* 1987;72(7):470–472.

The use of agents that decrease bone resorption, notably the calcitonins, diphosphonates (bisphosphonates), and mithramycin (plicamycin), has been shown to result in symptomatic and/or biochemical improvement in patients with Paget's disease of bone (osteitis deformans). The effects of short-term (6 months), low-dose (5 mg/kg body mass/d) etidronate disodium, a diphosphonate compound, on the clinical and laboratory manifestations of this disorder were examined. Marked symptomatic improvement was noted in 70% of patients, while biochemical parameters of bone turnover, namely serum alkaline phosphatase level (44%) and urine hydroxyproline excretion (56%), decreased significantly ($P < 0.001$). A technetium-99m bone scan revealed an impressive reduction in uptake of isotope in 50% of patients. The drug was well tolerated, and no adverse reactions (clinical, biochemical, or hematologic) were evident. It is concluded that short-term, low-dose etidronate disodium affords a convenient and effective therapeutic alternative in patients with symptomatic Paget's disease. (18 references)

153

Mulder, H.; Schop, C.; Koster, J. C.

Influence of pharmacologic doses of calcitonin on serum osteocalcin concentration in patients with Paget's disease of the bone. ***Acta Endocrinol (Copenh)*** **1989;120(6):721–723.**

The effect of continuous infusion of calcitonin on serum osteocalcin concentration was studied in 14 patients with Paget's disease. In all patients serum osteocalcin was initially increased. Within 24 hours calcitonin gradually reduced serum osteocalcin, a marker of osteoblastic activity. This means that inhibition of the function of the osteoclasts by calcitonin results in inhibition of the osteoblasts within 24 hours in patients with Paget's disease. (9 references)

154

Nagant de Deuxchaisnes, C., et al.

New modes of administration of salmon calcitonin in Paget's disease: Nasal spray and suppository. ***Clin Orthop*** **1987;(217):56–71.**

The activity of various doses of a nasal spray and of a suppository of salmon calcitonin was compared to that of a placebo and to the parenteral route of administration in volunteers. Both new modes of administration were found to be active on the kidney (and the suppository was found to affect bone turnover as well). The parenteral route proved more effective, but the nasal and/or rectal route had no systemic side effect and minimal local intolerance. The nasal spray was used at 200 units daily in 15 patients with Paget's disease and at 400 units daily in another 9 patients; both trials lasted 1 year. The two regimens affected bone turnover, and the higher dose was more effective than the lower one. In another trial, still in progress at the time of publication, a 300-unit suppository was given to another 12 patients. At the third month of therapy, the parameters of bone turnover were significantly depressed. Both new modes of therapy were able to improve the focal bone balance of the osteolytic lesions motivated on sequential roentgenograms. Systemic side effects were absent and local side effects were minimal. Only 1 patient interrupted the nasal spray therapy, and none interrupted the suppository therapy. (31 references)

154a

O'Doherty, D. P., et al.

A comparison of the acute effects of subcutaneous and intranasal calcitonin. *Clin Sci* 1990;78(2):215–219.

The acute effects of intranasal and subcutaneous calcitonin were studied in 40 patients with active Paget's disease of bone. Patients received a single dose of either 400 units of calcitonin delivered as a nasal spray; or 1, 10, or 100 units of subcutaneous calcitonin; or placebo. Subcutaneous salmon calcitonin, administered at doses of 1, 10, or 100 units to 9 patients with Paget's disease of bone, induced a dose-dependent fall in the serum calcium. This calcium-lowering effect was not seen in a second group of 9 patients receiving placebo. The lower doses of calcitonin had significant effects, which were more pronounced in patients with lower rates of bone turnover. Four hundred units of calcitonin administered as a nasal spray induced effects qualitatively similar to those seen with subcutaneous calcitonin, with an efficacy equivalent to approximately 30 units of subcutaneous calcitonin. The bioequivalence of calcitonin given by intranasal insufflation is low compared to that by parenteral administration. The intranasal route may be more appropriate for managing patients with disorders associated with low bone turnover. (27 references)

154b

O'Doherty, D. P., et al.

Treatment of Paget's disease of bone with aminohydroxybutylidene bisphosphonate. *J Bone Mineral Res* 1990;5(5):483–491.

This study examined the effects of aminohydroxybutylidene bisphosphonate in 30 patients with Paget's disease of bone, administered as an intravenous infusion for 5 consecutive days. Treatment (5 mg/d intravenously) induced marked suppression of biochemical indexes of disease activity. Urinary excretion of hydroxyproline fell to 50% of pretreatment values within 2 weeks and was followed by a similar, but later, decline in the serum activity of alkaline phosphatase. Disease activity remained suppressed throughout the 6 months of observation, and only 1 patient showed biochemical signs of an early relapse. Symptomatic improvement was noted in 27 of the 30 patients. Bone biopsies, undertaken in 10 patients, indicated no adverse effects on mineralization. Transient falls were noted in the total white cell count, particularly in lymphocyte and neutrophil fractions, and were associated with short-lived fever in 3 patients. The authors conclude that short courses of intravenous AHButBP provide a promising treatment for active Paget's disease of bone. (42 references)

155

O'Donoghue, D. J.; Hosking, D. J.

Biochemical response to combination of disodium etidronate with calcitonin in Paget's disease. *Bone* 1987;8(4):219–225.

The biochemical responses to salmon calcitonin (SCT: 100 MRC units three times a week) and disodium etidronate (EHDP: 400 mg daily) administered alone and in combination for 6 months were compared in 72 patients with symptomatic Paget's disease of bone unresponsive to simple analgesic agents. SCT produced a 53% reduction in alkaline phosphatase (AP) and a 38% reduction in 24-hour urinary hydroxyproline excretion (HYPRO). The response to EHDP was not significantly different: 56% reduction in AP and 48% reduction in HYPRO. Their use in combination produced a significantly greater reduction: 71% in AP ($P < 0.002$) and 69% in HYPRO ($P < 0.0001$). In those who remained symptomatic with increased disease activity, treatment for longer than 6 months had an unpredictable effect and normal bone turnover was rarely achieved. Once therapy was withdrawn, AP and HYPRO increased rapidly in those given SCT alone, returning to initial levels within 6 months. More sustained control of disease activity was achieved in those given EHDP either alone or with SCT, but the combination retained the advantage obtained during treatment. Combinations of SCT + EHDP may find a place in the treatment of very active Paget's disease. (25 references)

156

Perry, H. M. III; Droke, D. M.; Avioli, L. V.

Alternate calcitonin and etidronate disodium therapy for Paget's bone disease. *Arch Intern Med* 1984;144(5):929–933.

The efficacies of salmon calcitonin and etidronate disodium were compared in the therapy of Paget's bone disease in 37 patients. Nineteen patients, who received etidronate for 6 months, had a mean alkaline phosphatase reduction to 53% of initial values. Bone scintophotographs results improved in 12 and were unchanged in 7. Symptoms improved in 11 subjects, were unchanged in 7, and worsened in 1. Twelve of these patients, who were then treated with calcitonin for 6 months experienced continued improvement in alkaline phosphatase values to 36% of initial values. All bone scintophotograph results improved compared to those of initial studies. Symptoms of 7 patients continued to improve symptomatically; 5 described no change. Eighteen individuals were treated initially with calcitonin for 6 months. During therapy, the alkaline phosphatase level fell to 76% of initial values. Bone scintophotograph findings were worse in 2 patients, did not change in 7, and improved in 9. Eleven patients reported improvement in symptoms and 7 reported no change. Seventeen of these patients were then treated with etidronate for 6 months; they had a decrease in alkaline phosphatase levels to 64% of initial values. When compared with the results of initial tests, those of bone scintophotographs were worse in 3, exhibited no change in 5, and improved in 9. Three patients reported improvements in symptoms, 4 noted no change, and 10 reported increasing pain. The reason for the poor response to initial calcitonin therapy and/or subsequent etidronate therapy is not apparent. The authors conclude that patients fare better when treated with an etidronate calcitonin sequence than those treated with a calcitonin-etidronate sequence. (20 references)

157

Preston, C. J., et al.

Effective short term treatment of Paget's disease with oral etidronate. *Br Med J* 1986;292(6513):79–80.

Twelve patients with Paget's disease of bone were treated with high doses of disodium etidronate for 1 month and compared with patients given treatments for longer periods. The effects of treatment for 1 month with etidronate 20 mg/kg/d were indistinguishable from those of 6 months' continuous treatment with the same dose but significantly better than those of treatment with 5 mg/kg/d in suppressing biochemical indexes of disease activity. Treatment for 1 month was associated with transient osteomalacia but sustained suppression of bone resorption. Short-term treatments with high doses of disodium etidronate may maximize suppression of disease activity but decrease exposure to unwanted effects. (9 references)

158

Ralston, S. H., et al.

The effect of 1 alpha-hydroxyvitamin D3 on the mineralization defect in disodium etidronate-treated Paget's disease—a double-blind randomized clinical study. *J Bone Min Res* 1987;2(1):5–12.

A double-blind randomized study of 29 patients with symptomatic Paget's disease was conducted to compare the clinical, biochemical, and histomorphometric responses to 3-month treatment with placebo (10 patients), low-dose disodium etidronate (EHDP) 5 to 7 mg/kg/d) (10 patients), and low-dose EHDP plus 1 alpha-hydroxyvitamin D3 (1 alpha D3). 0.5 μg/d (9 patients). In placebo-treated patients no significant changes were observed in symptoms, biochemistry, or bone histomorphometry. Histologically apparent mineralization defects developed after 3 months of therapy in 90% of patients in the EHDP group, compared with 45% of patients in the EHDP/1 alpha D3 group. In 19% of the patients treated with active medication, the mineralization defects in pagetic bone were accompanied by histologic evidence of continued osteoclastic resorption. The development of mineralization defects was not related to serum levels of vitamin D metabolites, alkaline phosphatase, or intestinal calcium absorption but did correlate with the occurrence of hyperphosphatemia during treatment, which was most marked in patients treated with EHDP alone. Although mineralization defects were less frequent in the EHDP/1 alpha D3 group, these patients also responded less well symptomatically, thus limiting the potential usefulness of this drug combination in Paget's disease. (17 references)

159

Reginster, J. Y., et al.

Biological and clinical assessment of a new bisphosphonate, (chloro-4 phenyl) thiomethylene bisphosphonate, in the treatment of Paget's disease of bone. *Bone* 1988;9(6):349–354.

Several bisphosphonates have been used as therapeutic agents for Paget's bone disease. (Chloro-4 phenyl)thiomethylene-bisphosphonate (CIPsMBP) has recently been shown to have significant antiosteoclastic activity, whereas an effect of CIPsMBP mineralization was only observed at high doses. The authors tested this drug for 6 months in 23 pagetic patients distributed in three groups. Group 1 ($n = 5$), receiving 200 mg/d, showed a decrease of serum alkaline phosphatase (SAP) to 42% ± 4% ($P < 0.01$) of initial value (100%) while hydroxyprolinuria/creatinuria ratio (OH/Cr) dropped to 69% ± 8% of baseline. In 4 patients receiving 400 mg/d, SAP improved to 48% ± 9% of initial value ($P < 0.01$) and OH/Cr to 40% ± 3% ($P < 0.01$). In the last group ($n = 14$), who received 200 mg/d for 3 months and 400 mg/d thereafter up to the sixth month, SAP decreased to 53% ± 4% and OH/Cr to 62% ± 6% of initial value ($P < 0.01$). Clinical improvement was significant from the first month of treatment. No resistance (mean decrease of SAP lower than 30%) was recorded, and no radiologic or clinical evidence of mineralization defect appeared. Clinical and biologic tolerance was excellent throughout the study. (22 references)

160

Reginster, J. Y., et al.

One year's treatment of Paget's disease of bone by synthetic salmon calcitonin as a nasal spray. *J Bone Mineral Res* 1988;3(3):249–252.

The effectiveness of synthetic salmon calcitonin (SCT) administered as a nasal spray was assessed via clinical, biologic, and radiologic variables in 17 previously untreated pagetic patients over a 1-year course of therapy. The results showed a highly significant decrease of serum alkaline phosphatase (S-ALP) ($P < 0.05$ after 1 month of treatment) and of urinary hydroxyproline/creatinine ratio (OH/Cr) ($P < 0.01$ after 1 month of treatment). For the whole group, the mean decrease in S-ALP was 37% ± 4% (SEM) after 6 months ($P < 0.01$) and 31% ± 5% after 1 year ($P < 0.01$). The mean fall in OH/Cr was 35% ± 6% (SEM) ($P < 0.01$) and 37% ± 7% ($P < 0.01$) after 6 and 12 months, respectively. None of the usual side effects of SCT was reported, and local tolerance was excellent throughout the study. (25 references)

161

Rico, H., et al.

Biochemical assessment of acute and chronic treatment of Paget's bone disease with calcitonin and calcium with and without bisphosphonate. *Bone* 1988;9(1):63–66.

Response to acute and chronic administration of calcitonin and calcium and of bisphosphonates (EHDP) was evaluated in 14 patients with Paget's bone disease who were grouped on the basis of homogeneous disease activity as appraised by bone involvement and alkaline phosphatase and hydroxyproline levels. At first, 100 MRC U of calcitonin followed 4 hours later by 500 mg of elemental calcium was given for 10 days; a significant ($P < 0.001$; paired and unpaired Student t test) reduction in alkaline phosphatase (−25%) and hydroproline (−55%) was observed. Subsequently, 5 mg/kg/d of EHDP was given for 20 days. Both parameters increased to levels similar to basal values. These increases were significant ($P < 0.001$ for the paired and unpaired Student t tests) compared with those obtained after calcitonin administration; alkaline phosphatase rose by +27% and hydroxyproline by +135%. After this, patients were divided into two groups (A and B). Group A was treated with calcitonin and calcium, at the dosage indicated for 10 days a month for 6 months. Group B continued with the same protocol with the addition of EHDP for the 20 days during which calcitonin and calcium were not given. The results of 6 months of treatment showed that calcitonin was more active and suggested that EHDP diminishes hormonal effects. These results also demonstrate a short-term absence of EHDP activity. (31 references)

162

Singer, F. R.; Wallach, S.

Paget's Disease of Bone: Clinical Assessment, Present and Future Therapy. **New York, Elsevier Science Publishing Co, 1991. Available from Elsevier Science Publishing Co., 655 Avenue of the Americas, New York, NY 10010.**

This book contains a compilation of papers presented at the Symposium on the Treatment of Paget's Disease, sponsored by the Paget's Disease Foundation, that was held in New York City in October 1989. The aim of this volume is to present a current assessment of available therapeutic intervention in Paget's disease. Topics covered include radiology of Paget's disease; biochemistry of Paget's disease; pathology of Paget's disease; indications for treatment; porcine, salmon, and human calcitonin therapy; resistance to calcitonin; etidronate disodium therapy; APD therapy; new bisphosphonates; novel forms of treatment; plicamycin therapy; response to treatment; arthritis management in Paget's disease; and surgery in Paget's disease.

163

Spencer, H.; Kramer, L.; Wiatrowski, E.; Lender, M.

Fluoride therapy in metabolic bone disease. ***Isr J Med Sci*** **1984;20(5):373–380.**

Multiple forms of treatment are used for osteoporosis, Paget's disease of bone, and osteogenesis imperfecta. Because of the effect of fluoride (F) on bone, these bone conditions may benefit from F therapy. In the present study, the metabolic effects of two dose levels of F (20 and 45 mg, given as sodium flouride) were studied on calcium (Ca) and F metabolism in patients with osteoporosis, whereas the effect of the 45-mg dose was studied in patients with Paget's disease. In patients with osteoporosis, the retention of F increased with increasing F intake, indicating F deposition in bone. However, only the 45-mg dose decreased urinary Ca excretion. F did not decrease fecal Ca excretion, indicating that the intestinal absorption of Ca did not improve during F therapy. This was confirmed in 47 Ca absorption studies. The duration of F therapy was 3 months with the 45-mg dose. Clinically, the patients experienced relief of bone pain, and the onset of this change coincided with the decrease in urinary Ca. The 3-month course of treatment was sufficient for alleviation of clinical symptoms for many months and even years. In patients with Paget's disease, F supplements decreased urinary Ca and also produced relief of bone pain. F therapy for osteogenesis imperfecta resulted in decreased fracture incidence. (59 references)

163a

Stumpf, J. L.

Pharmacologic management of Paget's disease. *Clin Pharmacy* 1989;8(7):485–495.

The author reviews the pathogenesis, clinical features, indications for therapy, and current pharmacologic management of Paget's disease. Overactive bone resorption leads to accelerated formation of disorganized, weak bone. Pain and fractures are common clinical features. Neurologic, cardiovascular, metabolic, and neoplastic complications may also be reported. Because most patients are asymptomatic, the disease is often detected during routine roentgenography or laboratory tests. Primary indications for pharmacologic intervention include bone pain, neural compression, immobilization hypercalcemia or hypercalciuria, cardiac failure, and orthopedic surgery. Recurrent or nonhealing fractures and rapidly progressing complications are additional indications. Drugs used in the management of Paget's disease include calcitonin, etidronate disodium, and plicamycin. Although these agents are efficacious, each has disadvantages. Clinical resistance to animal calcitonins may develop, and the cost of therapy may be prohibitive. Etidronate may induce osteomalacia. The use of plicamycin is limited by potentially severe toxic efforts. Dichloromethylene and aminohydroxypropylidene are promising diphosphonate (bisphosphonate) compounds but are still under investigation. In those patients who are unresponsive to single-agent regimens, combination therapy may prove effective. Although many individuals with Paget's disease do not require pharmacologic therapy, calcitonin and etidronate are the agents of choice when it is indicated. (103 references)

164

Stutzmann, J. J.; Petrovic, A. G.

Diphosphonates for otospongiosis. *Am J Otol* 1985;6(1):89–95.

Diphosphonates (DPPs) (bisphosphonates) have proved useful in recent years in the medical management of certain disorders of bone metabolism, especially in Paget's disease, in which bone turnover rate is accelerated. Since patients suffering from Paget's disease often are affected simultaneously, and mostly bilaterally, by evolutive otospongiosis, a quantitative organ culture study was undertaken to assess the turnover rate of otospongiotic bone removed surgically from such patients, before and during treatment with three different DPPs. The results indicated that (1) such treatment strongly restrained otospongiotic bone formation, mineralization, and resorption; and (2) the diphosphonate-induced decrease in otospongiotic bone turnover rate resulted in a rate similar to that in individuals not affected with Paget's disease. The differences in the effects produced by the three DPPs are discussed. The findings seem to be full of promise, encouraging further investigations. (17 references)

165

Thiébaud, D., et al.

A single infusion of the bisphosphonate AHPrBP (APD) as treatment of Paget's disease of bone. ***Am J Med*** **1988;85(2):207–212.**

Eleven patients with mild but symptomatic Paget's disease and 1 patient with very severe disease were treated with AHPrBP administered as a single intravenous infusion of 60 mg over 24 hours. Follow-up with clinical and biochemical evaluations was performed over 6 months for all patients and over 1 year for 7 patients. Clinical improvement and normalization of biochemical parameters were observed in all patients except 1 with extremely severe disease. On average, plasma alkaline phosphatase activity fell progressively and significantly from 256 ± 29 U/L (mean ± SEM) to 97 ± 6 U/L after 6 months, and to 102 ± 11 U/L after 1 year (normal: less than 120 U/L). Urinary excretion of hydroxyproline decreased within 7 days to normal (from 4.3 ± 0.5 μmol/L of glomerular filtrate [LGF] to 1.7 ± 0.2 μmol/LGF; normal: 2.2 μmol/LGF). Thereafter, it remained within the normal range until 1 year (1.8 ± 0.2 μmol/LGF after 6 months and 1.9 ± 0.3 μmol/LGF after 1 year). Side effects were negligible. Two patients noted only a transient increase in body temperature. When bone scintigraphy was repeated after 6 months, it revealed a marked decrease of the activity of the disease. Because of the important and sustained inhibition of bone resorption induced by AHPrBP, a single infusion of 60 mg of the bisphosphonate leads to a rapid decline in activity and a long-standing remission of moderate Paget's disease, without significant side effects. (45 references)

166

Thiébaud, D.; Jaeger, P; Burckhardt, P.

Paget's disease of bone treated in five days with AHPrBP (APD) per os. ***J Bone Mineral Res*** **1987;2(1):45–52.**

Aminohydroxypropylidene bisphosphonic acid (AHPrBP [previously APD]) is a potent inhibitor of bone resorption. Since it remains in bone for a long time, and since it was not found to impair bone mineralization, it could be administered at a high dose over a short period. Therefore, 11 patients with symptomatic Paget's disease were given AHPrBP orally at 1,200 mg/d for 5 consecutive days. Controls were performed after 1 month in all patients, 6 months in 8 patients, and 1 year in 4 patients. Clinical improvement and biochemical remission were observed in all patients, except in 1 who had a severe case of the disease. Side effects were negligible. Disease activity at bone scintigram decreased over 6 months. Plasma alkaline phosphatase activity fell progressively and significantly from 210 ± 26 U/L (mean $\pm$ SEM) to 103 ± 10 U/L after 6 months (normal: less than 120 U/L). Urinary excretion of hydroxyproline decreased immediately and became normal (normal: less than 2.3 μmol/L of glomerular filtrate [LGF]) as a mean at day 5 (from 4.6 ± 0.4 μmol/LGF to 2.1 ± 0.3 μmol/LGF). Thereafter it remained within the normal range (2.0 ± 0.2 μmol/L at day 180). Plasma calcium and phosphate concentrations fell transiently between days 4 and 15, whereas plasma parathyroid (PTH) levels increased over this period. In conclusion, a short course of AHPrBP given per os at high dose induces a rapid decline in activity and remission of moderate Paget's disease, without significant side effects. (46 references)

167

Turek, S. L.

Paget's disease, in *Orthopaedics: Principles and Their Application*, ed 4. Philadelphia, JB Lippincott Co, 1984, pp 734–743. Available from JB Lippincott, East Washington Square, Philadelphia, PA 19105. (215) 238-4200

Paget's disease is a very common idiopathic chronic condition of the skeleton occurring in patients past middle age. It is characterized pathologically by partial or complete involvement of a single bone or multiple bones by exaggerated rates of resorptive and osteogenic activity, leading to bony thickening and deformity. Clinically, this may cause pain, bone deformity, deafness, susceptibility to fractures with trivial trauma, and such complications as secondary osteoarthritis, sarcomatous degeneration, referred pain and nerve entrapment syndrome, and, in extensive disease, high-output cardiac failure. This book section reviews the pathology, pathophysiology, clinical picture, complications, roentgenographic findings, laboratory findings, and treatment. Principles of surgical management of the pagetic patient are discussed as they apply to correction of long bone deformity, total hip replacement, repair of fractures, and spinal involvement in Paget's disease. (34 references)

168

Vega, E.; Gonzalez, D.; Ghiringhelli, G.; Mautalen, C.

Intravenous aminopropylidene bisphosphonate (APD) in the treatment of Paget's bone disease. ***J Bone Mineral Res*** **1987;2(4):267–271.**

The authors studied the effect of intravenous administration of the bisphosphonate APD in nine patients with Paget's bone disease. The medication was given in a daily dose of 25 mg for 7 days in 0.9% saline infusion over 2 hours. At the end of treatment a significant decrease in the levels of serum calcium and phosphate was observed. The urinary excretion of calcium decreased markedly, and the serum levels of the midmolecule parathyroid (PTH) fragment increased from (mean ± SE) 85 ± 11 to 122 ± 16 pg/mL ($P < 0.05$). A marked and rapid decline in the hydroxyprolinuria was observed, from 297 ± 61 mg/24 h to 194 ± 51 mg/24 h ($P < 0.01$); meanwhile the serum alkaline phosphatase level decreased from 102 ± 22 to 84 ± 21 KAU ($P < 0.05$). The effect of ADP on suppression of hydroxyprolinuria varied markedly from +1% to −81% and was negatively related to the basal hydroxyprolinuria ($R = 0.90$; $P < 0.001$). The duration of the bone turnover suppression was short. A relapse greater than 30% in hydroxyprolinuria was observed in six of eight patients 2 to 3 months after APD withdrawal. The short-term intravenous administration of ADP is a useful means to suppress the activity of Paget's bone disease rapidly. However, further studies should determine the optimal dose, the length of treatment, and the need to associate oral therapy to induce a prolonged remission. (22 references)

169

Vellenga, C. J., et al.

Quantitative bone scintigraphy in Paget's disease treated with APD. ***Br J Radiol*** **1985;58(696):1165–1172.**

Half-yearly bone scintigrams of 27 patients with Paget's disease, who were treated with the bisphosphonate APD, were evaluated. Uptake of ^{99m}Tc-Sn-EHDP was determined by computer analysis. All patients reached clinical and biochemical remission, usually within 6 months. The scintigraphic uptake dropped steeply during the first 6 months and only slightly during the second 6 months. The decrease in uptake was proportional to the original uptake and averaged 80% of this value. The residual 20% persisted, although clinical and biochemical remission was attained. The scintigraphic results obtained with APD agree with our earlier findings for patients in remission after treatment with a combination of calcitonin and EHDP. Eight patients suffered a recurrence after discontinuation of

APD. In all cases scintigraphic deterioration also occurred, usually simultaneously or 6 months before the recurrence. In two patients with scintigraphic deterioration a recurrence could not be confirmed during this study. The scintigraphic deterioration presented as one of the three patterns seen after combination therapy. (32 references)

170

Vellenga, C. J.; Mulder, J.D.; Bijvoet, O. L.

Radiological demonstration of healing in Paget's disease of bone treated with APD. *Br J Radiol* 1985;58(693):831–837.

Twenty-three patients with Paget's disease received the bisphosphonate APD and were examined radiologically every 6 months. Because routine roentgenographic procedures were followed, a number of the radiographs were not fit for comparison. The radiographic technique and the positioning of the patients are critical since both could lead to artifacts. All patients reached normal biochemical levels, usually within 6 months. Of the 23 patients 11 showed definite improvement in radiologic outcome in one or more lesions; probable improvement was seen in another three. Where films were comparable, it could be seen that 30% of the 65 individual lesions definitely and 20% probably improved; 50% did not change, but deterioration was never encountered. Osteolytic lesions in the long bones are most suitable for the evaluation of radiologic changes, and follow-up of these lesions during treatment should be most rewarding. (29 references)

171

Wade, J.; Liang, M. H.; Stern, S.

Management of non-inflammatory musculoskeletal disorders in the elderly. *Compr Ther* 1988;14(6):38–43.

This paper discusses the management of three important types of non-inflammatory musculoskeletal disorders in elderly patients, including Paget's disease of bone (osteitis deformans), a focal disorder of unknown cause. This disorder is initially characterized by excessive bone resorption, culminating in an altered pattern of lamenellar bone associated with increased vascularity and fibrous tissue in adjacent marrow. Management involves the use of antiinflammatory agents or etidronate disodium (a diphosphonate [bisphosphonate]). Management of various complications is discussed. This report also discusses the diagnosis and management of osteoarthritis and osteoporosis. (12 references)

172

Walton, K. R.; Green, J. R.; Reeve, J.; Wootton, R.

Reduction of skeletal blood flow in Paget's disease with disodium etidronate therapy. *Bone* 1985;6(1):29–31.

Fourteen patients with Paget's disease of bone were treated with disodium etidronate in doses of 5 to 7 mg/kg/d. Skeletal blood flow (SBF) was measured by the modified 18F clearance technique of Wootton et al. (1976) before treatment and again during treatment. In 10 patients restudied 3 to 4 months after the start of therapy, SBF had fallen by a mean of 21% of the initial value, and the individual differences correlated well with the individual reductions in serum alkaline phosphatase ($R = 0.77$; $P < 0.01$). The results were similar to those seen in an earlier study in patients treated with calcitonin. However, in contrast to previous findings with calcitonin, no early reduction in SBF was seen in six repeat studies performed at the end of the second week of treatment. (12 references)

173

Yates, A. J., et al.

Intravenous clodronate in the treatment and retreatment of Paget's disease of bone. *Lancet* 1985;1(8444):1474–1477.

The effects of short courses (5 days) of intravenous clodronate (300 mg daily) were studied in 31 patients with active Paget's disease of bone. The diphosphonate (bisphosphonate) induced a striking reduction in biochemical indexes of disease activity, which was sustained for at least 6 months after withdrawal of treatment. Apparent resistance to further treatment in patients previously treated for Paget's disease was an artifact due to complete relapse before retreatment. There was no significant difference in the degree of suppression of alkaline phosphatase activity between the patients given intravenous clodronate and 45 patients given clodronate 1.6 g daily by mouth for 6 months. Short-term intravenous clodronate provides a useful alternative strategy for the treatment of patients with Paget's disease. (28 references)

174

Ziegler, R.; Mine, H. W.

Paget's disease of bone: Treatment with calcitonin, in Cecchettin, M., Segre, G. (eds): *Calciotropic Hormones and Calcium Metabolism: Proceedings of the 5th International Congress on Calciotropic Hormones and Calcium Metabolism. Venice, Italy, 28–30 April 1985.* New York, Excerpta Medica, 1986, pp 123–129. Available

from Elsevier Science Publishing Company, 655 Avenue of the Americas, New York NY 10010. International Congress Series, Number 679. ISBN: 0444807713.

Since 1973, the authors have treated about 100 patients with Paget's disease of bone with calcitonin. This paper evaluates 60 cases with respect to efficacy, side effects, and future use of this treatment. The authors conclude that calcitonin is a very effective symptomatic drug for long-term treatment of Paget's disease. There are no contraindications against calcitonin therapy. However, disease activity relapses sooner or later after administration of the hormone eases. (8 references)

AUTHOR INDEX FOR BIBLIOGRAPHY

Numbers are citation numbers for abstracts, not page numbers.

SUBJECT INDEX FOR BIBLIOGRAPHY

Numbers are citation numbers for abstracts not page numbers.

Index